# Racketeer for Life

Christopher—

I hope you enjoy
this little bit
of pro-life history

Joe Scheidler
June 1, 2020

# Racketeer for Life

Fighting the Culture of Death from
the Sidewalk to the Supreme Court

A MEMOIR BY JOSEPH M. SCHEIDLER
WITH PETER M. SCHEIDLER

EDITED BY JOHN F. BRICK

TAN Books
Charlotte, North Carolina

The following is a memoir. To protect the privacy of certain nonpublic figures, in some cases, names have been changed, slightly altered, or surnames not given.

Cover design by Caroline Kiser

ISBN: 978-1-61890-850-6

Published in the United States by
TAN Books
P. O. Box 410487
Charlotte, North Carolina
www.TANBooks.com

Printed and bound in the United States of America

*To my wife, Ann, who led me into the pro-life movement,
and for Monica, who gave me hope in the darkest hours of the battle*

# CONTENTS

# ABBREVIATIONS

American Civil Liberties Union (ACLU)

American Law Institute (ALI)

Americans United for Life (AUL)

Chicago Transit Authority (CTA)

Clergy Consultation Service (CCS)

Delaware Women's Health Organization (DWHO)

Federal Communications Commission (FCC)

Freedom of Access to Clinic Entrances (FACE)

Freedom of Choice Act (FOCA)

Friends for Life (FFL)

Illinois Right to Life Committee (IRLC)

Indiana University (IU)

Knights of Columbus (K of C)

Ku Klux Klan (KKK)

National Abortion Federation (NAF)

National Association for the Advancement of Colored People (NAACP)

National Association for the Repeal of Abortion Laws (NARAL)

National Conference of Catholic Bishops (NCCB)

National Organization for Women (NOW)

National Right to Life Committee (NRLC)

Officer of the Day (OD)

People Expressing a Concern for Everyone (PEACE)

People for the Ethical Treatment of Animals (PETA)

Pro-Life Action Network (PLAN)

Pro-Life Nonviolent Action Project (PNAP)

Racketeer Influenced and Corrupt Organizations Act (RICO)

Religious Coalition for Abortion Rights (RCAR)

Single European Act (SEA)

Society for the Preservation of the Unborn Child (SPUC)

Southern Illinois University (SIU)

United States Department of Health and Human Services (HHS)

US Catholic Conference (USCC)

Women Exploited By Abortion (WEBA)

# PUBLISHER'S NOTE

TAN Books is honored to publish this memoir of a true American hero. For more than forty years, Joe Scheidler has dedicated his life, time, treasure, and talent to the pro-life cause, often at great personal cost to himself and his family.

While his efforts and resolve have been unstinting and unyielding, and his tactics at times controversial, Joe Scheidler has never advocated violence, the claims of his opponents notwithstanding. To the contrary, as a profoundly moral and religious man, he has consistently repudiated it based on the principle that a good end does not justify an immoral means. We at TAN are proud to stand with Joe, both in his steadfast opposition to abortion and his rejection, in no uncertain terms, of violence in the struggle to end this great moral evil.

May God bless all of those who dedicate themselves to the pro-life cause; may He bless all mothers and expectant mothers; may He bless all children in and out of the womb. And may God bless His good and faithful servant, Joe Scheidler.

# AUTHOR'S NOTE

This is the way I remember it—the more than four decades of legal abortion and the fifty years of moral decay that led to the January 22, 1973, disasters known as *Roe v. Wade* and *Doe v. Bolton.* This is the way I remember the early years that prepared me for the raging battle to save the lives of the unborn. It is, of course, an abridged history, but it is filled with my memories of the fight against abortion and the effort to turn our national culture away from the ugly, violent narcissism that makes legalized abortion possible. This is the way I remember the people I worked with and planned with and went to jail with. This is the way I remember the enemy we are still fighting.

Our office in Chicago is filled with files upon files from decades of work—old newspapers, flyers, news bulletins, press releases, court transcripts, and photographs. I used all the tools at my disposal to check, double-check, and recheck my facts to tell the most accurate story I could. I reviewed more than six thousand transcripts of my hotlines—daily recorded phone messages each a few minutes long. I pored over back issues of our *Action News* monthly, reread old newspapers and magazines, studied volumes of court documents, interviewed scores of activists and friends, and viewed miles of taped news reports and video footage of our activities. I gave a dozen drafts of my manuscripts to people who were also there, to find out what they remembered.

But memory is a funny thing. It takes impressions of the stories we find ourselves a part of, like metal in soft wax. Our memories hold the shape of things that were, but they can't capture the things themselves. While researching my own past for this book, I've often been surprised at what I'd forgotten, or that what happened wasn't quite the way I remembered it. Everything in this book is as accurate as I could make it, with the help and dedicated diligence of my wife, Ann, and my son Peter.

But this is still a memoir. It is *my* memoir: my recollections, my reflections, my impressions, my own story in a vast and intricate history.

Now I invite you to join me on my journey.

Yours for life,
Joseph M. Scheidler
National Director
Pro-Life Action League

## Chapter 1

# Sorry I Missed You

In the spring of 1987, I was in northern California to meet with local and national pro-life leaders and to speak at a rally. Early one morning, before the meetings began, I visited the newest branch of the Feminist Women's Health Centers, a clinic in Redding. I hoped to talk with the new administrator there, but the clinic was closed, its windows dark and the door locked. I flipped over one of my Pro-Life Action League business cards and wrote, "Sorry I missed you." I signed my initials—JMS—and wedged it in the door.

I met with the leaders and spoke at the rally, but I wasn't able to stop back at the clinic before I left town. But I did see that business card again—eleven years later in federal court. It was March 1998, and I was on trial in downtown Chicago for violating federal racketeering laws. In the first week of a seven-week trial, that card was displayed for jurors on a screen as big as a billboard, while Dido Hasper, founder of the Feminist Women's Health Center, testified to being scared when she arrived at her Redding clinic and found my card. The plaintiffs alleged that my card constituted a death threat, part of a pattern of conspiracy and extortion against the nation's abortion providers and their clients.

Early in my activist career, I regularly visited abortion clinics, asking to speak with the physician or the administrator, hoping to learn why they got into the business and to try to talk them out of it. Over time, I realized that many are not happy—abortion is a grisly line of work. Some abortion providers responded to an outsider's concern. I tried to persuade them to use their talents to build up society, not add to its many miseries. Strange as it seems, I've seen people quit the business after a compassionate encounter with a pro-lifer, some even right on the spot.

As I sat in that courtroom, seeing my card on that screen and trying to puzzle out how my message could be read as a death threat, I found myself wondering how I wound up there. How did a guy from Hartford City, Indiana, population seven thousand, end up a defendant in a federal racketeering trial? Chicago has a long history of mob bosses. But me? I didn't know the first thing about running a national crime syndicate. But here I was, sitting in the Dirksen Federal Building at the defendant's table, watching a jury study my handwriting, and hearing my life's work described as a wild, decades-long crime spree.

This is how it happened. In 1973, when the Supreme Court's abortion rulings were announced, I was working as an account executive with a public relations firm in Chicago. Within a few months, I'd left that job to work full time on the pro-life cause, some on my own and some part-time with the Illinois Right to Life Committee (IRLC). By January 1974, I was working as the director of the IRLC.

In those early days, most pro-lifers thought lobbying and debating were the best place for the movement's energies. I believed in direct action, and I eventually had to found my own group, the Pro-Life Action League, for like-minded activists. There was no manual for how to be a pro-life activist. We tried a variety of tactics to save lives and to keep the issue before the American public.

After more than a decade of trying different approaches, learning what worked and what didn't, adjusting our strategies against stifling pro-abortion campaigns, other pro-life groups started asking how to implement some of our tactics. So in 1985, I published *CLOSED: 99 Ways to Stop Abortion*. Most of the *99 Ways* were techniques I'd tried myself. Some I'd only heard of, and a few were ideas that nobody had tried yet. The title font looked like stencils, the sort of thing you might see spray painted on a shuttered storefront. The idea was to expose the macabre realities of the abortion industry, to educate readers about the lives of the unborn, and to offer tangible, practical alternatives for unplanned and unwanted children. If we could take away clinics' customers, we would drive clinics out of business.

When *CLOSED* was published, my father-in-law, an attorney, recommended I place my home in a land trust in case I was sued. I took his advice. A year later, when I was picketing the National Abortion Federation (NAF) convention in Kansas City, a man emerged from the hotel, picked me out of the small crowd, and handed me an envelope. It was a notice that I'd been named in a lawsuit brought by the National Organization for Women (NOW).

I didn't think much of it. NOW had filed the suit in Delaware under federal antitrust charges. Legal injunctions and even false charges were nothing new, and they hadn't deterred us before. This new gimmick of calling the pro-life movement an anticompetitive conspiracy to restrain trade seemed like quite a stretch. But regardless of how baseless their case was, we had to answer the charges.

My wife Ann's brother-in-law, Ken Theisen, was a lawyer, and she asked him if he ever worked in antitrust law. He hadn't, but he had a friend, Tom Brejcha, who had just briefed an antitrust case before the Supreme Court. So we set up a meeting.

My first impression of Tom was not good. He was too quiet. I thought we needed an aggressive attorney, and Tom just didn't seem forceful enough. But when Tom said, almost inaudibly, "I win cases," I heard a confidence in his voice that impressed me. Tom set to work on the case, along with young lawyers from Americans

United for Life (AUL) Defense Fund. We applied for and were granted a change of venue from Delaware to Chicago. Soon after, Tom's law firm dissolved. They wrote off the charges incurred for his services, which by then were about one hundred thousand dollars. Tom moved to the firm of Abramson & Fox and continued representing me in the case.

NOW evidently recognized the weakness in their antitrust case, and in 1989, they added charges under the Racketeer Influenced and Corrupt Organizations (RICO) Act, alleging that I was masterminding the movement of civil disobedience against abortion clinics that was sweeping the nation, and Tom Brejcha became an expert in racketeering law.

That same year, Planned Parenthood took out a full-page ad in newspapers and magazines across the country, including *Time* and *Newsweek*. It was a picture of me at a rally in Atlanta, bearded and wearing my fedora, with the caption, "Should a woman's private medical decisions be made by a man with a bullhorn?"

The picture came from a picket outside a clinic in an old mansion set back from a sidewalk in downtown Atlanta. I asked if anyone there would be willing to march with me past the front of the clinic. The first volunteer was a boy about ten years old, and that encouraged others to follow. The police were called, but they allowed us to continue our march across the property, and nobody was arrested. As we marched past the clinic door, someone on the other side snapped the picture.

I never set out to craft a signature look, but that's what happened. The beard started as a joke—I had a boss in the 1960s who told the staff she could do anything a man could do, so all the men grew beards. I wasn't a hat-wearer either, until my dad, Matthias Herman Scheidler, died in December 1974 and I returned to Hartford City for his funeral. I went into his room and found his Alpaca coat and felt hat at the foot of his bed. It was a brutally cold day, so I put on the coat and picked up the hat—an exact fit. I wasn't nearly as good-looking as Dad, but people said I looked like him, and that was a compliment.

I wore his hat back to Chicago, and I've worn one like it ever since. People recognize me by my hat and beard at pickets and rallies, and pro-life groups have raised funds by auctioning off my hat several times. After seeing the ad, a supporter wrote to me, "If Planned Parenthood will spend thousands of dollars to print your picture in *Time*, you know you've made it."

The RICO case went on for two more years. Finally, in May 1991, Federal Judge James Holderman dismissed the racketeering allegations as "nonsense." As for the antitrust allegations, Judge Holderman cited numerous interviews in which abortion industry spokespeople bragged that pro-life activism hadn't made a dent in their business.

Not discouraged by Holderman's handing us a victory, NOW turned to the Appellate Court. But in June 1992, the United States Court of Appeals for the Seventh Circuit unanimously upheld Judge Holderman's ruling.

The very next day NOW filed their appeal to the Supreme Court. President Clinton's Justice Department submitted briefs supporting NOW's case. The court rejected their antitrust allegation but agreed to hear arguments on the RICO charge. So in December 1993, I found myself at the Supreme Court for the oral arguments in *NOW v. Scheidler*.

Tom Brejcha and staff attorneys at the AUL recruited the author of the RICO statute, Notre Dame law professor Robert Blakey, to affirm that the district court had rightly dismissed the RICO charges. But we were asking Blakey to argue against his own law. If he made too forceful a case, there was a chance that RICO itself could be found unconstitutional. He failed to convince the court, which ruled unanimously to let the case proceed.

The following summer, Tom's boss, Jim Fox, invited Ann and me to lunch at the Wrigley Building on Michigan Avenue. I assumed we'd talk about the case and I'd have a chance to thank him for letting Tom spend so much time on it.

Jim knew Tom Crowley, Ann's father, who had passed away a few years earlier, so we reminisced about him for a while, but Fox soon got down to business. He quoted a line from St. Paul's letter to Timothy: "A laborer is worthy of his hire." I thought he was talking about the League and saying that our cause was so important that he was glad to support us.

But that is not what he meant. Tom was the laborer, and we were there to talk about money. The AUL wasn't paying for Tom's work, he said, and Abramson & Fox was not interested in offering its services pro bono. Jim told us we owed his firm $240,738, and he expected a first installment of $40,000 by August 1.

Jim seemed uncomfortable as he told us this, and I suspected that his partner, Floyd Abramson, was behind the firm's decision. Jim did offer to contact the Knights of Columbus (K of C) on our behalf, thinking they could be a source of funding, but he soon learned that the K of C wasn't interested in getting involved with our court battle.

So we had five weeks to raise forty thousand dollars or NOW would succeed in driving us into bankruptcy. We worked frantically, sending out letters and making phone calls, trying to raise the money to make this first installment. We came up short, but we scrambled together enough to keep Abramson & Fox at bay for a while.

The following spring, Clarke Forsythe visited our office to tell me that the AUL didn't have the resources to handle trial expenses and was pulling out entirely. They pledged a final amount of fifty thousand dollars to help with what we owed. Tom stayed on the case, but the bills continued to mount.

Finally, late in 1997, just months before the trial was set to begin, Abramson & Fox gave Tom an ultimatum: quit the case or quit the firm. Soon afterward Tom went home and told his wife, Debbie, that he'd resigned from the firm.

"Well, go back and unresign!" she urged. But the resignation was deemed final, and fortunately Tom stuck with us. Debbie unretired from her teaching career, and against so many odds, I managed to have Tom Brejcha with me when the trial finally started early in 1998. We got to work establishing a pro-life law firm in Chicago, but the timing was so tight that for the first days of the trial, Tom was listed as a member of Ken Theisen's law firm. Then the state approved the charter for our new firm—The Thomas More Society—and by the time I was being reintroduced to that business card from the late '80s, I was officially represented by the Thomas More Society and have been ever since.

"Sorry I missed you." The irony of the message really struck home as I sat at the defendant's table in the Dirksen Federal Building that March day. Not only had I missed talking with any of the staff at the Feminist Women's Health Center, but my intended message—a compassionate connection—missed its mark. It meant what it said. If I could have talked with Dido Hasper, we could perhaps have shared a human moment. Perhaps I could have even helped her get out of the lethal business.

"Sorry I missed you" speaks to our whole society. Those of us who got involved in the pro-life movement in the early days thought it would take just a few years to reverse course and bring Americans to their senses. We were convinced that, with the right tools and the right people, we could remind the nation that self-determination should never come at the cost of killing another innocent, sovereign self.

Newcomers to the pro-life movement can only experience much of what we did in those early days, when you could walk into a clinic and leave your card, through stories like the ones in this book. I've been at this work for nearly half a century, and I'll be at it as long as God continues to grant me life. But there are activists to come I'll never meet, more women and men who will carry the work forward. I'm sorry I missed you. I hope you enjoy reading these tales of activism from before your time. I hope you find inspiration in them.

To those who champion abortion as a right, I'm sorry we missed you. We were on the same street, and we didn't connect. Our literature never found its way into your hands. We were on the same corner, and perhaps our pictures were too graphic, and perhaps I didn't reach out. We missed each other in medical schools, outside voting centers, and at the clinics.

There are millions of unborn children who have never been read to, will never learn to read, and will never see this or any other book. Over the years, we've saved many, but not enough. To the victims we couldn't save, I also say, "Sorry I missed you."

## CHAPTER 2

# A Calling

It was a beautiful afternoon in the fall of 1972, and I was looking forward to watching the Notre Dame football game on television. But my wife, Ann, had other plans. She'd promised a friend that she would join her at a rally at the Civic Center in downtown Chicago. So I reluctantly gave up on my plans to watch the Fighting Irish. We loaded our three sons into the car and headed downtown.

This was a few months before the Supreme Court would hand down its abortion ruling. Abortion had been legalized in a few states but was still illegal in Illinois. In the late 1960s, there were efforts to change state prohibitions on abortion and introduce new statutes that allowed it for the "hard cases," such as rape or incest, or when the mother's health was at risk. A small but growing branch of this movement wanted a total repeal of abortion laws: abortion on demand, for any reason. As this call for after-the-fact birth control grew, some state right-to-life organizations were founded to oppose it. The National Right to Life Committee (NRLC) was established in 1968, and in response, the National Association for the Repeal of Abortion Laws (NARAL) was founded the following year. Their intention was "repeal," not reform: Their goal was to make abortion a right. After *Roe*, rather than disband, this group simply changed the words behind their acronym and became the National Abortion Rights Action League.

But that was still to come. An abortion "reform" law had been proposed in the Illinois legislature. At the time, Illinois was a strongly pro-life state, and a repeal effort wasn't making any headway in the General Assembly. But the IRLC organized a rally to galvanize opposition to the effort. This was the event Ann and the boys and I were going to that fall afternoon.

As we entered the plaza, a young lady handed me a pamphlet titled *Life or Death*. On the back was a small picture of a black garbage bag full of babies aborted in a Toronto hospital. One face in the picture stopped me dead in my tracks—the baby in a corner of the plastic bag looked like my son Eric's baby picture. The shock of recognition made abortion suddenly personal. Here was a bag full of dead babies. These were real children whose only crime was being unwanted.

I was riveted. I paid close attention to the speakers at the rally. One of the most compelling was the majority leader of the Illinois House of Representatives, Henry Hyde. That night I couldn't sleep. Over the next few weeks, I started studying abortion and the right-to-life movement.

Some people have vivid memories of when they first became aware that infants could legally be killed in the womb. For me, the *Life or Death* pamphlet was an epiphany, but of course, I'd been aware for years that there was such a thing as abortion. I can't recall exactly when it was that I learned that such a thing did occur. Still, I do have early memories of being preoccupied with the safety of young children. The first child I can remember grieving for was one I didn't even know.

In May 1927, ten weeks before I was born, Charles Lindbergh landed the *Spirit of St. Louis* at Le Bourget Airport in Paris. The historic transatlantic crossing made Lindbergh an instant superstar on both sides of the Atlantic. In my preschool years, Lindbergh was featured often in the papers and on newsreels. The media covered his marriage to debutante Anne Morrow, their purchase of a home in East Amwell, New Jersey, and the birth of their first child, Charlie Jr., a little boy with blond curls. The Lindberghs seemed to be the living ideal of the perfect American family.

When I was four years old, Charlie Jr. was kidnapped. Someone, the reports said, had put a ladder up to the second-story nursery window and snatched him from his crib. My hometown of Hartford City was so small that we almost never heard newsboys shouting headlines, but the kidnapping brought out a special edition, and I remember the newsboys on the streets shouting, "Extra! Extra! Read all about it—Lindbergh baby kidnapped!"

I'm the third of six siblings. I have two older sisters, but I was a big brother to my sister Elly, who was two at the time. I remember worrying that someone would try to kidnap her. Six months after the Lindbergh abduction, my brother Bob was born, and I worried for him too. As the big brother, I felt I had to protect them both.

I was too young to realize that kidnappers target children whose parents can afford a hefty ransom. Lindbergh paid the ransom, but six weeks later, Charlie Jr.'s remains were discovered a few miles from his home. He had died of a massive skull fracture. There was speculation that he may have been dropped from the ladder, but whether his death was accidental or intentional, the kidnapper demanded the money just the same. Charlie Jr. died so someone could get rich.

The Lindbergh tragedy planted the first seeds of my concern for vulnerable children. But eventually my anxieties about kidnapping passed, and I settled into a comfortable, secure routine: a loving family, playing cowboys and Indians, attending a tiny Catholic grade school—in short, typical Midwestern small-town life.

Hartford City had no Catholic high school, so after grammar school, I attended Hartford City High. In those days, there was no ban on prayer in schools, and on Monday mornings, our homeroom teacher would ask students about the services they'd attended on Sunday. It was interesting to discover that the Baptist preacher, the Lutheran minister, and the Catholic priest often covered similar themes.

The Japanese attack on Pearl Harbor on December 7, 1941, came during my freshman year. The fighting was still going on when I graduated, so I joined the navy. I was stationed at Camp Peary Naval Base in Williamsburg, Virginia, and assigned to the base police.

My job at Camp Peary was to guard sailors on work duty for minor infractions, such as overstaying their leave. Occasionally a sailor would go around collecting money for an abortion for a friend's girlfriend—it was always "for a friend." Of course, when they asked me, I refused. Abortion was illegal, and any practicing Christian knew that abortion was a serious sin. Still, I didn't try talking these guys out of it. It was someone else's problem.

After my stint in the navy in 1946, I went to the University of Notre Dame on the GI Bill. Notre Dame was very Catholic in those days, and it was a great time to attend a men's college, since so many students there were mature men who had served in the war. Few were looking for a four-year extension of their adolescence. Nearly everybody on campus seemed to have a goal, and their faith was central to that goal.

Many of the teachers were Holy Cross priests, and others were former military chaplains from various orders who were finishing their education, earning higher degrees, and paying off part of their tuition by teaching. I was taught by Dominicans and Jesuits, as well as Holy Cross religious. In addition to Sunday Mass, we were encouraged to attend three other Masses each week. Religion was an important part of the curriculum. Many religious vocations came out of those classes.

I majored in communication arts, which was bolstered by courses in theology and philosophy. All three reinforced each other. Central to each was the belief that truth existed and could be known. Making up something and calling it truth did not make it so. Our goal was to find truth. We were taught that the object of the will is the good—truth in action. All are called to seek what is good and assess their behavior accordingly. Catholic education was about applying clear, logical reason to that assessment. The beauty of Catholic thought resonated with me during those years. I audited Latin and took Greek with the seminarians, wondering if I might be called to the priesthood. In those days, it was common for young Catholic men to consider the priesthood. I had two cousins and three uncles who were priests. My brother Bob would enter the seminary as would my brother Jim, and several of my closest college friends considered the priesthood as well.

My graduation year, 1950, was celebrated as a Holy Year by the Church. Three schoolmates and I spent the summer bicycling through Europe. Rome was our final destination. During part of the trip, we went our separate ways, and I traveled on my own to Bavaria. One day I biked to Dachau to visit the Nazi concentration camp. I had planned to spend the night in the quaint, medieval Bavarian town, but being at the camp was overwhelming. The Reich's policy of human slaughter had been conducted under a system of laws. I couldn't sleep so near to the site of so much death, so I biked back to Munich.

When I got back, I went into a phone booth and looked up my last name in the phone book. There were eighteen Scheidlers listed. They had been there while Dachau was operating. What did they do? I wondered. Did they try to stop the trains, to stop the killing? I told myself that if anything like this were to happen in America,

I would do something—but I didn't expect that two decades later I would have to make just such a decision.

After my trip to Europe, I came home to look for a job. I had won an award from the *South Bend Tribune* while studying journalism at Notre Dame, so I went to the *Tribune* and asked for a job. They hired me, and I started work on the desk editing copy for our four daily editions.

I soon started writing as a reporter. One of my early stories featured a man whose mother was robbed at gunpoint while bringing home money from the family store. She screamed, and her son rushed out to the porch and was shot. The thief fled without the money, and I wrote up the son as a hero, saving both his mother and the family income. But I hadn't interviewed him, and the next day, he came to see me at the *Tribune*.

"Why did you make me out a hero?" he asked. "Coming out and putting myself in the line of fire? I just came out to see why my mom was screaming—I got shot by accident. Now the insurance company won't cover me!"

I had to write a retraction. That taught me a lesson: just the facts. That's what our professors had been trying to teach us, and I thought I'd learned it. Perhaps journalism wasn't my calling after all. I worked for the *South Bend Tribune* for a year, wondering all the while about the lingering draw to the priesthood.

In the summer of 1951, I decided to enter the seminary. Because I had studied philosophy and theology and already earned a bachelor's degree, I was accepted into a one-year accelerated program at Our Lady of the Lake Seminary in Syracuse, Indiana. My brother Bob was there, and we roomed together. I did some intensive study of Greek and Latin, became enamored of Gregorian chant, and joined the schola.

From Our Lady of the Lake, I went to the major seminary at St. Meinrad in southern Indiana, run by Swiss Benedictines. After finishing philosophy and one year of theology, my spiritual director encouraged me to join the monastery. I wasn't eager to switch to the monastic life, but he said he believed my vocation to the priesthood depended on my becoming a monk. So in the summer of 1954, I joined the order. After a year as Novice Joseph, I took the monastic name Frater Gregory, after St. Gregory the Great, who codified the Mass in the sixth century and for whom Gregorian chant is named.

There was much about monastic life that I liked, but what attracted me most to the priesthood was serving the Lord and his Church by working in a parish. However, the closer I came to ordination, the more I became aware of serious doubts about my calling to the priesthood.

I talked over these doubts with my spiritual advisor, and he sent me to Michigan City, Indiana, to see a psychiatrist who specialized in vocational concerns. I doubt if his methods would meet with approval today, but that day in 1958, he injected me with a dose of sodium pentothal—truth serum—and started asking a raft of questions. At first they were trivial—what foods I liked, my favorite pastimes, what I liked to read. Then he asked, "If your mother were dead, would you become a priest?" I answered him matter-of-factly, "No." It was considered a great honor for a mother to have a son ordained, and perhaps that was what had kept me in the seminary so long. When the truth serum wore off, the psychiatrist told me, "I don't think you have a priestly vocation."

I left St. Meinrad shortly after that, but I wasn't ready to give up on the priesthood. I went to work with my cousin, Father Leo Piguet, the chaplain at the St. Thomas Aquinas Newman Center at Purdue University in West Lafayette, Indiana. I taught religion at the local Catholic high school, directed the parish choir, and taught Christian initiation classes for converts. And I enjoyed working in a parish.

I also began to devour the secular press, reading up on all the news I had missed for several years: Elvis, the Corvette, the hydrogen bomb, the McCarthy hearings. A new morality, if you could call it that, was taking over. And it wasn't just secular society that was changing—Pope John XXIII had announced that he would soon convene the Second Vatican Council. As a devoted Catholic, I was worried that my Church might abandon some of my favorite traditions.

At the end of the semester at Purdue, my bishop sent me to St. Mary's Major Seminary in Norwood, Ohio, to make a retreat in preparation for ordination to the subdiaconate. Life as a parish priest had seemed the right path for me. But while on retreat, I realized that the doctor in Michigan City had been right. I did not have a priestly vocation. I went home and broke the news to my parents. My mother cried. My dad said he had never wanted to be a priest himself.

I went back to teaching at Central Catholic High in Lafayette and joined the art department of the Catholic weekly, *Our Sunday Visitor*. In the fall of 1959, I got a call from my former journalism teacher at Notre Dame, Ed Fischer, with an offer to join the Notre Dame faculty—a dream job dropped in my lap. I had loved Notre Dame during my undergrad years and relished the opportunity to return to the campus.

I taught classes in journalism, layout and design, and public speaking. For the speech classes, I brought in a reel-to-reel machine—state of the art at the time—to record student speeches. I'd then schedule students to come to my office and critique their own talks. Playing their voices back for them was the most effective way of eliminating pauses and other verbal tics. My classes were full, and at the end of each semester, we would hold a banquet in the basement of Franky's, a local hangout, and the best speakers would provide our entertainment.

I stayed at Notre Dame for three years, but I was teaching on a bachelor's degree and needed a master's to stay on the faculty. I enrolled at Marquette University in Milwaukee for a one-year master's program, but when I returned to Notre Dame, I was disappointed to learn that the teacher who replaced me had been such a hit with the department that my old position was no longer open.

I was free to go wherever I wanted, and I set my sights on Chicago. I'd lived in small towns my whole life, and I was eager to move to a big city. One of the strongest draws away from the priesthood was my desire to have a family, and I didn't want to raise my kids in a tiny hamlet that they'd be eager to leave when they grew up. While looking for a teaching position, I reflected that I'd attended an all-male school (Notre Dame didn't go co-ed until 1972) and had been in the navy, seminary, and monastery—a world populated exclusively by men. I decided I needed a change, and so I applied only to Catholic women's schools. I was hired by Mundelein College to teach journalism and religion, including a class called "Redemptive Incarnation." I also handled marketing and PR for the college, designing their brochures and programs.

While I was in my first semester at Mundelein, the whole world changed. I was in my office looking through the newspaper and listening to my little Philco radio when a news flash came over that President John F. Kennedy had been shot in Dallas. Mine was one of the only radios in the building, and people began crowding into my office. Soon we got the news that the president was dead.

Something was jarred loose in America with Kennedy's assassination. The optimism surrounding the Kennedys energized the nation. Then suddenly, he was gone, and the world changed. Vietnam heated up. Ghetto riots started. The youth movement began openly celebrating rebellion. The country seemed to falter.

All authority was being challenged, and the Church in America was no exception. Mundelein asked me to go out to San Francisco to attend workshops with some "new theologians." I'd read their work and knew I wasn't interested—some of it was blatantly heretical. One of my colleagues went instead and brought back some ideas that were at odds with Church traditions. That was not for me.

The Mundelein faculty ate lunch in a college cafeteria with the quaint name of the Tea Room. It was here I'd often see a pretty blonde girl going from table to table, visiting with classmates. She was the student council social chairman, a junior named Ann Crowley. I also saw Ann at noon Mass at Madonna Della Strada on the nearby Loyola University campus, which we both attended frequently.

I lived just a block from Mundelein, so it was common for me to be on campus in the evening, grading assignments or doing PR work. One evening I headed down to the auditorium where there was a rehearsal for a variety show. Ann was in the chorus line with nine other girls. At the beginning of the routine, they had their backs to the audience, then they all turned around in unison, pointed to the audience, and said, "Hey you!" It looked like Ann was pointing right at me. But it couldn't be—she was just a kid, and I was facing middle age. But that "hey you" stuck with me.

When Mundelein started courting "new theology," I started looking for another place to teach. I was offered a position at Marian College in Indianapolis. Indianapolis wasn't as impressive as Chicago, but most of my family lived there, and it would be a place where my reverence for tradition would still be respected. I was all set to take the job when I came into my Mundelein office and found a pink note on my desk that read, "Don't go." It wasn't signed, but I knew it was from Ann.

I called Marian and canceled my contract, then went downstairs and told the Mundelein administration that I would stay on for at least another year. Ann's sister, Mary, had attended my theology class while visiting colleges, and she remembered me when I called to ask Ann to dinner. Ann later told me that when she told Mary it was Mr. Scheidler on the phone, she said, "Oh Ann, if he asks you to marry him, say yes!" We started dating the summer after Ann's junior year. The nuns thought that was sweet.

When I had left the seminary, my mother descended into a deep depression. My youngest brother Jim had already left the seminary, and it was clear that Bob was not going to be ordained. I was Mom's last hope of having a priest in the family. But it was meeting Ann that finally brought her out of her depression. If there was a woman out there who could be such a perfect match for me, then I really couldn't have had a calling to the priesthood after all.

In the summer of 1965, Ann and I got engaged. I proposed at Buckingham Fountain on Chicago's lakefront. She was twenty-one, and I was thirty-seven, so when we went back to her house that night, I expected her father to reject the match. But he approved, and we were married that September.

It was interesting timing. As I was making a serious commitment in my personal life, America seemed to be losing its sense of commitment. The sixties were in full swing. Movies, music, plays, and novels reflected the changing attitudes toward a hedonistic, materialistic bent. I recall going to see a popular film in 1966, *Alfie*, starring Michael Caine. It's a story of a London playboy who refers to his girlfriends as "it" instead of "she." There was one scene that stands out as particularly somber. One of Alfie's lovers has an illegal abortion in her apartment. Alfie comes in and sees the dead baby in the kitchen sink. He breaks down in tears. The camera never reveals the infant, only Alfie's reaction. It's the only moment in the film when the hedonist reveals a human side, when he says to a friend: "You know, it does bring it home to you what you are when you see a helpless little thing like that lying in your hands. He'd been quite perfect. And I thought to myself, 'You know what, Alfie, you know what you've done? You murdered him.'"[1]

The scene struck me. But abortion was still, for the most part, off my radar. Shortly after our first anniversary, Ann and I brought home our first child, Eric. Mundelein did not pay enough to raise

---

1    *Alfie*, directed by Lewis Gilbert (1966; Hollywood, CA: Paramount Pictures, 2001), DVD.

a family in a big city, so I took a job with the city of Chicago in public relations. This was the time when the Great Society programs were being enacted, and I worked for Mayor Richard J. Daley with a program that addressed gangs and other problems in the poorer neighborhoods. Our department was trying to get kids into baseball leagues and art programs instead of gangs. It was my job to publicize the things we were doing. It was frustrating work. Many of the city's outreach programs looked good on paper but didn't really accomplish much.

Ann and I were living in the one-bedroom apartment near Lake Michigan that had been my bachelor pad in my Mundelein days. It got pretty crowded once Eric came along in 1966, so when our son Joey was born the next year, we had to start looking for a house. The city required employees to live within the municipal limits, so we picked out a nice Georgian in a quiet neighborhood called Edgebrook.

Not long after we were settled, a former colleague from the mayor's office, Mike Sitrick, recruited me to Selz, Seabolt and Company, a downtown advertising firm. I started as an account executive that fall. I had some interesting accounts, and I enjoyed designing ads for Marlite Paneling, Shakespeare Fishing Tackle, and Tolibia Cheese for a while.

Then *Roe* came down.

CHAPTER 3

# Raw Judicial Power

On January 23, 1973, I was home from work with the flu, so I wasn't paying attention to the news. The following day, I read about Lyndon Johnson's death and the impending end of the Vietnam War, then turned to the court's abortion rulings that had been announced the previous day.

I was already sick, but reading about the court's decision made me feel even worse. In those days, there were four Chicago dailies—the *Tribune*, the *Sun-Times*, the *Daily News*, and *Chicago Today*. As a PR executive, I read them all. Each covered the *Roe* ruling and the court's decision to divide pregnancy into three stages, decreeing that no state could prohibit abortion in the first trimester. Abortion could be regulated in the second trimester, but only in ways designed to safeguard the woman's health. Only in the third trimester could states try to safeguard the lives of the unborn.

Of the four newspapers, only the *Daily News* devoted any real attention to *Doe v. Bolton*. Their editorial focused on a line from that ruling about regulating late-term abortions, stating that "the medical judgment may be exercised in the light of all factors—physical, emotional, psychological, familial, and the woman's age—relevant to the well-being of the patient. All these factors may relate to health. This allows the attending physician the room he needs to make his best medical judgment. It is room that operates for the benefit, not the disadvantage, of the pregnant woman."[1]

The *Daily News* pointed out that by letting the abortion decision rest on emotional and familial factors, the *Doe* ruling enacted abortion-on-demand throughout the full term of pregnancy in all fifty states. No unborn child was safe. No state government or national legislature—much less fathers—had the authority to protect them.

As I read, I thought about our unborn child, five months in the womb. Initial reporting about *Roe* made it seem that her life might still be protected under law. The *Doe* ruling made it clear that it was not.

The twin rulings struck me as a suicide note for our country. Our claim to be the land of the free and home of the brave, to be refuge for the tired and the poor, now seemed a ghastly sarcasm. The huddled mass of dead babies in the picture on the flyer at the Civic Center rally was a reality now enshrined in law. The slaughter of the innocents in Bethlehem was two millennia ago. And the Nazi atrocities were horrifying, but that was under a dictatorship. But now the United States of America had stripped away its most cherished unalienable right—life—from its most vulnerable population. I felt like a foreigner in my own country. We had embarked on a program of destroying our posterity. I remembered the eighteen Scheidlers in Munich and my promise to fight.

I returned to work, but I'd lost interest in my clients. I became preoccupied with the issue of abortion, hunting everywhere for pro-lifers, attending meetings, and reading everything I could find on abortion.

---

1    "Court Rules on Abortion," *Chicago Daily News*, January 24, 1973.

I read the full text of the Supreme Court's rulings. Justice Harry Blackmun authored both opinions. In *Roe*, he wrote, "We need not resolve the difficult question of when life begins."[2] Any elementary biology student knows that life begins at conception—the question is when *personhood* begins. Blackmun sidestepped, spending several pages on the history of abortion and abortion law around the world. He noted that abortion and infanticide were common in ancient Rome and that the Hippocratic Oath, which included an abortion ban, had never been taken seriously by ancient physicians.

My own historical research showed what Blackmun had left out of his opinion. For example, as medical licensing was developing in the 1870s, there was a strong women's rights movement in America. Leaders across the nation condemned abortion as a barbaric crime against women and children. When states started regulating medical practice, abortion bans were among the first statutes passed. By 1900, every state had passed laws banning abortion except in cases where it was deemed necessary to save the life of the mother.

It was in 1962 that the abortion issue broke into the wider national consciousness. The host of the children's program *Romper Room*, "Miss Sherri" Finkbine of Phoenix, Arizona, had taken thalidomide tranquilizers that her husband, a teacher, purchased while chaperoning a class trip to England. When Miss Sherri read an article linking the pills to birth defects, she told her doctor, and he counseled her to end the pregnancy. He set up a meeting with the hospital review board, which approved the abortion.

Moved to warn other women about thalidomide, she told her story to the *Arizona Republic*. What she didn't realize was that the review board was breaking the law. Arizona law permitted abortion if the *mother's* health was endangered—that wasn't the case here.

---

2    All quotations from court decisions have been taken from publicly available sources.

When the magazine revealed her identity, the story generated a lot of publicity, and the hospital canceled the abortion. She and her husband flew to Sweden to end the pregnancy. In August 1962, her story was on the cover of *Life* magazine.

I remembered reading the story, and I knew she made the wrong decision, but I had no idea that this story was already being used to push for changes to state abortion laws. The American Law Institute's Model Penal Code of 1962 redefined abortion so that it would not fall under "homicide," which allowed hospital review boards to approve abortions more broadly than ever before. Under these guidelines, abortion was permitted if the baby might be deformed—or if the child was a result of rape or incest.

From 1967 to 1970, thirteen states enacted such laws, each requiring that a woman seeking an abortion reside in the state where it would be performed. New York passed a more liberal law in 1970, eliminating the review board and granting abortion on demand up to twenty-four weeks gestation at the doctor's discretion. Unlike the "reform" laws in other states, New York had no residency requirement, in effect legalizing abortion for any woman able to travel there. In his *Roe* opinion, Blackmun cited the New York law as proof that legal abortion was safe for the mother. He opined that the rationale for the late-1800s abortion bans no longer existed.

The *Roe* decision focused specifically on the Texas abortion law, but the ruling effectively struck down all the abortion bans still on the books of most states. *Doe v. Bolton* was aimed at the American Law Institute's (ALI) legislative reforms, specifically one passed in Georgia regarding the hospital review boards authorized to make the life-or-death decisions for the unborn. Under the ALI guidelines, if a doctor thought a patient should have an abortion, he had to make an argument for necessity strong enough to convince enough doctors on the board. After *Doe*, doctors could make those determinations themselves. Now all a woman needed to obtain a legal abortion anywhere in the United States was an abortionist willing to take her money.

In order to strike down all the nation's abortion laws, Justice Blackmun had to find something in the Constitution that gives a woman a right to terminate a pregnancy. He found that in the "right to privacy"—but of course there is no such right in our founding documents. I read that Blackmun had been the attorney for the Mayo Clinic in the 1950s, so he had to be aware that when treating a pregnant woman, the doctor is caring for two patients. Yet throughout *Roe* and *Doe*, Justice Blackmun uses the word *patient* in the singular. For Blackmun, the unborn baby ceased to exist.

The privacy right Blackmun used to justify his rulings was not his own invention. Justice William Douglas set the precedent in 1965 with *Griswold v. Connecticut*, the case that struck down state laws banning contraceptives. Douglas wrote that the First Amendment's freedom of religion, the Fourth Amendment's right to freedom from warrantless searches, and the Fifth Amendment's right to remain silent together constituted a "penumbra" of a right to privacy. The word derives from Latin for "nearly a shadow." It's the hazy part on the edges of a shadow where light is partially obscured. A partial eclipse casts a penumbra. Streetlights do too. And that's the word the court chose when establishing a constitutional right to privacy: a shadow of laws that somehow permits a right to kill the unborn.

Reading about the rulings, I couldn't decide which was most shocking, that Justice Blackmun had composed such nonsense or that seven justices had accepted it. But I wasn't surprised to find just how closely abortion decisions were linked with the birth control cases. *Griswold* had granted married couples access to contraception in 1965, and in 1972, *Eisenstadt v. Baird* declared that birth control had to be made available to single people as well. Justice William Brennan wrote in his *Eisenstadt* opinion that "if the right of privacy means anything . . . it is the right of the individual, married or single, to be free from unwarranted governmental intrusion into matters so fundamentally affecting a person as the decision whether to bear or beget a child."

Justice Brennan circulated his opinion to his fellow justices on the same day the court heard oral arguments in the *Roe* and *Doe* cases. *Eisenstadt* was about contraception, so Brennan was on the mark when discussing a decision to *beget* a child. But he went further, stating that the government had no role in the decision to *bear* a child. For him, the oral arguments in the abortion cases would be a mere formality. He already knew how he would vote.

The one thing that kept me from total despair was that the decisions were not unanimous. Two justices had dissented: Byron White and William Rehnquist. Justice White's dissent was powerful:

> I find nothing in the language or history of the Constitution to support the court's judgment. The court simply fashions and announces a new constitutional right for pregnant women and, with scarcely any reason or authority for its action, invests that right with sufficient substance to override most existing state abortion statutes. The upshot is that the people and the legislatures of the 50 States are constitutionally disentitled to weigh the relative importance of the continued existence and development of the fetus, on the one hand, against a spectrum of possible impacts on the woman, on the other hand. As an exercise of raw judicial power, the Court perhaps has the authority to do what it does today; but, in my view, its judgment is an improvident and extravagant exercise of the power of judicial review that the Constitution extends to this Court.

It was good to know that there were still bastions of logic and reason on the court. As Justice White pointed out, abortion did not come to America through the democratic process. It seemed to me at the time, and it still does, that if the American people could see the reality of what this right actually entails, they would demand that the court reverse these outrageous decisions.

One other hopeful detail was provided by Justice Blackmun himself. "If this suggestion of personhood is established," he wrote at the end of the *Roe* opinion, "the appellant's case, of course, collapses." It was clear that a major thrust of the pro-life movement would have to be proving the personhood of the unborn.

CHAPTER 4

# Going Full Time

W hen I was six years old, I attended the ordination of my cousin, Russell Scheidler, at Notre Dame. Ordination ran in my family. Of the ten children in my father's family, two of the eight brothers became priests. I had several cousins who were priests, and my mother's brother, Leo Pursley, became the bishop of Fort Wayne–South Bend.

That day at Notre Dame, because I was small, I was allowed to sit in the choir stalls bordering the sanctuary with my godmother, Frieda Scheidler. The altar at Sacred Heart has a towerlike structure with a dozen angels stationed on it. I knew they were angels by their wings, but these angels were different—they were holding spears. I asked Aunt Frieda why these angels looked like soldiers. "That's what they are," she said. "They fight Satan."

When Father Russell celebrated his first Mass in Greensburg, Indiana, my grandparents hosted a reception for him at their home in Millhousen. In the living room, there was a large painting of a knight on horseback stabbing a dragon. I asked Aunt Frieda about the painting. "That's Saint George," she told me, "slaying the dragon, the devil." I thought, *Angels are soldiers, saints are soldiers—this must be a Church for soldiers.*

After *Roe* came down, Ann and I started looking for groups who would take a stand on this issue. The IRLC had been founded in the late 1960s, when the ALI's abortion reform legislation had been introduced into the Illinois General Assembly. The IRLC had done good work in the state. They were the group that organized the Chicago rally where I'd first seen the *Life or Death* pamphlet. Shortly after *Roe* and *Doe* were decided, Ann and I went to an IRLC meeting. We expected it to be packed. It wasn't.

The rulings were announced in late January. Not long after that, my brothers and I had a winter family get-together at Pokagon State Park near Angola, Indiana. We all had small children, and we all went tobogganing. After a few runs, it started raining hard, so we went into the lodge and visited. I couldn't stop talking about the abortion decisions. My brothers wondered if I'd come somewhat unhinged—they couldn't understand my preoccupation. I think that perhaps because of our upbringing, they assumed abortion would remain a rarity, used only by people on the social fringe. But—as I tried to explain that day—I felt that abortion would win a much wider following.

I felt that what was most needed to bolster our nation's collapsing moral character was strong and persistent leadership. I expected that leadership to come from the Catholic Church. Here was a blatant evil with the federal government's seal of approval. Surely the bishops had to react, and forcefully. I thought they might even do something as dramatic as calling for a nationwide tax protest. Imagine what could have happened if the American Catholic leadership had called on their flocks to withhold financial support from the government.

To their credit, the bishops did release a strong condemnation in a pastoral message three weeks after *Roe* and *Doe*. The court, they wrote, had relegated the unborn child "to an inferior class of human beings, whose God-given rights will no longer be protected under the Constitution of the United States." They called the opinions "erroneous, unjust, and immoral" and declared that "bringing about a reversal of the Supreme Court's decision and achieving respect for unborn human life in our society will require unified and persistent efforts. But we must begin now—in our churches, schools, and homes, as well as in the larger civic community—to instill reverence for life at all stages. We take as our mandate the words of the Book of Deuteronomy: 'I set before you life or death . . . Choose life, then, that you and your descendants may live.'"[1]

The message was encouraging, and I waited to see the "unified and persistent effort" they had described. I went to talk with the priest who ran the Respect Life office at the Archdiocese of Chicago. I was shocked to discover that he didn't share my zeal. He told me frankly, "You're a little too enthusiastic, too aggressive for the Church. The Church moves slowly. It has a lot of other problems besides abortion." If I wanted to see something done about defending life, he suggested, I should plan to do it on my own.

I spent my lunch hours doing research at the IRLC offices. That's how I heard about a dinner where Father Paul Marx would be the keynote speaker. A Benedictine monk from St. John's Abbey in Minnesota, he had been fighting abortion long before *Roe*. His book charting the legalization movement, *The Death Peddlers*, was published in 1971.

The Archdiocese of Chicago gave away free tickets to the banquet, but nonetheless the room was almost empty, which made me feel

---

1    National Conference of Catholic Bishops, "Pastoral Message of the Administrative Committee," National Conference of Catholic Bishops, February 13, 1973, http://www.usccb.org/issues-and-action/human-life-and-dignity/abortion/upload/Pastoral-Message-of-the-Administrative-Committee.pdf.

even more alone in my concerns. But it gave me the opportunity to have a private conversation with Father Marx after his talk. He went up to his room and came down with two jars containing carefully preserved fetuses, one at twelve weeks and the second at eighteen. I was amazed at how developed they were, their tiny fingernails already visible. As I gazed at the jars, I asked Father Marx, "Why does abortion bother me so much, when it doesn't seem to matter to most people?"

"It's a calling," he answered. "You are blessed with a special calling to fight this evil."

For so much of my life, I'd thought I had a calling—to the priesthood, to journalism, to teaching. But I knew Father Marx was right. Abortion was a special kind of evil, and I knew I absolutely had to do something about it.

A few days later, Paul Fullmer, one of my bosses at the PR firm, called me into his office. He'd noticed how much my zeal for advertising had waned and how passionate I had become about abortion.

"Joe, have you given any thought to doing pro-life work full time?" he asked.

"How would I survive?" I asked.

"You have PR experience," he said. "Build up a clientele that will support you."

Paul offered to keep me on at half salary until our fourth child was born so that we could keep our maternity benefits. Our third son, Peter, had been born in 1969, and I was beginning to think the Lord was giving me a monastery all my own. But then on May 31, 1973—the last day our insurance would cover—our first daughter, Catherine, was born.

Here I was with a wife and four children, a mortgage and no job, but with a firm sense that I had to accept my calling to challenge this tragic national mistake. I'd spent more than a decade preparing for a vocation, honed skills in debate and argument, and worked as a publicist and organizer. And now I had a cause that would demand all my energy and such talents as I had. I was entering my true vocation: pro-life activist.

Ann's dad, attorney Thomas Crowley, helped me set up a non-profit organization that I ran from my back porch: the Chicago Office for Pro-Life Publicity. I thought at the time that publicizing the humanity of the unborn and the medical and psychological threats abortion posed to the mother would be the most powerful tools in combating the terrible turn the nation was taking.

In the spring of 1965, *Life* magazine had published Lennart Nilsson's amazing photos of life in the womb, but less than a decade later, the courts had declared our society free to forget what these pictures taught. I saw it as my job to deliver a refresher course on the humanity of the unborn, and we had new photos to add to the discussion.

Dr. Jack Willke, a pro-life pioneer from Cincinnati, had collected a host of images of abortion victims and infants who survived premature births. He made these available in a slideshow for pro-lifers' use. His 1971 *Handbook on Abortion* sold more than a million copies of the first issue, and he produced the *Life or Death* pamphlet that made an indelible impression on me. Dr. Willke understood that if Americans never saw the brutality involved, we were doomed. I was certain these visuals could be used to show others how critical the issue was.

One of my first plans to inform the public was to buy ad space in the local newspapers. Clinics were opening all over the Chicago metropolitan area, and the newspapers were carrying their ads, so I wanted to place notices about the reality of abortion right where the clinics were advertising. I composed an ad describing fetal development and the dangers of abortion, encouraging mothers to choose life. I included my address and invited readers to send a donation to support the Chicago Office for Pro-Life Publicity.

I submitted the ad to the *Sun-Times*, since that paper ran nearly a full page of clinic ads, more than any of the other newspapers.

The editors required me to substantiate every claim I made with extensive footnotes. With all the extra type, the ad cost more than one thousand dollars—a lot of money in the early '70s. But when I picked up the *Sun-Times* on the first day the ad was to run, it wasn't there. I went to their office to find out why it was missing. A worker in the composing room found my plate with the ad hidden in a drawer. It had been scratched with a large X. Someone working there didn't like it. I got my money back and ran the ad in the *Chicago Tribune*. The ad generated almost no revenue.

Since newspaper space was so expensive, I decided I had to aggressively pursue all the free press I could get. I constantly wrote letters to editors. I called radio stations to encourage them to do a show on abortion, telling them I'd be glad to come in and argue the pro-life side. I called in to shows that were already discussing abortion. I did telephone interviews. I wrote short articles for various publications. I passed out flyers. I found out where the clinics were so that I could try to talk to women going in or visit the doctors. But it was all very disorganized. I was doing much of this work from home, and we had three small boys and a baby girl. My older children remember having to keep quiet while I did radio interviews over the phone.

By 1974, I'd made something of a name for myself in print and on the radio and TV, and the IRLC had noticed. At first they hired me to do freelance PR work, paying me for doing a seminar on fetal development, for doing a radio show, or for taking part in a debate, all on an hourly basis.

I'd often go out to speak to church groups to help pro-lifers organize. One snowy night in the winter of 1974, I went to speak to a group in Blue Island, Illinois. When I got there, I was disappointed—they had coffee and brownies for scores of guests, but because of the storm, only three people showed up. I suggested that we four sit around the table and have a discussion.

One woman asked what the IRLC needed most. I mentioned our need for more adequate office space, and she said that her husband, a retired lawyer, had an unused office in the historic Monadnock Building at Dearborn and Jackson in downtown Chicago. They offered us that space rent-free. It was a wonderful offer, and we took it. I'd been annoyed that almost nobody showed up for my talk, but one of the three that did come gave us a free headquarters.

By the time I was organizing marches and pickets, getting the IRLC a lot of media exposure, Dr. Bart Heffernan, a respected cardiologist and one of the original founders of the IRLC, was diagnosed with a heart condition. Knowing he had to cut back on his pro-life work, he asked the committee to hire me as full-time director. I was doing so many seminars and interviews that I was practically working full time anyway, so the committee agreed. The salary was less than half of what I'd earned as an account executive at Selz, Seabolt and Company, but there was no danger that I'd lose interest in my work.

I was constantly on the lookout for activists, and I found a number of people who felt the way I did. In addition to the IRLC, there were the Illinois Citizens for Life, Birthright, the AUL, and many neighborhood pro-life organizations. There were about thirty pro-life groups in the Chicago area, and I got to know them all. If I heard that a clinic was opening up, I'd call the leaders of various groups, and we'd form a sizable picket or rally on short notice.

I did a lot of speaking in those early years, and it soon began to dawn on me that since I was organizing much of the activism in Chicago, like it or not, I was becoming a leader in the pro-life movement.

The *Chicago Sun-Times* continued to carry their full-page abortion ads, so I printed a flyer that said the *Sun-Times* supported abortion, and a group of daring friends helped me post flyers in their lobby. We got thrown-out several times but kept going back.

If there were any employees there who hadn't known their paper was serving the abortion cause, they knew it by the time they left the building.

I learned through a contact at the *Sun-Times* that two young men in the advertising department were Catholic. I invited them out to lunch at the Little Corporal, a restaurant near the *Sun-Times* offices. Over lasagna, I told them that by taking abortion ads, they were helping promote a grave moral evil.

"There's a full page of abortion ads in the *Sun-Times* almost every day. You've got to do something to make up for that. You've got to stop advertising abortion, period. For your own good as well as others."

They nodded politely, but I didn't seem to be getting through. So in the middle of their lasagna, I pulled out a pack of color photos of aborted babies, some dismembered, others burned with saline. I tossed them in the middle of the table. They almost gagged. It was a dirty trick, but it was effective.

They looked carefully at the pictures; then one of them said, "We'll do something."

"I'm counting on you," I told them.

I didn't hear from them for about a week, so I called one of them and asked if they'd discussed the matter with their boss.

"Yes," he said. "We can't get the paper to drop those ads, but we're going to give you a free ad. You can run your ad whenever the abortion ads run—and you can use any wording you want. It will be on the page with the abortion ads."

No pictures would be allowed, but it was a good offer. We filled the space with facts about fetal development. One day it would read, "Your baby's tiny hands are formed six weeks after conception. He can feel pain by seven weeks. Don't abort your baby." The next day it read, "Your baby can move at six weeks after conception. Fingerprints are formed by eight weeks. Don't abort your baby." The abortion ads all had the word "abortion" in bold letters. Our ads always had "baby." With half as many letters, "baby" was twice as large as "abortion," and it stood out. We always included our office phone number in each ad.

Decades later, in January 2015, at a March for Life in Palatine, Illinois, Ann and I were sitting in St. Theresa Church listening to a speaker recount how his girlfriend had an abortion in the mid-1970s at age fourteen. It was his child. The following year, she was pregnant again. But this time, while looking for a clinic in the *Sun-Times*, she came upon the IRLC ad. She called the number and reached a young woman—my assistant, Laura Canning—who not only counseled her to keep the baby but agreed to go with her when she broke the news to her parents.

This is exactly why I had placed the ads, but it never occurred to me some women would mistake the IRLC for an abortion clinic. I was astounded when we began getting calls from women wanting to schedule abortions. One day in 1976, a salesman, Tom Bresler, came to our office to sell us a coffee service. While he waited in the office, he overheard Laura Canning on the phone with a woman who had called to schedule an abortion. As Tom listened, Laura managed to talk the woman into keeping her baby.

When I came out of my office, Tom told me what he'd heard. "Laura does that all the time," I said. "She's good at it."

He was so impressed that he lost interest in trying to sell us coffee, which was fine, since we wouldn't have been able to afford it anyway. Now he wanted to help with our mission. He offered to pay our rent, but when I told him that we were already set in that area, he started looking for some other way to help. A Jewish convert to Catholicism, Tom was troubled by the *Roe* decision but didn't feel he could do much about it. The Supreme Court had ruled, and abortion on demand was now the law. But the day he tried to sell coffee to a small nonprofit, he found a pro-life vocation.

In 1977, Tom got a group together at his north suburban home, and the following year, they opened a crisis pregnancy center, Aid for Women, nearby. In those days, Michigan Avenue had more clinics than any other street in Chicago. In 1981, Tom opened a second Aid for Women office on Michigan Avenue. These centers helped thousands of women choose life over the years, and they all got started because a coffee salesman overheard a life saved over the phone—and a wrong number at that!

By spring of 1974, I was working full time for the IRLC, leading pickets and protests, issuing press releases, doing television and radio interviews and editorials, and emerging as a leader in the pro-life movement.

## CHAPTER 5

# God So Loved the World

The phone tree method I was using to gather crowds for pickets and protests was effective, but even by the spring of 1974, there were so many pro-life events happening and so much news to get out to activists that a phone tree and monthly newsletter were inadequate. I had to find another way to circulate information.

When I worked for Chicago's public relations department, our office received a complaint about a neo-Nazi telephone line laced with racist commentary. We tried to stop it, but it was a private line, so we were powerless to shut it down. As long as this neo-Nazi wasn't making outgoing calls, however disgusting the message was, we couldn't do anything to keep him from putting out his messages. People called it. The content was ugly, but the concept was clever. I decided to use the same system to keep pro-lifers informed.

As director of the IRLC, I established a daily hotline. Our first recording was May 23, 1974. If we had a rally or a picket planned, it would be on the hotline. I'd clip newspaper stories every day and discuss them on the hotline with a pro-life perspective. The delivery was fast—there was usually a lot of information to cram into what I tried to keep to a three-minute message. If a big story was developing, I might update it two or three times a day.

The *National Right to Life News* did a story on our hotline, and soon we were getting calls from across the country. Other pro-life groups started their own call-in lines, and some would call for my message, record it themselves, and put it on their own hotlines. By the time we were getting five hundred calls a day, we had to add a second phone machine so all our callers could get through. With the advent of the Internet and social media, the hotline has become outdated, but every time I suggest discontinuing it, I get enough calls to encourage me to update it at least once a week. Not everybody has an iPhone. Feel free to give it a call: 773-777-2525.

Dr. Bart Heffernan approved of how I was increasing public awareness of abortion, and Dennis Horan, one of our attorneys, liked my approach to educating the public through direct action. Whenever I saw an opportunity to promote the cause, I would launch a program to do it. I assumed that most of the board was satisfied with my work, and I took their permission for granted. But a few of the board members saw matters differently.

Starting in 1972, the Catholic Church designated the first Sunday of October as Respect Life Sunday, and the IRLC got a statement each year from then mayor Richard J. Daley to promote the day. I thought the message they prepared for him to sign was weak, since it had no specific reference to the unborn. So I wrote up a more forceful statement about respecting human life from conception onward. I ran it over to City Hall for the mayor's signature. Later, when the board saw my statement, some said it was too strong and that Daley wouldn't sign it. One board member even told me that if I asked the mayor to sign my version, he'd see to it that I was fired.

"Too late," I replied, showing him my copy with Daley's signature.

The mayor's office hosted a health fair at City Hall each year, and we were offered a booth. A few weeks before the fair, my assistant, Laura Canning, had taken our display to a local college campus. A friend of one of the board members saw the booth and complained that the picture of the garbage can full of babies—the one from the Toronto hospital that made such an impression on me—was too graphic to be used. The board considered this objection and voted against having the Toronto picture on display. I thought this picture was one of our strongest tools. More than any other piece of evidence, that was the one that brought me into the pro-life movement. It was the centerpiece of the booth.

So ignoring the board's vote, I set up the display the way I had designed it, with the Toronto picture in the middle and a film about fetal development that ran in a loop. It drew a bigger crowd than any other booth at the fair. A pro-life nurse volunteered to work in uniform at the booth to help counter the notion that the medical community favored legal abortion. When I stopped by City Hall to see how things were going, the nurse was trembling—the picture was gone. "What happened?" I asked.

"Some man jumped into the booth. He grabbed the picture and threw it." I looked. It was some distance away, lying against a wall. A piece had broken off the corner, but it looked fixable. "Can you describe him?" I asked. She pointed across the lobby. "He's right there." It was an IRLC board member.

Just then, Mayor Daley stopped at our booth. News photographers were hovering around, and one of them said, "Let's get a picture of you right here looking at the exhibit." That evening's *Sun-Times* had a picture of the mayor in front of our booth, with a big empty space where the abortion picture had been. Maybe that photo wouldn't have been used if our Toronto picture had been in the background. But maybe it *would* have—and I was incensed that we missed the opportunity to get that image into the mainstream media.

This was becoming a problem for me. Too many members of the IRLC board seemed afraid of alienating anyone. I wasn't particularly concerned about risking alienating people. We couldn't compromise our effectiveness. Thankfully, other pro-life activists felt the same way. Planned Parenthood also had a booth at the health fair, and we noticed at one point that it was unmanned. Some pro-lifers saw this as their cue to help Planned Parenthood pack up for the day. The story later circulated that someone had stored their exhibit some blocks away—in a dumpster.

I found opportunities to promote the pro-life cause everywhere I went. One morning in March 1979, I was driving down Devon Avenue looking for a billboard that someone had alerted me to. It wasn't that far from my home. I was surprised to think that I'd probably passed it dozens of times without seeing it. Finally, there it was, the side of a three-story building, taking up at least half of the wall: ABORTION in letters four feet tall with a phone number. It faced traffic coming from the east. I parked and went to talk to the building manager.

"That sign out there is promoting a grave evil," I told him.

"Yeah, I know. I'm embarrassed it's there," he said. "Some medical clinic rented the space—I didn't know it was going to be an abortion ad."

"When is their contract up?" I asked.

"It's already expired."

I explained who I was, and he offered to let me rent the space to put up a pro-life ad.

"Well, you've already been giving the clinic free advertising since their ad is still there, haven't you? We'd only have to change two letters to make it read 'Adoption.'"

"You can do that free of charge," he said. "But you'll have to paint it yourself."

As it happened, the clinic's phone number on the sign was only a couple of digits different from the number for Preserving Human Dignity, a pregnancy assistance center. It looked like it would be an easy job.

That afternoon, a young law student named Pat Trueman turned up at our office. He'd just finished his first year of law school, which had been so demanding that he'd made a bargain with God. If He'd help Pat make it through the first semester, Pat would devote himself to pro-life work. He came to see me in the middle of his second semester to follow through on that pledge.

"Well, that's good," I said, "because tomorrow I'm going to paint the side of a three-story building that has a pro-abortion ad on it. We're going to make it a pro-life billboard, and I might need some help. Here's the address. But you probably won't show up."

"Why do you say that?" he asked.

"We get a lot of volunteers with good intentions, but they usually don't show up. But you've got the address."

The next morning, I borrowed an extension ladder and got a couple gallons of fast-drying paint—white and black. I really thought I'd be alone, but I'd underestimated Pat Trueman. Soon he was fighting the wind, holding the ladder while I changed a *B* to a *D*. I was happy to have him there—if I'd have been alone, the ladder might have blown over.

After I finished the *D*, we needed to move the ladder to turn the *R* into a *P*. My car was in the way, so I threw my keys down to Pat so he could move the car. I started down as he backed up, but the bumper caught on the ladder, nearly dragging it out from under me. I caught the rails and slid down like a monkey on a string, miraculously keeping all the paint in the bucket.

Fortunately, that was the only time Pat Trueman ever came close to killing me. Having changed ABORTION into ADOPTION, all we had left to do was change a few digits in the phone number. When we were done, the sign looked pretty good.

Pat came to our house for dinner so often that he started calling Ann "Mom." We hosted his law school graduation party at our house. He was planning to head back to Buffalo, Minnesota, where he had a job lined up with a local firm, but I hoped to keep him in Chicago working with the pro-life movement.

At that time, Dennis Horan was on the board of the AUL. He wanted the AUL to have a legal arm. He and I sought the help of my uncle, Bishop Leo Pursley, who was then president of the Catholic weekly, *Our Sunday Visitor*. We were able to secure a twenty-thousand-dollar grant from *Our Sunday Visitor* to establish the Legal Defense Fund for the AUL, and they asked Pat to be the head of the Defense Fund. Pat later served in the Justice Department prosecuting pornographers, and in recent years headed up Morality in Media, an antiporn group.

While still working with me at the IRLC, Pat helped out with numerous late-night activities. We had hundreds of posters of the Toronto picture with the text "Abortion Kills Babies" printed on cheap, mealy paper. Twelve of us would break into pairs and blanket downtown Chicago. One carried a bucket of soapy water and the other a paste made from water, flour, and Elmer's glue. We'd race around the Loop, cleaning grime off the lampposts and pasting two signs as high as we could reach on each post. Since the paper was grainy, it was almost impossible for pro-abortion advocates—or the city—to tear them off.

Pat and I are tall, as were our other helpers. We'd balance on the bases of the lampposts to paste up our posters. We covered the whole Loop in a single night, then reunited at an underground restaurant called Plato's. Since we returned all covered in grime, we named ourselves the Dirty Dozen.

We got artistic with some of our public relations efforts too. In those days, when a new building was going up, the plywood fencing around the construction site was left blank. Those panels would eventually be discarded anyway, so we took big plywood squares and jigsawed out three-foot square letters, making stencils to spell out "Abortion Kills Babies." We fitted each stencil with two hooks so we could hang them on the construction fencing. They were impressive, readable from over a block away. Pro-abortion activists would come out at night and change the message to "No Abortion Kills Women." Then we'd go back and change it to the original. We went through a lot of spray paint.

The City Office of Special Events used to spray large white squares on the corners of major intersections to advertise upcoming events. When an event was over, they'd paint over the wording that announced it, leaving a fresh white square. We'd come out at night with specially prepared stencils to fill those squares with pro-life messages.

We were using all manner of techniques to get the message out. Every Thursday, we'd leaflet an area of downtown Chicago. Initially, we fanned out to be on as many corners as possible, but when we converged to reload on leaflets, we noticed that when we were together in a group, more people took our flyers. We discovered that we could hand out a lot more flyers by concentrating in one area than we would by spreading out. We adopted a new plan of group distribution.

In June 1977, I was invited to speak at the NRLC convention at the Hyatt Hotel in downtown Chicago. I was to give two talks: one on lobbying and the other on dealing with a hostile media, scheduled back to back on Sunday morning. The day before, I got some news about St. Joseph College in Rensselaer, Indiana. I knew the school—one of my uncles, Father Albin Scheidler, of the Missionaries of the Precious Blood, had taught at St. Joe's for many years. He had supervised the work to enlarge the Lourdes grotto on campus. Another of my uncles, Benno Scheidler, had died the previous fall and willed a large grant to the college.

I learned that St. Joe's had invited Indiana Senator Birch Bayh to be its commencement speaker. Bayh headed the Senate Judiciary Committee. A week after the *Roe* and *Doe* decisions, Senator Lawrence Hogan introduced a Human Life Amendment to Bayh's committee to nullify the rulings, and other versions soon followed. Bayh was able to keep all these efforts stalled in his committee. He initially claimed to support the pro-life effort, but in 1976, he publicly told Planned Parenthood that he was on their side. When Senator Jesse Helms moved to bring the Human Life Amendment to the full Senate for a vote, Bayh blocked the motion. And he was scheduled to speak at St. Joe's graduation.

It was going to be a busy Sunday.

As soon as I found out about Bayh's appearance, I called St. Joe's and spoke with the provost, alerting him to Bayh's anti-life position and asking that they withdraw the invitation. I'd heard that some faculty were boycotting the graduation, but there was no organized protest of Bayh's appearance—yet. I told them if they permitted Bayh to speak, I would be at the graduation. They wouldn't withdraw the invitation, so I asked to be allowed to take the podium to explain how the senator's position was at odds with Church teaching. They denied that request too.

I finished my talks at the Hyatt at noon and left for Rensselaer with Jack Ames, a Baltimore activist attending his first NRLC convention, and Chicago pro-life stalwart Greg Morrow. We raced down to Gary, Indiana, to pick up Father Ted Mens, a dedicated pro-life pastor, and headed to St. Joe's. We got there just as the procession was starting. I asked Father Charles Bannett, the college president, if I could offer a few words from the podium. He refused.

The ceremony was in the gymnasium. The bleachers were pulled out, and chairs lined the floor. We climbed to the very top row of the bleachers and sat down. I had a bullhorn in a sack. When Senator

Bayh began to speak, we all stood up. I pulled out the bullhorn and said, "You, Birch Bayh, vote to kill babies."

I continued for a while, and the crowd began to boo. To his credit, Bayh said, "This man has a right to speak. Let's listen to what he has to say." But the booing grew louder. The crowd moved away from us on both sides, then parted as we began walking down the bleachers.

When I got to the bottom of the stands, I was met by campus security, local police, and state troopers. One faculty member, who introduced himself as the head of the school's finance committee, recognized my name and spoke with the police. I think when he heard the name "Scheidler," he remembered Uncle Benno's unexecuted will or possibly Father Albin's long tenure at St. Joe's. In any event, he asked us to leave the campus, but he didn't push for my arrest. I convinced him to let us visit the chapel Uncle Benno had paid to refurbish and say some prayers at Father Albin's grotto.

Father Albin earned the nickname "K.O." Scheidler at that grotto in 1931. One of the students responsible for carrying the stones started slacking off, and Father Albin told him to get back to work. The young man mouthed off, and my uncle socked him. The grotto got finished pretty quickly after that. That was a different time, of course, and it seemed that St. Joe's was losing that fighting spirit. But the next year, St. Joe's invited Louise Summerhill, founder of Birthright International, to be their commencement speaker.

The day after my visit to St. Joe's commencement, parents started calling the IRLC to try to get me fired for disrupting the ceremony. Dr. Heffernan had moved to Florida for his health, and I had only a few allies left on the IRLC board. Within a year of my trip to Rensselaer, I was fired. The committee assembled a long list of things I'd done that they disapproved of, and interrupting St. Joe's graduation was at the top of the list.

When I started at the IRLC, the organization had five thousand members. By the time I left, we were up to twenty thousand. Most of that increase, I believed, was a result of my more aggressive methods. I knew there were many members who joined because it was dedicated to direct action—even impolite action—to save the unborn. As it became clear that I'd be leaving the IRLC, some of the board members who approved of my activism joined me to found a new organization, Friends for Life (FFL).

Like the IRLC, the FFL would have a board of directors. Father Charles Fiore, O.P., a Dominican priest from Oak Park, was my codirector. We agreed that neither of us would be members of the FFL board. Father Fiore was a zealous pro-lifer and a dynamic speaker, always experimenting with new methods to help fund the organization.

But the FFL eventually developed many of the same problems that had plagued me at the IRLC. Here, too, the board had members too concerned with projecting a respectable public image. While I was director of the FFL, the *Chicago Sun-Times* quoted my take on activism: "You can try for fifty years to do it the nice, polite way, or you can do it next week the nasty way."[1] Some of the board doubted that the nasty way was appropriate for a group with such a friendly name. Eventually, the board voted to fire me. And within the year, the FFL closed its doors.

Clearly, I needed to found my own pro-life organization. And I needed a name that left no doubt as to our activist mission: the Pro-Life Action League. We were 100 percent pro-life, totally committed to direct action. I chose a slogan to show we weren't just about making speeches and collecting petitions: "Because action speaks louder than words."

Once again, my father-in-law helped us incorporate as a nonprofit. Legally, a nonprofit needs to have a board of directors, but

---

1   Pamela Zekman and Pamela Warren, "Meet the Abortion Profiteers," *Chicago Sun-Times*, November 28, 1987.

I had become wary of large groups trying to control my activism. I knew I needed freedom from a troublesome board, and the legal minimum was a three-member board. Ann and I were two. Rosie Stokes, a friend I had known since college, became our third, and every vote the Pro-Life Action League board ever cast has been unanimous.

Tom Roeser, who was a board member of the IRLC and a founding member of the FFL had once asked me to keep the FFL board informed about my plans. "These ideas come to me in the middle of the night," I had told him. Furthermore, if they denied permission, I couldn't comply. If the IRLC board had tried to bar me from confronting Birch Bayh, I'd have ignored them too.

A few years after the FFL folded, Tom Roeser told *Chicago Tribune* reporter Linda Witt, "We fired Joe, but Joe was really right. . . . The only thing that could work was a desperate, uncoordinated, hit-the-streets movement that goes to the very brink of uncivility, embarrasses people, makes them uncomfortable. And Joe's the very guy to pull that off."[2]

For a while, I worked from home, as I had in the days of the Chicago Office for Pro-Life Publicity, but I was looking for an office. I found one a block from my house, and as soon as we'd done our first fundraiser, we moved in. Behind my desk, I hung a plaque, a gift from some fellow activists: "God so loved the world that He didn't send a committee."

---

2    Linda Witt, "Man with a Mission," *Chicago Tribune*, August 11, 1985.

CHAPTER 6

# Give Us Barabbas

Gloria was pregnant.

Her husband, Michael, said he was worried about overpopulation and about the environment and wasn't ready to be a father. He stormed out of the house. Gloria was conflicted, and she talked with her mother, Edith, about an abortion.

"Gloria, no. You wouldn't do a thing like that?" Edith asked.

Gloria asked Edith whether she thought a woman should have that right.

"Well, when I'm sitting here watching them women talk about it on TV, I guess it's yes," Edith answered. "But when I'm sitting here with my own daughter, who's carrying my own grandchild—oh, Gloria, I'm already in love with that baby."

"Well, so am I," Gloria said. "But the baby isn't here, and Michael is, and I don't want to lose my husband." She started to cry.[1]

Her father, Archie, came downstairs to see what was happening. He tried to comfort her. Shortly afterward, Michael came

---

1    "Gloria's Pregnancy," *All in the Family*, season 1, episode 6, aired September 8, 1975 (Norman Lear/Tandem Productions).

home. He'd come to his senses and decided they should keep the baby.

This episode of *All in the Family* aired in September of 1975, two and a half years after *Roe*. We were relieved that CBS had Gloria and Michael choose life, and the following day I directed my hotline callers to congratulate CBS for this episode.

But that wasn't the only time a CBS sitcom had an abortion theme. Two months before the Supreme Court's rulings were announced, the lead character in *Maude* was pregnant at age forty-seven. The show was set in New York, and throughout the episode, characters reminded the audience that abortion was legal there. Maude's adult daughter advocates passionately for killing her younger sibling, emphasizing women's freedom to do as they please with their bodies and criticizing Maude for being old-fashioned. "When you were young," she says, "abortion was a dirty word. It's not anymore."

The first episode ended in a cliffhanger. Maude's decision would come at the end of the next episode. She chose abortion. In the final conversation, Maude's husband, Walter, assures her, "For you, Maude, for me, in the privacy of our own lives, you're doing the right thing."[2]

That line about privacy is central. The oral arguments in the *Roe* and *Doe* cases took place just weeks before "Maude's Dilemma" ran. Questions of whether there is a constitutional right to privacy and whether it confers a right to abortion were the key issues in those arguments, but that kind of jargon likely wouldn't come up in a personal conversation about abortion. *Maude's* writers were making a case to the nation as directly as Sarah Weddington, *Roe's* lawyer, had made to the Supreme Court, and on the same grounds. They weren't just presenting a controversial issue; they were taking sides on it.

---

2  "Maude's Dilemma" Pts. 1 & 2, *Maude*, season 1, episode 9, aired November 14 and 21, 1972 (Tandem Productions).

The summer after the *Roe* and *Doe* rulings, CBS reaired the *Maude* abortion episodes. By then, pro-life groups were active all over the nation and picketed a number of CBS stations. Abortion was still a dirty word to most Americans, and the public outcry over presenting it as a suitable topic for a sitcom led many CBS affiliates to preempt the rebroadcasts and may have been one reason the *All in the Family* episode, which aired in 1975, had a pro-life outcome.

Our Chicago protests didn't convince our local CBS affiliate, Channel 2, to drop the *Maude* episodes, but they earned us some airtime. I suggested that if they were going to promote abortion, they should give us equal time to promote the pro-life message. I was invited to make two separate appearances on the talk show *Common Ground*, hosted by Warner Saunders.

In the first program, I appeared opposite Dr. Theodore Roosevelt Mason Howard, who ran Friendship Medical Center on the South Side. He advertised "lunch-hour abortions." I'd met Dr. Howard some months earlier when I called him and set up a meeting. T. R. M. Howard was a hunter, and his office was adorned with some of his prey. A mounted cougar stood next to his desk, behind which was a stuffed mountain goat that resembled a lamb. I remember thinking to myself, *He hunts children, too.*

Dr. Howard was a big man, very welcoming—charming, in fact. During our meeting at his office, we talked about hunting and taxidermy. When I brought up the topic of abortion, he didn't want to talk about it beyond the usual line: It was a woman's right, and he did a good job in a profession that had too many quacks.

Warner Saunders was an extremely fair host, and I was able to present a lot of information on fetal development. At one point, I teased Dr. Howard about having a stuffed lamb in his office, that it seemed wrong for a man to shoot a lamb, and what that revealed about his profession. He took it well. We both knew it was actually a mountain goat, but he got the point.

Saunders and I struck up a good relationship, and after that, any time he wanted to do an abortion story, he'd invite me down to his studio. My experience with *Common Ground* was much better than another of my earliest TV appearances, when I was on Irv Kupcinet's show. He had a daily piece in the *Sun-Times* called "Kup's Column" and a late-night TV show. Both were syndicated nationwide. Kupcinet had briefly been a host of *The Tonight Show* years before Jack Parr or Johnny Carson. *Kup's Show* had a huge viewing audience, and it was a big deal to be on his program. His other guest that night was writer and political commentator Gore Vidal. I was looking forward to this program. I was certain I knew far more about abortion than either Kup or Vidal.

I assumed Vidal and I would have a debate, with Kup moderating. Instead, Kup was clearly on Vidal's side, and the two dominated the show. I had scarcely any opportunity to present information on fetal development or the arguments against the Supreme Court rulings. Their touchstone was "nobody really knows when life begins," ignoring basic biology and selling Justice Blackmun's lie.

I had scientific retorts to their smokescreens, but I had hardly any chance to present them. I realized afterward I'd been too polite. I had to be more forceful to get my point across—from now on, no more Mr. Nice Guy.

Of course, I've had the opposite experience too: too much help from my host. When I was on *Hannity and Colmes*, each time the pro-choice guest made a point, Sean Hannity challenged her. He was using all the usual pro-life arguments, but I started wondering why he'd bothered to invite me on if he was determined to do all the talking.

Fox's Bill O'Reilly rarely allows his guests to finish a sentence. The one time I saw O'Reilly struck speechless was when he interviewed Jill Stanek, a nurse at Christ Hospital in Oak Lawn, Illinois. She described a late-term baby dying in her arms and the hospital's policy of shunting these infants off to a soiled linen closet to die. That produced the longest spell of dead air on O'Reilly's program ever.

I appeared on *The O'Reilly Factor* in 2003, at the very hour Paul Hill was executed for the 1994 shooting of Florida abortionist John Britton. I told O'Reilly that there were three murders: a doctor murdering babies, Hill's murder of Britton, and the state of Florida murdering Hill. He took offense at my calling Hill's execution murder, suggesting I might lead people to think shooting abortionists is justified. I didn't intend that, but O'Reilly was invested in making it appear that I did, perhaps to make the segment more sensational. I said afterwards that I'd never accept another invitation to be on *The O'Reilly Factor*. But later I did. I've read his books. I hope he reads mine.

In 1982, I was a guest at a conference in Colorado: the Aspen Film and Television Seminar, hosted by the American Film Institute and the Aspen Institute for Humanistic Studies. Representatives from several special interest groups were invited to discuss how certain social issues were addressed in the media. The three major television networks were represented, as were the National Association for the Advancement of Colored People (NAACP) and La Raza. Playboy's cable division was also there, as was the Gay Media Task Force and a number of other groups. I was attending at Judy Brown's request as a representative of the American Life League. There were about thirty-three guests and a team of presenters at the conference.

We were gathered around tables arranged in a large square. The first speaker launched into an attack on traditional morality, criticizing religious beliefs and praising the trend that faith in God and the Ten Commandments were already being disregarded by the masses. No one was allowed to interrupt, but you could raise your hand and they would take your name. When the speaker was finished, you could ask your question.

"Is there anything immoral or pornographic enough," I asked him, "that you wouldn't show it on TV or in the movies?"

"What do you mean by immoral?" the speaker asked. "Who decides what's moral?"

About the only absolute the speaker acknowledged was opposition to censorship—any censorship. The La Raza rep pointed out that the media would be their own censors, the ones telling the public what was right and wrong. If people don't like what's on TV, the argument went, people can just turn it off. "They can just turn it off" became the catchphrase for the conference.

Throughout the conference, I felt that I was in some neo-pagan world. The conference campus didn't help, with its strange obelisks and weird bronze and stone sculptures all over the grounds. The people behind much of our televised news and media were constructing their own moral universe. I wondered if they'd lost touch with the "people" they claimed to entertain and inform, or if I had. I found the experience so oppressive that I sought out a church in Aspen and started going to an early Mass. It helped. At the end of the conference, I headed for home, feeling that I had some idea of how a soul feels getting out of Purgatory.

In 1983, I contributed to a book by two sociology professors, Arthur Shostak and Gary McLouth, who were studying male involvement in abortion. They were working with thirty abortion clinics to conduct surveys of more than a thousand men who had been involved with abortion, including those who accompanied their wives or girlfriends to the clinics, as well as those who did not, because they either didn't know about the abortion, were told not to come, or refused to go. The book was called *Men and Abortion*.

In the interview, I learned that one area the authors intended to study was whether an abortion could strengthen a couple's relationship. I wasn't happy with how my interview went, so I wrote up my thoughts on the issue and sent it to the authors. When the book was published, I was surprised to see that they printed every word I had sent them. They gave me four pages in a chapter on activism. These are my concluding paragraphs.

> The only way a man should be brought into the abortion decision is as an advocate for the unborn child. As the father, he should want his child to live. To talk about "making a hard decision together" is too bizarre to discuss. Picture the parents of a three-year-old discussing plans to kill their child, and deciding that this decision would be "life-enhancing." Abortion is the murder of a younger child, and "discussing abortion" is plotting a murder. You can play with semantics until you find a nice sounding excuse, but the facts remain. It is almost 1984, and we are set for "doublespeak," using words to mean what we want them to mean, using illogical conclusions as though they make sense, and calling good evil, right wrong, and life death.
>
> Through it all, there will remain a few who know the difference, who are not taken in by the twisted semantics of the age. And these few will know clearly that society is living a lie. We will hear your arguments that confuse and impress the many, and we will know that you are living a lie. And we will not even have to condemn you. You will have condemned yourselves.[3]

On the pro-abortion side, the activism chapter included excerpts from abortion rights activist Bill Baird, the self-styled "Father of Abortion Rights." Baird has some claim to that title. It was his Supreme Court case, *Eisenstadt v. Baird*, that brought about the court's assertion of a right to decide whether or not to bear a child.

---

3    Arthur Shostak, Gary McLouth, et al., *Men and Abortion: Losses, Lessons, and Love* (Westport, CT: Greenwood Press, 1985).

In the Gospel of John, when Pontius Pilate interrogates Jesus about whether he is the King of the Jews, Jesus replies that he came to testify to the truth. Pilate's response, "What is truth?" contains a critical lesson. The question suggests that truth is esoteric if not unknowable, and if that is the case, "truth" is relative. Pilate's next move is revealing: Though he openly admits he finds no guilt in Jesus, he accedes to the will of the crowd. When truth is up for grabs, what is left but popular opinion?

What led the crowd to turn on Jesus? The Jewish leaders, the "opinion-makers" of their day, told them what to think. So when Pilate offers to release a prisoner and gives the assembled crowd the choice between Jesus and Barabbas, the crowd shouts, "Give us Barabbas!" When Pilate asks what to do with Jesus, they answer, "Crucify Him!" On Palm Sunday, the congregation speaks these replies. We are the crowd. We are the ones who shout for Barabbas.

This tradition reminds us that the betrayal, denial, and crucifixion of Christ results from humanity's refusal to accept his divinity. Christians are called to be Jesus' disciples—and if we're not following him, we're denying him. Going along with the crowd is an attempt to avoid decision making. Pilate washed his hands to show the crowd that Jesus' death was not his fault. The cry for Barabbas is a collective shirking of the responsibility to choose what is right, of standing with the truth.

My fellows in Aspen claimed TV audiences could "just turn it off." Certainly some would. But more would not. Entertainment and news are crafted to represent the mainstream, the accepted norm. The media shape the culture even more than the culture shapes the media. A character, plot line, or opinion inserted here or there isn't enough to send most people reaching for their remotes. And of course, many simply don't mind the racier stuff. Others delight in it. Bit by bit, the cultural norm shifts, and the mainstream changes. The water in the pot gets a little hotter.

The name *Barabbas* comes from Aramaic, meaning "Son of the Father." This is the very name Catholics use to praise Jesus in the Gloria at Mass. But given a choice between the true Son and an imposter, the crowd demands the imposter. But the crowd was *advised* to ask for Barrabas. Their leaders, those who defined their cultural norms, told them what would be best for them. And the crowd followed.

Human nature doesn't change much. In 1973, the Supreme Court told us there was a constitutional right to abortion. Of course there is no such thing, but much of the crowd has followed *Roe v. Wade* as the law of the land. They are told and they choose to believe that abortion is good for women and for society. Too many simply don't choose to "turn it off."

CHAPTER 7

# Principles and Protests

When I worked in public relations for the city of Chicago in the late 1960s, my office was in the same building as the Chicago chapter of Planned Parenthood. I would occasionally stop in and look at their literature. I became friends with the head of their Chicago office. *Roe v. Wade* was still a few years off, and though I found a lot of their values alarming, at the time I didn't see what a threat Planned Parenthood was becoming.

After *Roe*, it didn't take long for Planned Parenthood to become the nation's biggest promoter and provider of abortions. Thus Planned Parenthood was often a target of pro-life protests. While much of their funding comes from government grants, they also depend on private and corporate donations, including support from Playboy Enterprises.

One Friday evening in 1980, Playboy hosted a fundraising party for Planned Parenthood at Hugh Hefner's mansion on North State Parkway in Chicago's Gold Coast. Ann was in Indiana visiting my sisters, so I took all the kids to a protest I was leading in front of the mansion. We had picket signs with a silhouette of a fetus. I brought our two red wagons for my daughters. I hitched the wagons together.

Sarah, age one, rode in the front wagon and Annie, who was four, was in the back.

Annie didn't like to stay in the wagon, so she climbed out and walked in the picket line, carrying one of the signs. At one point, I realized she wasn't with us. She had followed some guests through the gate and into the mansion—with her picket sign. She wasn't at the party long. A security guard carefully nudged her out of the party and sent her back to the group. We all cheered Annie for having the nerve to attend a party that clearly wasn't child-friendly.

In 1983, I was interviewed by Carol Kleiman at my office for an article in *Ms.* Magazine. She was a reporter for the *Chicago Tribune* but also wrote stories for other publications. I knew *Ms.* was no friend of ours, but I've always had a policy of taking virtually any interview I can get—you never know who you might reach.

Kleiman had her notepad out and had just started asking questions when our office got a call for her. After a moment on the phone, she dropped her pad and pen, looking stricken. Her son had been in a car crash and was at a nearby hospital. I drove her to the hospital in my car while an office volunteer, Marian Masella, followed in hers. When we got there, we learned that her son had some facial lacerations but that they weren't serious and there would be almost no scarring. We left Kleiman there with her own car and drove back to the office, where I noticed she'd left her notepad with its list of questions on her chair. Since we'd barely started the interview, I read the questions on her list, typed up answers to each, and sent sixteen pages of responses to her *Tribune* office.

When the story came out in *Ms.*, Marian and my secretary, Barbara Menes, were incredulous. "This is terrible!" said Marian. "You took her to the hospital! You answered all her questions! And there's hardly a word of truth in there. After all that, she's made you out to be some kind of monster!"

"What did you expect?" I asked. "It's not nearly as bad as I thought it would be. I think it's pretty tame." If the editors at *Ms.* wanted to cast pro-lifers in a bad light, that's what they did. After years of pickets and protests, you develop a thick skin. Worse than being insulted is being ignored.

In June of 1990, I learned from some Empire State pro-lifers that the *New York Times* was hosting a news media convention in Manhattan. I thought this would be a good event to leaflet. We wanted to remind the media moguls that we exist, that we promote the cause of life nationwide, and that we show up in the hundreds of thousands every year for the March for Life in Washington. So I flew to New York and met with a group of pro-lifers at the home of Eileen Cullaghan on Lexington Avenue on the Upper East Side. Our crew included Joan Andrews, who had spent two years in jail for her activism and was known in the movement as "St. Joan." Chris Slattery, who runs a network of crisis pregnancy centers in the New York area, was there as well, along with half a dozen activists. At this meeting, we put together comprehensive press packets to distribute to conference attendees the next day.

We rented rooms at the Sheridan Center Hotel on Seventh Avenue, where the conference was taking place, so that we couldn't be kicked out of the hotel. Our timing was perfect. We got to the conference just as the attendees were between sessions. They were practically swarming us to get our packets, and nearly every reporter took one. This was encouraging, because it was obvious that we were handing out pro-life literature.

After distributing our packets, we headed over to picket the *New York Times.* The *Times* was, and still is, militantly pro-abortion. Reporters from other outlets covered our picket, but the *Times* didn't even send a reporter.

Almost every reporter at the Sheridan had taken one of our packets. But the editors pull the strings and control the content. Carol

Kleiman could have written me up as a saint, but her editors at *Ms.* had the final say. And anyone who believes that a woman has a right to destroy her child for any reason isn't going to be particularly concerned about the truth.

While media heads have a lot to answer for in creating a society that accepts abortion, more disturbing is how many Catholic colleges and universities have fallen in line with the media message and turned their backs on the identity they claim to profess. Near the end of my tenure at Mundelein College, in a discussion on the school's character, the vice president made a comment that could serve as a motto for most Catholic schools: "The less Catholic, the better."

A Catholic college is not just a school with a saint's name and a campus chapel. It is a place whose mission is to teach Catholic principles. A truly Catholic education teaches no contradiction between faith and reason—the two must go hand in hand. The study of history, the sciences, indeed all subjects, leads the student closer to God, not farther away.

The most disturbing case of a Catholic university losing its way is the case of my alma mater, Notre Dame. Tour the campus today, and you'll see that the grotto and the basilica and the beautiful mosaic of Jesus as the Word of Life on the library are all still there. It still looks like a Catholic campus. But its broad embrace of secularism has greatly undermined its Catholic identity.

Much of this goes back to the presidency of the late Father Theodore Hesburgh, who became president of Notre Dame in 1952, two years after I graduated. When I was a student, he was the chaplain of Vetville, the housing establishment for married veterans set up after World War II. He was the most popular priest on campus. He served as vice president when I taught there in the early '60s. I always admired him.

Father Hesburgh had an amazing memory. When we dropped off my daughter Sarah at Notre Dame to begin her study there, we saw

Father Hesburgh on campus. Ann and I introduced him to
and he asked what residence hall she was moving into. Four y
later, at Sarah's graduation, we ran into him again. He congratulated
Sarah and told her, "I remember when you arrived and moved into
Walsh Hall." His ability to remember and connect with people aided
his impressive career.

Father Hesburgh was valued and respected far beyond Notre
Dame. In 1954, President Dwight Eisenhower appointed him to
the President's Science Advisory Committee and, when the US
Commission on Civil Rights was created in 1959, to that committee as well. He served as head of the Rockefeller Foundation,
and President Carter appointed him to an immigration reform
commission.

In 1967, however, Father Hesburgh hosted a conference in Land
O' Lakes, Wisconsin, for a number of academics from Notre Dame
and other Catholic universities. He led them in drafting the Land
O' Lakes statement on academic freedom in Catholic institutions of
higher education, which declared in part that "the Catholic university must have true autonomy and academic freedom in the face of
authority of whatever kind, lay or clerical." For the undergraduate
student, "there must be no outlawed books or subjects."

While Hesburgh's intentions may have been noble, by formally
rejecting *any* authority not its own, the statement opened the door
to a wholesale crippling of Catholic character in almost all the
prominent Catholic colleges. While still acknowledging the influ-
ence of the Church, the statement asserts a principle of total autonomy, making a university's Catholicism merely coincidental to the
religious tradition and the intellectual teaching of the Catholic faith.
The document was presented as evidence of Catholic colleges taking
the lead in support of academic freedom, but despite this optim
façade, it was in truth a repudiation of its own birthright and
regard for tradition in line with the social ferment of the lat

ong enjoyed its reputation as *the* Cath-
. The declaration that emerged from the
rence asserted that Catholic universities
:inual examination of all aspects and activ-
d should objectively evaluate them." But
l for persistent self-reflection, coming as it
did on the heels of the Second Vatican Council and the period of
confusion that followed, encouraged faculty to abandon Catholic
principles or, in some cases, to present their own inventions as
authentic Catholic thinking. Perhaps worst of all, the statement
invited Catholic universities to join Notre Dame in cutting off
their unique and distinctive Catholic character from their parent
Church.

In 1974, Father Hesburgh gave a talk in Denver addressing the
moral leadership of the Catholic Church on key issues, including
abortion. He talked about political realities and criticized "mindless
and crude zealots" who alienated others in the fight against abortion.
When I read that, I called Father Hesburgh, who assured me that he
didn't mean *me*. This was a couple of years before I interrupted the
graduation at St. Joe's, so he had no cause to refer to me personally
as a crude zealot—yet.

But of course he meant us, the activists. We *were* the zealots. But
we were neither mindless nor crude: We were the ones most mindful
of just how serious the issue is, the ones fighting to protect human
lives. I talked with Father Hesburgh about how the media was trying
to discredit us and how much we'd appreciate it if he would speak
positively of us.

In future comments, Father Hesburgh was never critical of pro-
life activism. In fact, when the *NOW v. Scheidler* RICO case was
about to go to trial, Father Hesburgh wrote a powerful fundraising
letter for us and offered to come to Chicago as a character witness. I
always appreciated that support.

I'll never give up on Notre Dame. When they do something disastrous, I'll join those who try to steer them back. In 1992, they awarded the Laetare Medal, an award given at commencement to a Catholic who has made some notable contribution to society, to Senator Daniel Patrick Moynihan, whose voting record was emphatically pro-abortion. We picketed outside the Joyce Athletic & Convocation Center the day of the ceremony. My niece Elsa was graduating that year, and inside the arena, my brother Dr. Jim and his wife, Maria, stood and turned their backs when Moynihan received his award.

In 1999, Notre Dame hired Senator Bill Bradley to give a lecture series. Bradley touted himself as the liberal alternative to Gore—he had pushed hard for abortion in the Senate. I attended a talk in Washington Hall at the start of his lecture series to ask him whether he stood by his pro-abortion voting record. He said it had been a difficult stand to take, but he stood by his record.

I urged Notre Dame to cancel the Bradley lecture series. When that failed, I hired an airplane to do several flyovers at Notre Dame's home football games with banners urging Bradley's dismissal. We leafleted the tailgate parties and carried pictures of abortion victims through the crowds. Even Bradley himself remarked how impressive our campaign was, and fortunately he kept his pro-abortion position out of his Notre Dame lectures. A group of pro-life students and I attended his final lecture and had a friendly farewell.

A decade later, in spring 2009, my son Eric called and asked me to guess who Notre Dame had chosen for that year's commencement speaker. "I'll give you one guess," he said.

"Not Obama!" I said. "It can't be." President Obama was certainly a historic president and an eloquent speaker, and Notre Dame has a tradition of asking newly elected presidents to speak at their commencements. But the president proudly maintained—and was, in part, elected for—his 100 percent pro-choice voting record. To honor him at Notre Dame with a speech and an honorary degree flew in the face of the University's professed Catholic character—but fulfilled what Father Hesburgh had initiated at Land O' Lakes in 1967.

When it became clear that Obama would be coming to Notre Dame, despite protests from the pro-life movement nationwide, the Pro-Life Action League rented two billboards outside of South Bend on the Indiana toll road, one for eastbound and one for westbound traffic. We wanted the text "Obama is pro-abortion," but the agency that owned the board insisted we use "Obama is pro-choice." We didn't have time to bring a censorship case to court, so we settled for "Obama is pro-<u>abortion</u> choice"—poor English, but it got the point across.

That year's Laetare Medal was awarded to Mary Ann Glendon, a Harvard Law professor and US ambassador to the Vatican. She refused it, citing President Obama's invitation. Unlike the 1992 graduation, when we'd been able to picket Moynihan's Laetare award on campus, Notre Dame refused to allow any demonstrators who didn't conform to their guidelines for docility to set foot on campus. The university claimed that since it is a private institution, there was no First Amendment violation.

Several hundred protesters were on hand for the graduation. Two busloads arrived from Chicago, and another came from Michigan. We had half a mile of abortion victim photos on display and a picket at the main entrance. In addition to protesting the president's speech, we were there to support the students and faculty who boycotted the ceremony. A separate commencement was held near the grotto, with a very moving rosary led by Father Frank Pavone of Priests for Life.

Eighty-eight pro-lifers defied the ban on protests by marching onto the campus. They were arrested. At first, the university was determined to pursue charges against the "ND88," which included veteran activists Father Norman Weslin, Monica Miller, Jack Ames, and Norma McCorvey, the "Roe" from *Roe v. Wade* who had become a pro-lifer in the 1990s.

That fall we sponsored another flyover at a home football game. This time the banner read, "Free the ND88." After two years of legal battles, Notre Dame begrudgingly dropped the charges.

As I wrote in my newsletter during the Bradley protest in 1999, "At Notre Dame, Our Lady still stands atop the golden dome. It is her university and she will have the last word. We offer our hands and hearts and voices in the cause of victory for her Son." That hope lies in the strengthening of Notre Dame's Catholic identity with such initiatives as the Center for Ethics and Culture, which strives to push the University into a leading role, rather than follow the crowd, and in hosting debates over contemporary ethical issues. The Institute for Church Life has worked for years, mostly through the theology and sociology departments, to emphasize the message of the Gospel in society. The Sycamore Trust was established in 2006 through the efforts of Bill Dempsey during the controversy over *The Vagina Monologues*. Though not an official Notre Dame entity, the trust works to promote university alumni to pressure their school to hold true to its professed standards.

Notre Dame's pro-life student group showed great dedication at the time of President Obama's appearance there, and shortly afterward, history professor Father Wilson Miscamble, C.S.C., founded Notre Dame Faculty for Life. Since then, the number of Notre Dame faculty and students attending the March for Life, led by current president Father John I. Jenkins, C.S.C., has increased dramatically.

Miscamble and others understand that it should be unthinkable for a Catholic university to invite a vigorously pro-abortion person to be a keynote speaker. Bishops have urged Catholic universities not to offer platforms to such prominent public figures. But still it happens over and over again. In fact, in 2016, Notre Dame awarded the Laetare Medal to Vice President Joe Biden and former Speaker of the House John Boehner. Biden, while proud to call himself Catholic, is outspoken in his support of abortion.

These invitations are not extended as a deliberate challenge to the Church's position on the sanctity of life, but the cause of the unborn is not on the leadership's radar. So it is the job of pro-lifers to set the record straight.

Probably the toughest demonstration I ever did was protesting at my own daughter's graduation.

All seven of my children attended St. Ignatius College Prep on Chicago's West Side. When my daughter Catherine graduated in 1991, the administration invited former Illinois governor Jim Thompson to deliver the commencement address. Before he became governor, Thompson was Cook County state's attorney, and I visited him in his downtown Chicago office in the mid-'70s. He didn't want to see the slides of aborted babies I brought, but I plugged in my projector and flashed the pictures on his wall. He saw what was at stake in political support of the "right to choose," but the presentation had no effect on him. Thompson racked up an impressive pro-abortion record in Springfield, vetoing every pro-life bill that came across his desk. The NRLC graded Thompson the most pro-abortion governor in the nation.

Catherine was born in 1973. She was the first of my children whose life was not deemed worthy of protection by our government. Her class of 1991 was the first high school graduating class to be missing a third of its members due to legal abortion.

I was dismayed to learn that Jim Thompson would be the commencement speaker, and I called the president of St. Ignatius, Father Donald Rowe, to discuss the invitation. My three oldest sons had already graduated, my daughter Annie was a sophomore, and Sarah had just been accepted to begin there in the fall. My youngest, Matthias, would enter Ignatius in 1995.

Father Rowe knew about my pro-life work. Had the administration considered Thompson's voting record when choosing a speaker, they might have vetoed him, anticipating a strong reaction from parents. But apparently the leadership didn't consider Thompson's strong support for abortion when they chose him, and Father Rowe said it was too late to make a change. I told him that I would hate to protest at my own daughter's commencement, but if Thompson remained the speaker, I'd have no other choice.

Ann and I would have protested Thomson's appearance at any other Catholic school, and it would not have been honest to turn a blind eye to St. Ignatius just because our own child was graduating. Father Rowe's response made it clear that I'd have to honor my promise.

The school included a notice in the graduation program saying that as governor, Thompson "took positions on many issues" and that a parent had contacted the school asking that he be disinvited. Their statement made no mention of which particular issue prompted the concern. Ours did. We printed more than a thousand copies of a flyer to distribute outside Orchestra Hall on the evening of the graduation. The cover read, "In memory of one million young people who will not graduate with their class—the class of 1991—because they were killed by abortion."

Our flyer contained statements by the American bishops, Pope Paul VI, Pope John Paul II, Mother Teresa, and Joseph Cardinal Bernardin about the sanctity of life and Catholic politicians' duties to defend it. There was a flattering picture of a younger Jim Thompson and a synopsis of his pro-abortion record as governor. On the back cover, we invited parents to pray for Thompson's "conversion to a recognition of the value of each human life, born and unborn," and to pray that Church leaders and educators adhere to God's command, "Thou shalt not kill." In a box at the bottom, it said, "Finally, we advise that when the former governor has completed his talk, you politely refrain from any applause in silent tribute to the thousands of boys and girls whom he failed to protect during his tenure as chief executive of Illinois."

Catherine was embarrassed that her parents were protesting out in front of Orchestra Hall with a dozen activists distributing this flyer before the graduation. She feared being booed when called to receive her diploma. When we were handing out the flyers, a mother of another graduate came up to me.

"How can you do this to your daughter?" she asked.

"I'm not doing it *to* her," I answered. "I'm doing it *for* her."

After distributing the flyers, Ann and I went into the hall and sat behind Cathy. When Thompson finished his talk, there was only scattered applause. When Cathy went up to get her diploma, no one booed. As we walked out of the auditorium, several teachers told her she should be proud of what her parents had done. We had discussed the protest with Cathy prior to the event, and she understood our dilemma. She can laugh about it now and has often told us that she was proud of our strong stand for life.

One of Catherine's religion teachers came up to us and said, "Thank God you were here. Your protest restored integrity to the ceremony. We tell kids to live by the high standards we teach, then we go and invite someone like Thompson to give the commencement address. But you should have made more noise!"

Another teacher, Father Robert Thul, summed it up in a letter after the graduation: "If we just turn out sharp graduates," he wrote, "uninterested in a mission to the world, then we've failed."

If I had a second chance with any of these protests, I'd do them all again.

CHAPTER 8

# Ten Thousand Words

My father owned a half-interest in the two theaters in Hartford City, Indiana, and the Scheidler kids spent nearly every evening at either the Orpheum or the Jefferson, watching most of the movies produced during the '30s, '40s, and '50s, until television took over. We got in free and could take friends with us. We had lots of friends.

One night, when I was about seven, I was coming out of the Jefferson Theatre when I was shocked nearly out of my wits. A display of wrecked automobiles, drawn on flatbed trucks, was passing in front of the theater. Each car was severely damaged, and mannequins from local department stores were draped over the doors through shattered windows. Streaks of red paint running down the sides of the cars warned of the consequences of reckless driving. The grim procession of twisted wreckage and crippled figures stuck in my mind. I think of them to this very day when I'm driving in fast traffic.

As an activist, I've often been the one presenting that kind of display. I want to keep the picture of a mangled baby in the public consciousness, so that when people hear "abortion" they don't think of abstract "choice" but the bloody reality of a dead baby. The picture from that 1972 *Life or Death* pamphlet stuck in my mind the way those mannequins did.

I built a prop years ago to carry in pickets and demonstrations modeled after those mannequins. It was a metal garbage can with body parts from plastic baby dolls draped over the rim. The body parts and the can were covered in red paint. It was a jarring display, and it actually drew more attention from photographers and passersby than the images of actual abortion victims.

In the summer of 2013, the Thomas More Society, the law group that represented us in the *NOW v. Scheidler* case, celebrated its fifteenth anniversary at the Crystal Gardens at Navy Pier in Chicago. The keynote speaker, Lila Rose, recounted the story of how she became a pro-lifer. At age nine, she found Dr. Jack Willke's *Handbook on Abortion* in her parents' bookcase. When she saw its photos of aborted babies, she asked her parents what they were. Lila recalled being horrified that they depicted something that was legal and common in America. That was the day, she said, when she became a committed pro-lifer.

I was fascinated to learn that Lila Rose, already a nationally known activist at half the age I was when I started my pro-life work, was drawn to pro-life activism by the very same images that had changed my life in 1972. Listening to her talk, I was reminded of another gathering years earlier, when I took a half-dozen of my activist friends to dinner at my favorite restaurant, a friendly Sicilian place called Monastero's. In the course of our conversation, I asked the others what moved them to full-time pro-life work.

As we went around the table, it became clear that whatever their initial disposition toward the pro-life cause, everyone's answer was the same: Their calling to activism was sparked through images. It was the pictures of the aborted unborn babies that got each of us involved and convinced us that abortion was a matter of life and death.

We won't bring Americans back to a respect for life without engaging them on a concrete, visceral level. Images achieve that. As the old Chinese proverb says, a picture is worth ten thousand words. That's why, from the very beginning—and against the advice of some of my favorite people—I've never shied away from showing the graphic images of abortion victims.

No social movement has succeeded without showing the evil they were trying to stop. The campaign to end child labor didn't gain traction until Lewis Himes and other photojournalists produced their pictures of young girls working long hours at looms and little boys covered in coal dust. Their photos helped bring about child labor laws.

Even before the era of photography, reformers relied on images. In his crusade to end the transatlantic slave trade, William Wilberforce brought chains and other restraints into the Houses of Parliament and took MPs and their wives to see a slave ship docked in London. It took more than twenty years, but Wilberforce finally convinced Parliament to ban the slave trade. As photographic technology improved, images of slaves scarred by lashings were circulated, and abolitionists on both sides of the Atlantic garnered even more support.

Historians suggest that the 1954 Supreme Court ruling in *Brown v. Board of Education of Topeka* and Rosa Parks's 1955 arrest spurred African Americans to take to the streets and boycott the busses in Montgomery in the mid-'50s.

But an event that energized civil rights activists occurred in the summer of 1955. Emmett Till, a fourteen-year-old African American boy from Chicago, was visiting relatives in Money, Mississippi, where he allegedly whistled at a white woman. That night, two men came to his uncle's home and abducted him, beat him to death, and dumped his body in a river. Several days later, Emmett's body was found and returned to Chicago for burial.

Emmett's mother insisted on an open casket. "I wanted the world to see what they did to my baby," she explained. Thousands came to view the body, and the line into the church stretched for blocks. Parents brought their children to impress on them the reality of racial injustice in America.

The men who took the boy were tried for murder. A week before the trial, *Jet* magazine and the *Chicago Defender* published photos of Emmett Till in his casket, his face horribly mangled and bloated. The pictures were seen all over the country. Weeks after an all-white jury acquitted the men, Rosa Parks was arrested, and the bus boycott— one of the first initiatives of the civil rights revolution—began. The catalyst was the use of graphic images.

Even pro-abortion activists have tried to use disturbing images to champion their cause. In April 1973, to celebrate the *Roe* decision, *Ms.* Magazine printed a crime scene photo of the body of Gerri Santoro, who died from an illegal abortion. In 1963, Santoro took her two daughters, left her abusive husband, and began an affair with a married man named Clyde Dixon. A year later, she learned that her husband was coming to see his daughters. Nearly seven months pregnant, she panicked at the thought of him finding out. She decided to abort the baby. Dixon had no medical training but tried to perform the abortion himself. He borrowed a medical textbook and some surgical instruments, and the two checked into a motel. When Santoro started to hemorrhage, Dixon fled the motel, leaving her to die alone. Dixon was convicted of manslaughter and sentenced to a year in prison.

The photo was published under a headline that has become a favorite pro-abortion slogan: "Never Again!" The picture of Gerri Santoro's bloody body on the motel floor became an icon, evidence that laws limiting abortion threatened women's lives. Abortion advocate Bill Baird sometimes used this photograph in his debates against me.

But the *Roe* decision did not make abortion safe. Health codes enacted to cover abortion clinics were challenged in federal court and, under the guidelines in *Roe*, struck down as unconstitutional. Abortionists were free to operate without any state oversight.

The pro-life cause faces a challenge that causes like civil rights and child labor did not: reticence from a typically eager media to publish evidence of injustice. The pro-life movement has been cast as reactionary, as if our agenda is not about protecting unborn lives but subjugating women. Pro-lifers sometimes even have a tough time convincing each other that the images of the aborted babies should be shown.

In autumn 1975, we got permission to set up a fetal development exhibit at Northeastern Illinois University. There was nothing gory in the display, which was designed to show the beauty of the developing human in the womb. Shortly after we put up the exhibit in the library, someone taped paper over the glass case. We suspected a pro-choice group was behind the blackout, so we decided to present something more vivid.

A dozen of us went on to the campus and handed out hundreds of the *Life or Death* flyers, which featured fetal pictures and the corresponding pictures of infants at the same stage of gestation aborted by suction, dilation and extraction (D&E), and saline. Eventually, campus security escorted us off school property.

Some hours later, we returned to the campus. People were talking about abortion: in the cafeteria, the hallways, the grounds. Some were heated debates. Others were quiet conversations. But we had clearly engaged those students. They saw something upsetting, and they needed to talk about it. In a country where that kind of government-sanctioned violence happens thousands of times each day, those conversations are necessary.

I've been a guest on more than a thousand talk shows, including several appearances on Phil Donahue's program. Phil and I almost became buddies. For one of his programs, he came out to film a clinic protest and captured footage of our graphic signs. We were only in one segment of the show, but the final program was pro-life, showing how we used the images and why victim photos are important.

But *Donahue* was on right after *Bozo's Circus*, and the producers were concerned some children would still be around the TV, and there would be Phil with a graphic abortion presentation. They rescheduled the show to a later time slot. The juxtaposition of going from a children's program to a segment on children being killed would have sent a powerful message. Still, it was a major development for us to get even a brief amount of air time to show the victims of abortion.

On another occasion, I was invited to New York to appear on ABC's *Good Morning America* with Charlie Gibson, one of the most liberal hosts on any network in those days. *Good Morning America* is a live show. During the commercial break right before my segment, I was talking with Gibson, and I took a picture out of my pocket of a baby's hand at five weeks gestation. It was a black-and-white photo of four tiny fingers, a palm, and a thumb. No blood, no gore. No abortion.

"No graphics," Charlie said.

"But this is just a baby's hand at five weeks. Look at how perfect it is."

"No graphics, Mr. Scheidler. If you try to show that photograph, we'll go to a commercial break."

When the segment began, Charlie introduced me as an anti-abortionist. I retorted that we liked to be called "pro-life" but that I'd accept "anti-abortion" even though I represented the Pro-Life Action League. Then I looked into the camera and said, "I have a picture in my pocket of the hand of a five-week-old fetus. It's perfect in every way. It looks like a baby's hand—it *is* a baby's hand. And Charlie won't let me show it. If I were to take this picture out of my pocket right now, Charlie would call for a commercial break."

Gibson was angry. He didn't want any evidence that abortion involves somebody other than a woman and her doctor. This is precisely why the photos are so important: To nearly everyone, the unborn are invisible. A simple photo like the one Charlie Gibson wouldn't let me show could save lives. We have to use images. We have to show people the reality: Abortion kills an innocent human being.

In the late 1970s, abortion clinics began renting ad space on the Chicago Transit Authority (CTA) train platforms. These were quickly painted over by pro-lifers, which generated media attention. I met with the CTA's director of advertising and convinced him that the CTA could get out of the controversy if it simply refused to accept clinic ads. They followed that policy for a few years, but in the early 1980s, Planned Parenthood filed a lawsuit to force the CTA to carry their ads.

If the CTA had to run the ads, we expected equal access to advertising. The Pro-Life Action League designed an ad to counter the Planned Parenthood ads. We didn't have the budget to pay for that kind of advertising, but we knew there would be media interest and saw an opportunity to publicize pictures of abortion victims.

We used a color picture of a baby from a find of seventeen thousand bodies in a storage container in California in 1982 publicized as "the American Holocaust." During the 1984 court hearings on *Planned Parenthood v. Chicago Transit Authority*, our ad with the picture of the late-term victim was entered as evidence. The text read, "When you think of Planned Parenthood, think of this. We think it's murder." The local media covered the hearings, and our proposed ads were shown by all the Chicago network affiliates and on CNN.

Ultimately, federal judge Milton Shadur ruled that the CTA had to carry Planned Parenthood's ads, but not ours. Still, the whole event gave us a forum to show the public the horror of abortion, if only for a few seconds on the evening news.

Sandy Kirkbride, the head of Voices for Life in Dubuque, Iowa, saw our proposed CTA ad on CNN. She contacted us to get some images for a billboard and looked at a series of pictures before settling on one of a baby who had been pulled out mostly intact but with his limbs twisted and with visible forceps wounds on his head. He had been laid out on two overlapping pieces of paper towel that formed a cross. The text of her billboard read: "Abortion, the <u>REAL</u> Violence. Help us stop it." It included the names and numbers of Voices for Life and the Pro-Life Action League.

I flew to Dubuque for the unveiling. The billboard had an immediate impact, engaging editors and eliciting interviews and invitations to talk shows. But the company that owned the billboard got so many complaints that they took it down within twenty-four hours.

In February of 1992, I got a call from my cousin Bob Rust in Greensburg, Indiana, telling me about a young man who wanted to run for public office and use graphic pictures in his campaign ads. Could I help him? Mike Bailey was planning to campaign for a seat in the Indiana state legislature so he could run pro-life ads showing Hoosiers the grim reality of abortion. Conventional wisdom held that the graphic ads would anger voters and result in his defeat, but Mike wasn't expecting to be elected: His candidacy was to be a public awareness campaign.

Mike came to my office, and we watched *The Hard Truth* from American Portrait Films. He chose some segments from that film for his ads but wondered whether the stations would run them. Shortly afterward, we learned that a Federal Communications Commission (FCC) guideline barred stations from censoring political ads from federal candidates unless the ads were obscene. I suggested that Mike seek a seat in the US House of Representatives rather than run for state office. FCC regulations would protect his ads and would let him show them in more markets.

His ads opened with a warning about how graphic they were. They ran in Indianapolis, Evansville, Cincinnati, and Louisville, and they caused such a stir that Mike and I were invited to Cincinnati to appear on *The Jerry Springer Show*. The tactic of using graphic abortion pictures in campaign ads was adopted by several other pro-life candidates throughout the country in subsequent years, including Missy Smith in her congressional race in 2010 and Randall Terry in a presidential run in 2012. His ads ran in thirty-two states.

The Democratic National Convention was held in Chicago during the 1996 presidential race, when Bill Clinton was running for reelection. We were determined to capitalize on the media coverage. The main picture we used was a three-by-five-foot poster of a baby boy killed at twenty-one weeks. Pro-lifers named him Malachi.

We blanketed Chicago with Malachi's picture during the convention. Wherever Clinton was, we were there with Malachi. Of all the protests that took place during the convention, ours was the largest and most persistent. At one event, police moved us away from the street where the president's motorcade would pass and shuttled us to an area away from the action. As soon as the police left, I told our group to leave the area and spread out along the motorcade route. Now that we were no longer congregated in a group, the police were unable to corral us into the isolated protest area. As the Clinton entourage came by, they passed dozens of our posters, spaced over hundreds of yards, bearing the mangled body of baby Malachi. Anyone at the convention saw our signs. The Clintons certainly did, but the media gave us almost no coverage.

A couple years after the '96 convention protests, Reverend Matt Trewhella and his Milwaukee group, Missionaries to the Preborn, started staging displays of this kind in Wisconsin. He called these "Show the Truth Tours." The media resolutely refused to show the public the truth about abortion. So Matt bypassed the media blackout and took the reality directly to the streets.

In July 1999, I drove to Racine, Wisconsin, to see how the Truth Tour was organized. As I entered the city limits, for half a mile into town, both sides of the road were lined with pictures of victims. Dozens of pro-lifers stood on the street holding their vivid images for passing motorists and pedestrians to see. It was a dramatic display. Matt also had a group of high school students passing out flyers all over town explaining why they were there with their signs. I was impressed and commended Matt on his professional deployment of the images.

We'd been showing pictures for years, but always in rallies or protests, not in just any public place. The Truth Tour concept, specifically targeting ignorance and willful apathy, was a new approach. As Matt explained, "When something is so horrifying that we can't stand to look at it, perhaps we shouldn't be tolerating it."

We decided to give it a try. Teaming up with Monica Miller's Citizens for a Pro-Life Society, we called our project "Face the Truth." It was more than a statement against the media blackout—it was a move against our society's deliberate blind spot that avoids confronting what the "right to choose" really means.

We launched the first Face the Truth Tour in 2000 at sites from southern Wisconsin to Gary, Indiana. It was an educational mission—both for the public and for us. Showing pictures of unborn babies in the womb and pictures of aborted babies at each trimester, we spent ninety minutes at three sites per day for ten days. At each site, we covered all four corners of major intersections with volunteers standing thirty feet apart with five-foot-tall signs. At each corner, we posted Beth Sweigard's portrait of Christ weeping over a tiny broken body in his hand and an American flag, which signifies our nation's original affirmation of the right to life and *our* constitutional right to show the truth.

At Morris, Illinois, one of our volunteers had a motorist point a gun at her. She assumed that was a normal occurrence and didn't bother to get his license plate. We've had people kick our signs, rip them out of our hands, toss paint on us, and throw garbage at us or even knives.

The Truth Tour offers an interesting window on society. It is a coordinated event, but not a rally or picket. There's no chanting or slogans. You're participating with many other people, but it's also a deeply solitary experience—there's a strong sense that you're standing alone for the sake of the unborn child. When someone yells obscenities, they look right at you, not at a crowd. Many Truth Tour volunteers are elderly people who pray the rosary while they hold their signs. People swear at them, flip them off, shout hateful or vile things. I can think of few other contexts where people feel justified swearing at senior citizens at prayer. We take solace in the words of Jesus: "If the world hates you, realize that it hated Me first."

Face the Truth Tours also show a hopeful side. Many motorists tap their horns and give a thumbs-up. Drivers have parked their cars, asked for a sign, and joined us. Some offer donations. Other have brought out coolers of drinks and walked along the line, handing them out.

But the greatest joy is when holding a sign saves a life. One July afternoon, a teenage couple was walking to an appointment for an abortion in downtown Chicago. They were discussing whether or not they were doing the right thing and decided to offer a prayer for guidance. Just as the young man asked God for a sign, they turned the corner and saw *dozens* of Face the Truth signs. They walked up to a volunteer and told her about their prayer for a sign and that they had decided not to keep their abortion appointment. Their child is alive precisely because we were there.

Some might call that a coincidence, but we have heard hundreds of stories like this over the years. These accounts have erased the last traces of any doubt that I first had when I drove up to see Matt Trewhella's tour in Wisconsin.

The Truth Tour concept has caught on across the country. Bob Newman runs a highly successful tour in Pittsburgh. Sunny Turner caught onto the idea in Tucson and ran them for years in Arizona. We urged Jack Ames of Maryland-based Defend Life to bring the idea to his state and the DC area, and he has held Face the Truth Maryland Tours since 2001. Ann and I joined Jack for his first tour, and Eric has joined Jack for several Maryland tours. Jack introduced the idea of Face the Truth T-shirts, which we adopted in 2002.

At the heart of the protection of freedom of expression is a ratification of the value of each individual. That's the central message of the pro-life movement, and it's one of the reasons that I consider the First Amendment to be sacred. It's one of the things I love most about America.

While we have a right to be out on the streets with our graphic images, we do make a lot of our fellow citizens unhappy. A common criticism of the Face the Truth Tour is that young children may see the pictures. I understand that concern, and I've thought and prayed about it a great deal. It's one of the reasons I was skeptical when I went to Racine to see my first Truth Tour.

I met a father there holding a sign. His young son stood next to him with his own sign. I asked, "What do you think about this? You've got your little boy with you, looking at this picture. Don't you get a lot of flak?"

"My kid needs to see this picture," he replied.

When children see a picture of an abortion victim, they react with compassion, not horror. One little girl in downtown Chicago during our Truth Tour in front of City Hall saw our Malachi sign, then looked up at her mom and asked, "Who did that to the baby?"

She didn't ask what happened to the fetus. She knew what she was seeing. Children are naturally pro-life. When pro-life parents tell their children that the pictures are shown to fight a terrible wrong, to stop people from hurting children, they're not traumatized. Parents who support abortion don't have this explanation—hence their anger and outrage.

Curiously, though, we've learned that it isn't so much the disturbing images that raise people's ire but the very idea that the unborn have a right to life. We occasionally hold Truth Tours where we don't show images of dead children, only large pictures of fetal development or of babies who have already been born. And still passersby curse us and call images of preborn life "disgusting." It's a fundamentally sick society when the image of a healthy infant developing in the womb is "gross."

We understand that pictures of dead children are disturbing. When we set up our signs at a major intersection, we place warning signs a reasonable distance away to let motorists know that graphic abortion victim photos are ahead. They can change their route if they feel strongly about avoiding the images for themselves or their children.

There is a perspective within the pro-life movement that the posters of abortion victims are insensitive to postabortive women and could trigger painful memories. Some Christians suggest that Jesus would never expose people to a scene of such brutality. Yet the cross, a horrific instrument of death, is the symbol of Christianity. Christ's bloody, beaten body hung for hours on display along a public road. Catholic churches are required to have a crucifix—not just a cross—at the main altar.

Once while in Maryland with Jack Ames's Truth Tour, a woman pulled up to tell us that our images were harmful to women. In the course of the conversation, she said that she'd been forced into abortion as a teenager but would never willingly have one again. We talked for a while about postabortion healing. Still, she said, these images weren't appropriate for everyone and that we should try to engage people in conversation.

"What made you decide to stop and talk to me?" I asked.

"I saw your signs."

## CHAPTER 9

# Right-Wing Bigots

In June 1981, I led a group of Chicago pro-lifers into a conference of the NARAL at the Conrad Hilton hotel. The meeting was open to the public, but early in the proceedings, NARAL leaders insisted that the pro-lifers be removed from one of the seminar rooms. As the four were led out, a crowd of about seventy pro-abortionists cheered and shouted, "Out! Out!" Some of them began a chant: "Racist, sexist, anti-gay, right-wing bigots, go away!"

We pro-life activists have our chants, and pro-choice counterprotesters have theirs. Sometimes they shout "born again" instead of "right wing." One of the other most common chants, in a nod to the strong role Catholics play in the pro-life movement, runs: "Get your rosaries off my ovaries."

It's odd to hear these two slogans chanted together. The term "born again" has strong Protestant associations—Catholics rarely use it. But from a pro-abortion perspective, pro-lifers, especially religious activists, are fringe fanatics.

During the Republican convention in Houston in 1992, while we were picketing a clinic, a male counterdemonstrator dressed as the pope shouted the rosary chant repeatedly in Pastor Ed Martin's face. "Let me explain something," Pastor Ed said. "I'm not Catholic, so I don't have rosaries. You're not a woman, so you don't have ovaries."

But the accusation of racism is especially specious. Minorities are far overrepresented in abortion statistics. African American and Hispanic people together make up a little more than 30 percent of the national population yet account for 55 percent of all abortions. Anyone eager to preserve white supremacy in this country would be delighted by those numbers. Racists argue that abortion keeps minorities from overrunning the country.

This is not, of course, a new idea—Planned Parenthood founder Margaret Sanger, despite her opposition to abortion, was an outspoken supporter of the eugenics movement. One reason she was so passionate about increasing access to birth control was to limit proliferation of America's nonwhite citizens, and in 1926, she was a guest speaker at a meeting of the Women's Auxiliary of the Ku Klux Klan (KKK).

That group is known as the second-generation KKK—the first were vigilantes intent on preventing former slaves from gaining the blessings of liberty following the Civil War. It disbanded when Union forces left the South in the 1870s, since, with no outside force to ensure former slaves' constitutional rights, there was no need to work undercover. After World War I, a new Klan formed, more generous with its hatred, targeting Blacks, immigrants, labor activists, political leftists, Jews, and Catholics. Whereas the first Klan was active primarily in the South, this new Klan spread throughout the country, claiming six million members by the mid-1920s.

The Klan was very active in Indiana, where my family lived. There wasn't much to rile up a bigot in Hartford City, but there was a large klavern in our town that was very active in the years before I was born. When the Klan had a parade, my mother later told me, they marched right past our house on Washington Street. For some of them, their white robes and pointed hoods weren't much of a disguise. Mom could identify many of the women by their shoes or by their gait and height.

The Klan professed to reject Catholics, but they were willing to do business with them. My father ran eight businesses in Hartford City and the surrounding towns, including the local ice company and bottling plant, so when the Klan had its rallies in Willman's Woods, they bought their ice and pop from him. That was how Dad found out who some of them were. He learned that our local barber was the Blackford County Klan secretary and found out that the barber kept a list of Klan members in his shop.

Late one afternoon, the story goes, Dad and my grandpa went to his shop. Dad got his hair cut, then hid in the back while Grandpa got a shave. When the barber closed up, Dad was still in the shop, and he rummaged around and found the list. The next day, he and Grandpa took it to a local newspaper editor who was no friend of the Klan. They sent an anonymous message to the barber that the editor had the list and would publish it on the front page unless the klavern disbanded.

That's how the Blackford County KKK was broken up. This happened the year before I was born, and I didn't hear the story until years later, but when I did, I was proud of my dad's audacity in the cause of justice.

But it wasn't as though the Klan breakup turned my hometown into a model of integration and tolerance. I only knew two Jewish families, both clothiers. Our suits always came from Stein's or Levy's. They were nice people to work with. Our piano tuner was a black man who came over from Marion, Indiana. We always visited a while after he tuned the piano, but he always left before sundown.

There was a tacit understanding in Hartford City that no black person could stay in town overnight. Oddly enough, one of the richest men in town and a leading citizen of Hartford City, George Stevens, was a light-skinned black man who passed for white. Stevens lived at the Hartford Hotel and held court in the lobby each evening. After Stevens died, some of his Hartford City friends went to Akron, Ohio, for his funeral. When they met his relatives, they learned that he had been defying that unwritten rule for thirty years.

We kids saw lots of movies at the theaters Dad ran, and I couldn't help but notice that blacks had minor roles in these films, either as maids, servants, or entertainers or as unsophisticated buffoons. Our piano tuner wasn't like that.

Each winter, we took a family trip to Florida, where I noticed blacks would step off of the sidewalk when we were walking toward them and insist that we cut in front of them in line at shops. It made me uncomfortable. It seemed out of place with what I understood about America and equality. I never got used to separate drinking fountains and segregated movie theaters.

When I joined the navy after high school and was stationed at Camp Peary in Williamsburg, Virginia, the military was still segregated, and there were black regiments stationed on the base. I enjoyed watching them march with their unique cadence call. Up North, whenever I'd take a bus, I preferred to sit in the back. I continued to do so when I'd visit Richmond on weekends, and the drivers would try to get me to move to the front. I never did. I didn't intend it as a political statement. I must have aggravated a lot of bus drivers raised in a racist society.

When I was teaching at Notre Dame in the early '60s, one of my friends, Rudy Pruden, an African American, joined the glee club. They performed all over the country, and when they toured the South, it was hard to find a hotel that wasn't segregated. Dan Pedtke, the club director, refused to stay at whites-only hotels. He arranged accommodations in private homes when the club traveled through the South. The glee club's little boycott might not have changed any policies, but we were proud that Dr. Pedtke refused to accept the Jim Crow tradition.

When the movement emerged to challenge institutional racism, I was happy to get involved. In 1965, while I was teaching at Mundelein College, Dr. Martin Luther King Jr. led his march from Selma, Alabama, to the state capital in Montgomery. They were protesting the glacial pace of civil rights reform and the harassment and violence meted out to demonstrators.

College students from all over the North were organizing pilgrimages to Montgomery to join the march, and Mundelein organized its own group. Ann was in her senior year and, as social chairman of the student council, was in charge of ordering the bus and securing faculty to go along. She had to make sure to get a bus with a toilet on board since there would be places along the way where it might not be safe to stop with an integrated group.

The student council asked me to go as a chaperone along with a few nuns. Ann had to stay behind for her senior comprehensive exams that week. We drove south with a busload of students, and a few of us joined the march as it advanced on Montgomery. We stayed at the edge of town with the other marchers on the campus of St. Jude's, a local Catholic church and high school, where there was a rally that night. Everyone was there—Dr. King, James Farmer Jr., Jesse Jackson, John Lewis. It was an impressive gathering. Harry Belafonte and Peter, Paul, and Mary performed that night, along with other musical groups.

During the afternoon, unaware of just how volatile the situation was, I strolled toward downtown Montgomery to see what was going on. About a mile from St. Jude's, I saw a man decorating his car with Confederate flags. He'd painted "Yankee go home" on the door. I stopped for a moment to watch him work on his car when I suddenly found myself surrounded by a group of men who had come quietly out of a tavern behind me.

"What are you doing here, Yank?" one of them asked.

"I came down to see both sides. I want to talk to everybody," I said. "I'm a former reporter. I teach journalism now, and I'm very interested in the civil rights issue." Of course, it was obvious that I'd been on the march—I had red mud on my shoes.

"Were you marching in that Selma thing?"

"Just at the very end," I said. I felt like Peter at the cockcrow.

Some of the guys had picked up rocks. I had visions of being dragged into the woods and strung up. Then a middle-aged man came out of the tavern. "Guys," he said, "let's not have any trouble." He didn't have a Southern accent. "Go back into the bar. I'm setting you up."

That worked for most of them. They all went back inside except one guy with a rock. He kept tossing it from hand to hand. The one with the car kept working on it. The man who offered to buy the round looked at the guy with the rock and then came over to me. "There's going to be trouble," he said. "I come from Pittsburgh, but I know these guys pretty well. I wouldn't go any farther away from the encampment than you are now. Don't look back, just walk—don't run."

I turned around and went back, nervous. The man decorating his car got in it and started following me, very slowly, as I headed back to the St. Jude campus. Once I got there, I turned to see if my stalker was still following. He was gone.

The next day, we all marched from St. Jude's to the Alabama state capitol. There was a huge turnout. We all sat down in the street and listened to Dr. King's speech. "The end we seek," he said, "is a society at peace with itself, a society that can live with its own conscience."

But that night, Viola Liuzzo, a white activist from Michigan who was in Alabama to help organize the march and rally, was attacked driving one of the black marchers, Leroy Moton, back to Selma via back roads. A car with four Klansmen overtook them and opened fire. Two bullets hit Liuzzo in the head. Moton was covered in blood, and he lay motionless. The killers thought he was dead too. They sped away, and Moton ran off to get help. But it was too late. Viola Liuzzo was dead.

We didn't hear about Liuzzo's murder until we were back in Chicago. Getting out of Montgomery had been tough. Police were arresting people for trivial infractions, like setting one foot in the crosswalk at a red light. Some people who stopped to buy a paper were accused of taking two or three for the price of one. Some Southerners were looking to detain people, to scare them, to make them want to leave and not come back south.

March organizers had told us not to stop until we were out of Alabama, but as we started back, we saw paper bags over interstate and street signs, covering just about every sign that could be helpful. Someone had it in for the Northern invaders. We were lucky our driver knew his way around or we might have wound up farther south. Nashville seemed to be the border, where we could safely stop to eat and gas up.

Liuzzo's killers were found soon after the shooting. It turned out that one of the Klansmen in the car was an FBI informant who turned in the other three. While they were awaiting trial, someone burned a cross on Liuzzo's lawn in Detroit. The first trial ended with a hung jury, and the three killers were released and honored at a Klan rally. They were acquitted at a retrial.

I thought about what Dr. King had said at the statehouse about society and its conscience. This crime wasn't just the work of a few Klansmen. There was a whole social system in place, a brutal national machine that condoned murder.

In my earlier trips to the South, I'd always got the sense that white Southerners were absolutely convinced of their superiority. The campaign of terror against blacks who challenged that idea had been effective up until then. I knew the system was based on fear, but this trip taught me that there was more to fear on the white side too—maybe even more fear than the people they were oppressing. Their lifestyle was collapsing, dying.

Outside that Montgomery bar, worried that a violent mob was forming around me, one of the fellows had said, "You don't know anything about our problems. We've got to keep Blacks in their place. If they ever take over. . . ." Somebody started shouting, and I never heard the end of his sentence, but the point was clear. Even the slightest acknowledgement of a black person's basic human dignity could destroy the whole system.

Years later, this same attitude surfaced in the abortion debate. If the unborn have any rights at all, pregnant women—all women—would be relegated to second-class status. This fear is so intense that groups like NOW defend even the gruesome practice of partial birth abortion as a basic right and fight against laws requiring hospitals to provide care for children born alive after an attempted abortion. They even file lawsuits to stop pro-lifers from holding funeral services for aborted babies. They will do everything they can to make sure that the murdered unborn are not recognized as human beings.

When *Roe* and *Doe* were handed down, I saw a parallel between a pro-abortion society and the Jim Crow South. The nation was deciding to limit its definition of who counted as a person and who was entitled to equal protection under the law. Just as we'd done in the civil rights movement, activists were going to have to agitate for the people who were discarded by their government. But unlike the civil rights movement, these victims could not stand up for themselves.

I'd seen the hatred that surfaces when people decide that respecting another person's humanity threatens their own sovereignty. I knew I'd see the same fury in the battle to protect the unborn. But I was grateful that I had the experience of marching on Montgomery and learning firsthand how a social protest movement can change lives and advance the cause of justice.

I knew there would be others who would join me. I also knew that the opposition would form its own groups to demonstrate against us, claiming that we hated women, wanted to oppress them, wanted to force them to risk their lives in illegal back-alley abortions. But I never thought I'd be called a racist.

## CHAPTER 10

# Your Name's a Lie

In 1960, Planned Parenthood's medical director, Mary Calderone, wrote, "Ninety percent of all illegal abortions are presently done by physicians. Call them what you will, abortionists or anything else, they are still physicians, trained as such; and many are in good standing in their communities. They must do a pretty good job if the death rate is as low as it is."

Nevertheless, the fear represented by the image of the back alley still turns up at counterdemonstrations in the chant: "Pro-life: your name's a lie—you don't care if women die."

The idea that we don't care if women die implies that we have no concern for the women choosing to abort. But that couldn't be more wrong. A true pro-life philosophy shares the assertion of early feminist and American suffragist Alice Paul, who called abortion "the ultimate exploitation of women." Half a century after Alice Paul wrote the text of the 1923 Equal Rights Amendment, the term "feminism" would be co-opted by a group of radical activists who advocated the legalization of abortion, a practice many still thought hurtful to women.

While attending a rally in Chicago's Daley Plaza in the fall of 2012, during the outcry over the Affordable Care Act requirement that all health care plans, including those offered by religious institutions, cover prescriptions and operations that violate those institutions' moral precepts about the sanctity of life, I heard another familiar rhyme. A counterprotesting group shouted from across the square: "Not the church, not the state, women must decide their fate." It was strange, I thought, to hear "not the state" when *we* were the ones asking the government to respect individual liberty and not force us to violate our consciences. Yet state intervention is celebrated when it comes to the only medical procedure accorded explicit constitutional protection.

Many assume that pro-lifers are hard-hearted and want people to suffer for their choices and their mistakes. Perhaps some are. For myself, as a Catholic, I take seriously the Gospel message of forgiveness and the call to comfort the afflicted. Over decades of activism, I've met many women so haunted by their abortion that I can honestly say that even if I were not convinced of the humanity of the unborn child, I'd still be in this fight simply because I've seen how devastating it can be to a woman who has chosen to end a pregnancy by abortion.

Over the years, I've met many women who grieve over their abortions, and we've talked about ways to reach out to postabortive women to offer them resources for help and support. We laid the groundwork in 1980 for a group called Women Exploited, which later blossomed into Women Exploited By Abortion (WEBA). With more than a hundred chapters across the country, WEBA provided counseling and encouragement for thousands dealing with grief.

I helped Nola Jones found Victims of Choice, which quickly went national. One of its particular missions was to train counselors who specialize in postabortion grief. Rachel's Vineyard, an organization with a similar mission, specializes in hosting retreats to address the spiritual needs of women after an abortion, and Project Rachel trains priests and laypeople to minister to both women and men. Silent No

More is also dedicated to the needs of women, but its mission is more focused on outreach in which postabortive women share their stories as a way to question the doctrines of "reproductive choice."

Postabortion counseling from a pro-choice perspective is dubious at best. The regret comes from a realization that a child has been killed—and if your ideology rests on denying the humanity of the unborn child, your counseling can only admit that the loss *feels* real. There can be no admission that it *is* real—doing so would be an admission of a serious wrong.

In the years after *Roe v. Wade*, grieving women seeking help from an abortion provider were more likely to find a sales pitch than grief support. We learned from former clinic workers that they are trained to market abortion, not counsel. When clinics started advertising in newspapers in the early and mid-'70s, the ads were filled with phone numbers for counseling services. In 1978, an investigation by the *Chicago Sun-Times* found that they were a marketing arm for a network of abortion clinics. Operators were paid by the clinics for every abortion that came through their referrals. As soon as they learned a caller was pregnant, they were trained to say, "When do you want to schedule a termination?" They'd never say, "Have you considered your options?" or any line resembling supportive counseling.

Planned Parenthood pays lip service to adoption as an alternative to abortion, but their statistics reveal just how little effort they put into it. Year after year, their own annual report reveals that for every referral Planned Parenthood makes to an adoption agency, they perform 150 abortions. Real counseling isn't going to come from people with a profit motive.

Even those who understand and sympathize with the pro-life cause can be a barrier to postabortion recovery. Few priests and ministers ever risk addressing the issue for fear of unrest and hurt feelings, but for many women, especially those who struggle to reconcile their own religious practice with the decision to abort, a church can still be a safe space for suffering and grief—if anyone will listen.

It can also be a place where the truth about abortion, if told bravely and openly, can keep others from having to cope with the same grief and regret. The alternative can be catastrophic. The suicide rate for postabortive women is three times as high as for women in general. In contrast, the suicide rate for women who have given birth is only half the national rate. Statistics for teens are even more grim: In the six months following an abortion, adolescent women are ten times more likely to attempt suicide than girls who haven't had an abortion.

Very occasionally, mainstream culture itself opens up a space for this kind of truth-telling. The 2007 film *Juno* has a scene where the lead character, a pregnant teen, is on her way into an abortion clinic. A classmate of hers stands alone in the parking lot, holding up a picket sign and chanting a pro-life slogan about all babies wanting to be born. She sees Juno and stops chanting. They exchange some small talk about school. As Juno heads to the clinic door, the girl with the sign yells a few facts about the baby's heartbeat and ability to feel pain. The camera is in front of Juno, and we see her rolling her eyes at these tired lines. Then the girl with the sign calls out, "And it has fingernails!"

Juno stops and turns around. "Fingernails?" she says. "Really?"

Inside the clinic waiting room, Juno becomes intensely aware of everyone's fingernails. People are drumming them on clipboards, filing them, painting them, biting them. She gets up and runs out of the clinic.

The way the fingernail line was delivered in *Juno* was hasty. It doesn't seem to be part of the pro-life girl's usual repertoire, but for Juno, that was the image that stuck with her and why she changed her mind.

It can be like that in real life too.

In the summer of 1985, I was in Dallas to give a talk at the Greater Dallas Right to Life convention and attend a large protest at the Routh Street Women's Clinic. I always think it is good to have a man of the cloth at rallies, so I called my cousin, Bishop Thomas Tschoepe of the Diocese of Dallas, and invited him to join us. The organizers at the rally outfitted a flatbed truck with a speaker's podium. After I gave a speech from the platform, I introduced Bishop Tschoepe to some of the pro-life leaders. They asked if he wanted to address the crowd, but the Bishop said he'd rather talk with the abortionist.

All during the rally, Winston Wilder, dapper in his three-piece suit despite the Dallas heat, was standing across the street from the clinic reading the imprecatory psalms, which are all about punishment and sin. He didn't have a bullhorn, but he didn't need one. Some of the protesters found him annoying—he was interfering with their songs. They knew that I knew Winston and asked me to tell him to quiet down. I didn't want to embarrass him, and I didn't think what he was reading was all that bad, considering. So I didn't.

The clinic was at the top of a hill, and Bishop Tom and I walked up and rang the bell. The clinic director came to the door, and we had a short conversation while Winston continued loudly reciting psalms below us. The conversation was brief—the director stuck to the usual "women need abortions" lines—then we went back and rejoined the group.

A few minutes later, a young girl came out of the clinic and hurried down the front steps. She walked over to Winston and gave him a hug.

"What's that for?" he asked.

"This morning, when I got up, I opened my Bible to a random page," she said. "I put my finger on the page and read a verse. It was from the Psalms. I was up there getting ready for my abortion and I heard you recite that very same verse. That was a sign. So thank you. Thank God you were here."

Simple gestures—even just being in the right place at the right time—can change lives. One frigid Saturday morning in December, I was driving through downtown Chicago, running errands. A bitter wind was driving in off the lake. I took a wrong turn and managed to get lost. After some time looking for a major street to get my bearings, I turned onto Grand Avenue. I hadn't planned on going to a clinic that day, but Grand Avenue took me past Concord Medical Center, a clinic I'd protested many times. There was one sidewalk counselor out there shivering in the freezing cold, so I parked, walked over to her, and tapped her on the shoulder.

"You go get a cup of coffee," I said. "I'll cover you for a while. But hurry back!"

She left, and I stood against the wall. A moment later, a cab pulled up. A girl got out of the cab and walked right past me. A little while later, she came back, very angry.

"Why are you blocking the building number?"—I was standing in front of the address—"I'm going in there."

"I'd really rather you didn't."

"Well, I am. I'm having an abortion."

"I hope you don't. Can we talk it over?"

"What business is it of yours?"

"I like you," I said. "And I love your baby."

"It's not a *baby*."

"How far along are you?" I asked.

"Eight weeks."

I always carried a little fetal model of a ten-week-old baby. I took it out of my pocket. "Not a baby?" I asked. "Look at this."

She looked at it, then looked at the ground. "Well, I hate its father."

"Hey, I probably do too. Let's go talk about him."

We went to the restaurant around the corner for some coffee and donuts. The counselor I'd relieved was there, finishing her coffee before heading back to the clinic.

The girl's hands were trembling. She started talking about all the problems that had led her to the clinic that morning. Her father, she said, was a minister and would be shocked that she was sexually active and upset when he found out she was pregnant. Her boyfriend was going to leave her unless she had an abortion.

"Let him," I said. "You don't want him anyway. A guy who would send you to have an abortion isn't someone you want to be involved with."

We talked about her problems, and after fifteen minutes, they didn't seem so daunting anymore. At the end of our conversation, she held up her hand and said, "Look, I'm not trembling anymore! I'm going to be a mother. This is going to be a wonderful Christmas."

Some counselors can try for years and never have a save, but on her first day at a clinic, a young woman named Carol had one. She didn't think she knew how to counsel anyone, so she planned to just go and pray.

There were two experienced counselors in front of the Albany Clinic in Chicago that day. A young woman arrived, but when the other two counselors asked to talk, she refused them. Carol went up to her and said, "If you're going to go ahead and do this, let me give you a hug first."

The young woman let Carol put her arms around her, then started sobbing. Carol waited until she had calmed down before offering to take her to a nearby crisis pregnancy center. They went together, and months later, the young woman gave birth to a beautiful daughter. Carol went to visit them in the hospital and overheard the young mother murmur to her child, "I can't believe I was going to abort you."

We hear stories from many counselors about people headed to a clinic already resolved to turn around if someone is there, anyone at all, who cares whether the baby is given a chance to live. Many unborn children are aborted simply because nobody was there. It's easy to become overwhelmed and discouraged in the face of how many lives abortion has claimed, but in those moments it's important to remember that simply being there can save lives.

In my experience, a woman going into a clinic has already rationalized away concern for the infant, so frequently the only way to convince her to pause is to appeal to her own sense of self-preservation. We research clinics and doctors and share any information we find about health code citations or malpractice suits with the people going in. Often, the fact that a woman is at a clinic in the first place means that it's likely nobody is adequately looking out for her welfare. "Supportive" boyfriends, husbands, or parents aren't putting her needs above theirs, and on some level, she knows she's not being cared for. The key is to get her to pause and decide not to walk into the clinic. After that, we can also try to protect the child. We call this the "Chicago Method," and it has saved many lives.

In 1992, Congress considered the Freedom of Choice Act (FOCA), a bill that would have made federal support for abortion official US policy. NOW organized a march in Washington in support of the bill, and we held counterdemonstrations.

We set up a "Cemetery of Innocents" next to the Washington Monument, where the NOW march was to begin. We designed the memorial to emphasize the impact abortion has on women and unborn girls. The cemetery included 2,200 white crosses set up by a Texas pro-life group, one for each baby girl abortion claimed each day. The Pro-Life Action League contributed 109 tombstones representing the documented cases of women who had died from complications of legal abortions up to that point.

Tim Murphy made the tombstones out of Masonite. Each was three feet tall, and on the front of each was the name of the woman, the date of her death, and the name of the abortionist who was involved in her death. Supporting documentation was provided on the back of each stone. Tim put up a fence around the cemetery.

As NOW demonstrators yelled at us from the other side of the fence, Tim noticed that one of them had slipped inside the fence. He was afraid she was going to knock the tombstones over, but she simply walked over to one of them, took out her camera, and snapped a picture. Tim went over to talk to her and asked why she'd taken the picture.

"She was a friend of mine."

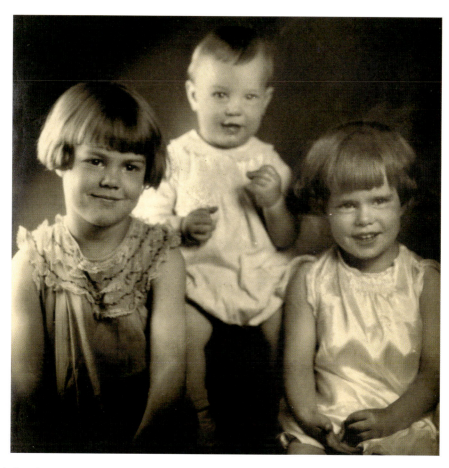

(*Above*) Sisters Mary Louise and Evelyn Ann with baby Joe, 1928. (*Below*) Joe with his sister Elly on the front step at home in Hartford City, IN, 1931.

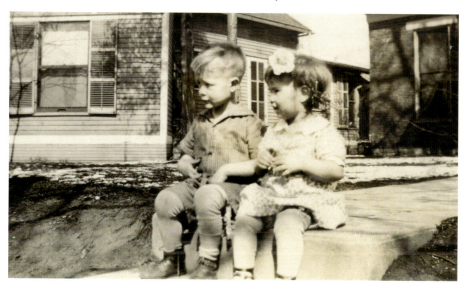

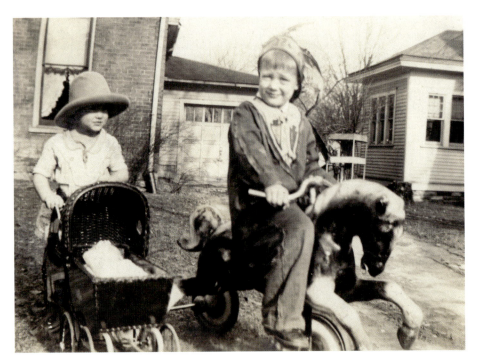

(*Above*) Sister, Elly, with her doll carriage and Joe riding "Tony Jr. Rex," 1932. (*Below*) Joe attends a tea party hosted by his sisters Elly and Evie, 1932.

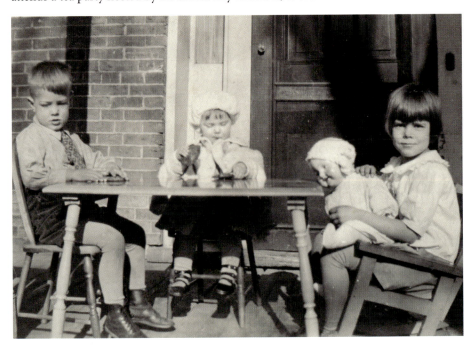

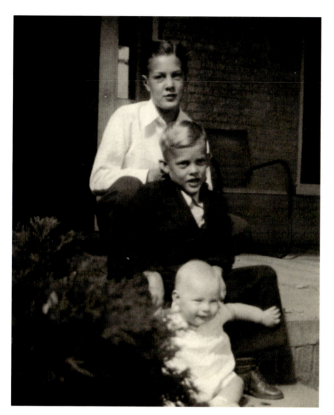

(*Left*) Joe with brothers Bob and Jim on the front step of their Hartford City, IN home, 1940. (*Below*) Joe in his aviator jacket in front of his home in Hartford City, IN, 1938.

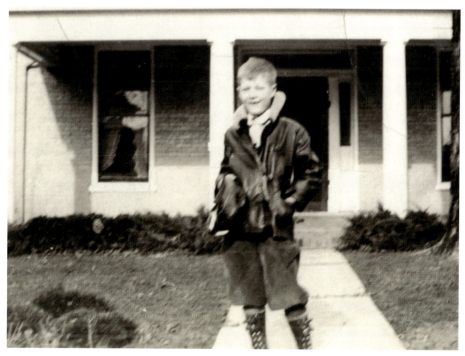

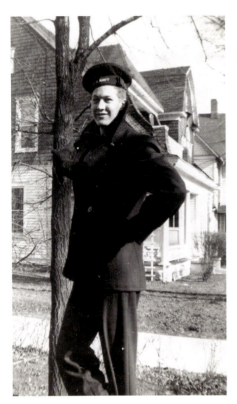

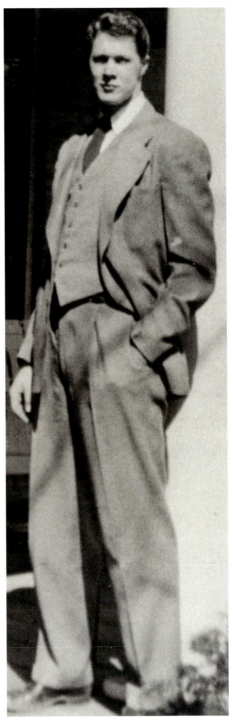

(*Above*) Seaman First Class Joe Scheidler, 1945. (*Below*) Joe with two St. Mary's students during his Notre Dame days, 1948.

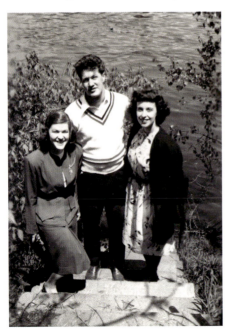

(*Above*) Joe during college days, 1947. (*Opposite*) Joe during his time teaching at Mundelein College, Chicago, 1963.

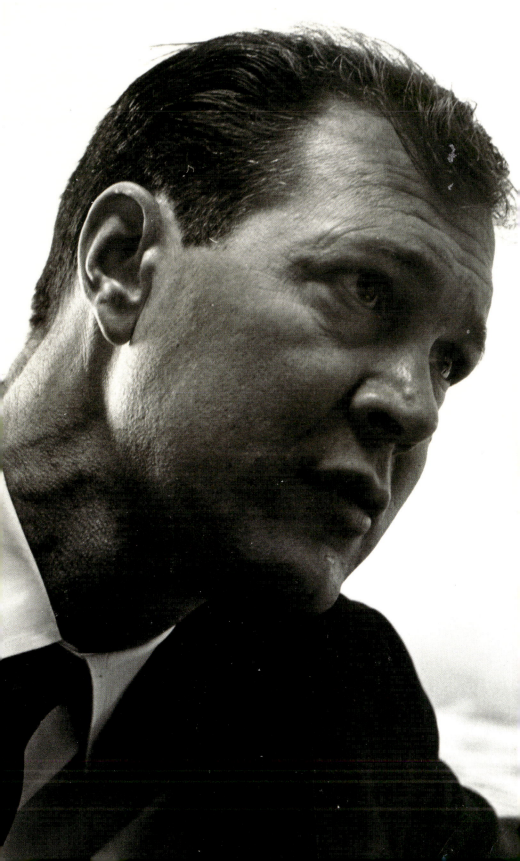

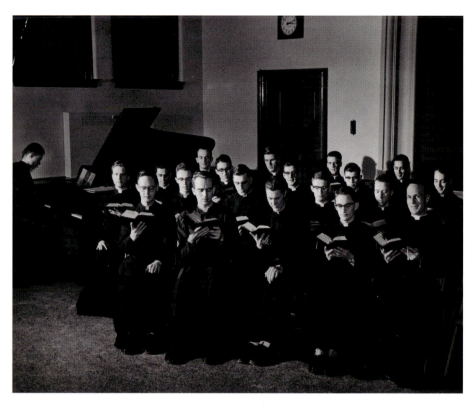

(*Above*) Joe (center front) in the Chancel choir of St. Meinrad Abbey, 1954.
(*Below*) Ann (center) in a variety show chorus line at Mundelein College, 1964.

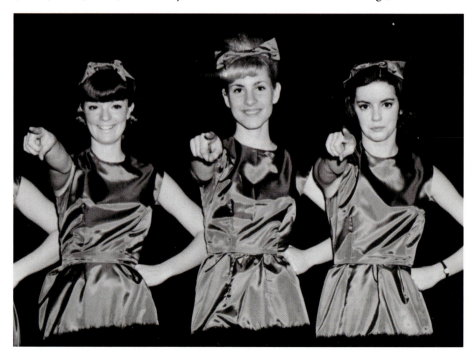

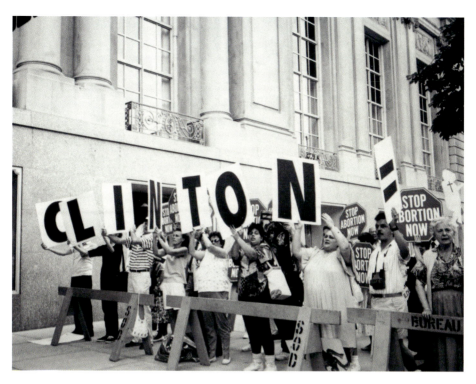

(*Above*) Picket of Bill Clinton, using large block letters, 1992. (*Below*) Joe putting his bullhorn to good use during a picket of Janet Reno in Chicago, May 1993.

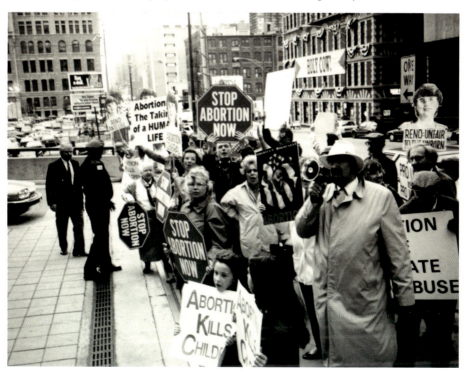

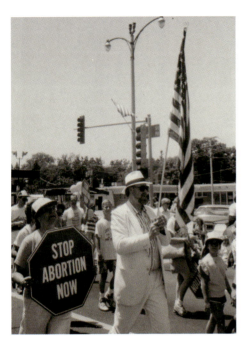
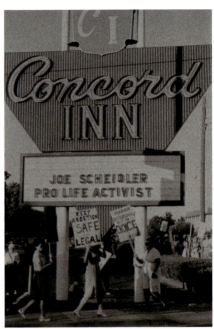

(*Left*) Joe marches in the Des Plaines, Illinois 4th of July Parade, 1989. (*Right*) Abortion supporters protest Joe's appearance at an event in California, August, 1985. (*Below*) Picket of Geraldine Ferraro with the 2 x 2 block letters, 1984. (*Opposite*) Picketing the Chicago Sun-Times, mid 1980s.

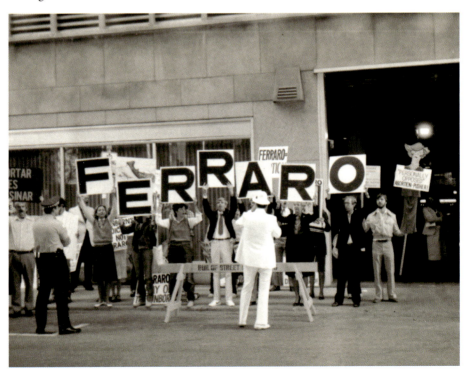

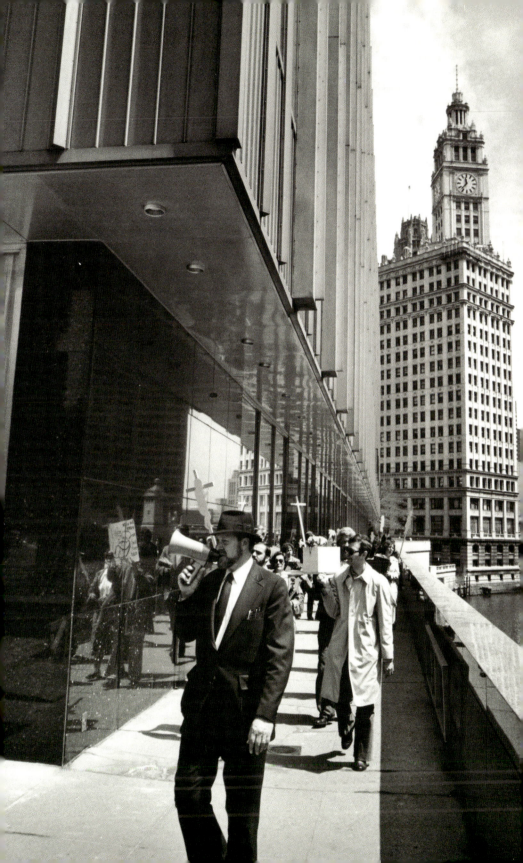

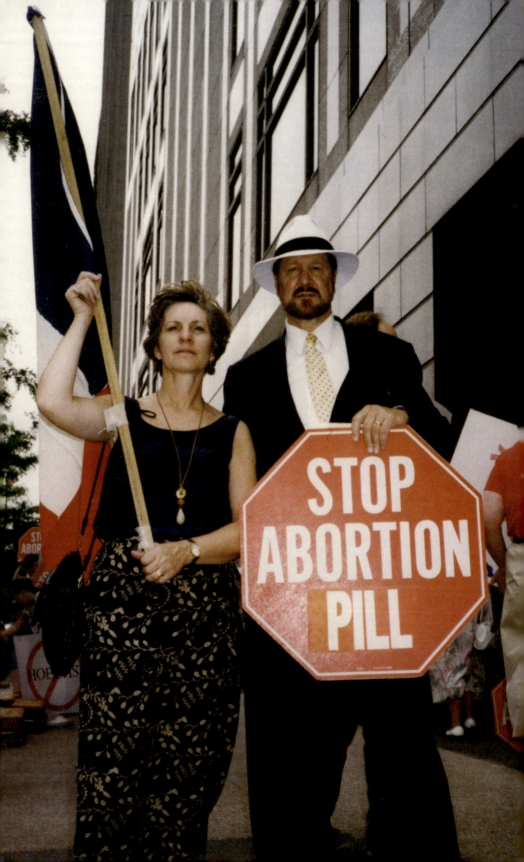

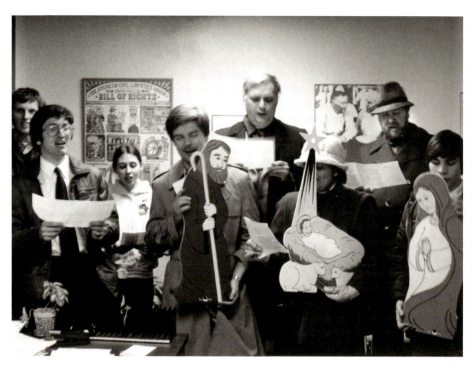

(*Opposite*) Ann & Joe Scheidler protest the introduction of Ru486 abortion pill at the French consulate in Chicago, 1991. (*Above*) Christmas caroling at ACLU office in Chicago, 1985. (*Below*) One of over 100 protests on the First National Day of Rescue, August 1980 (Chicago).

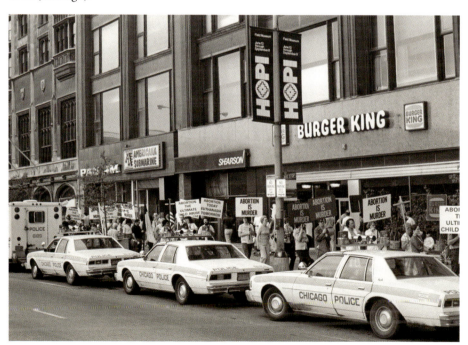

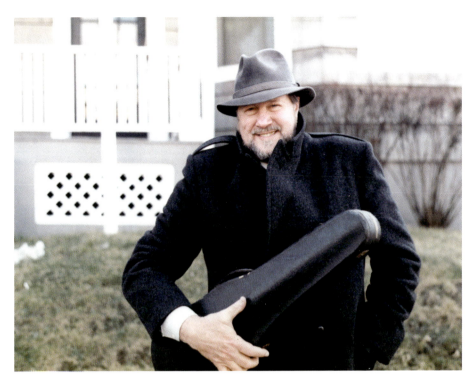

(*Above*) Joe in Binghamton, New York, posing with violin case. (*Below*) Tombstones of women killed by abortion, Wichita, Kansas, August 1991.

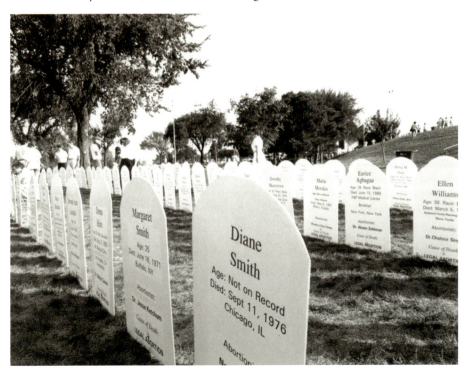

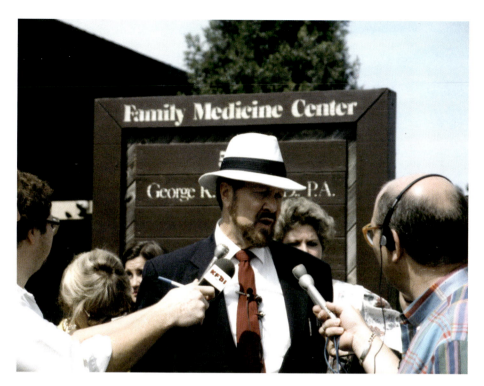

(*Above*) Joe answers media inquiries in Pennsylvania outside an abortion facility.
(*Below*) Joe uses his bullhorn to lead chants and direct a protest at Planned Parenthood.

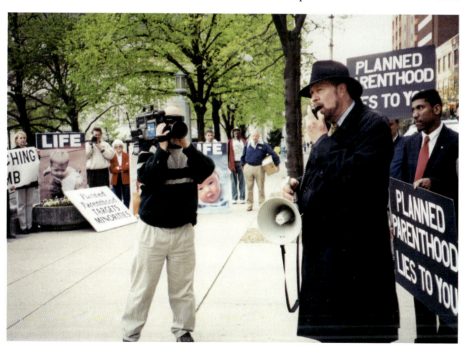

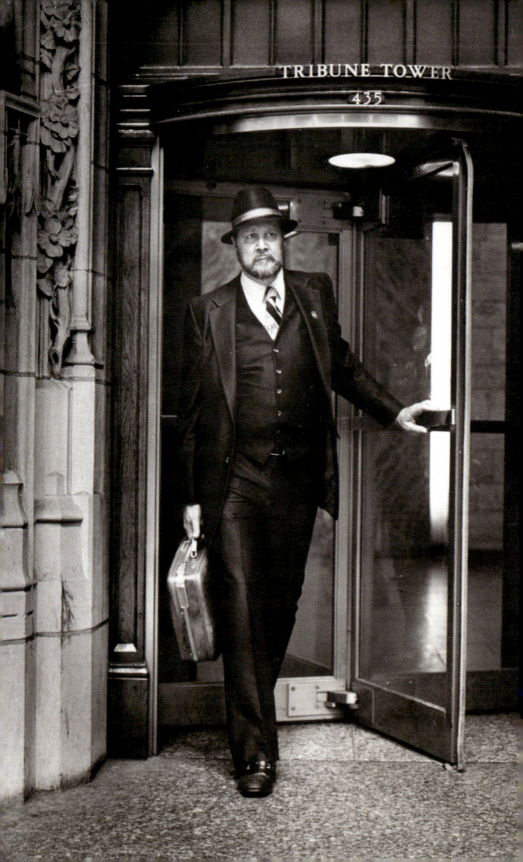

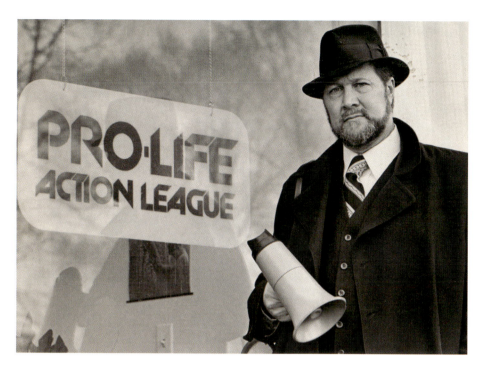

(*Opposite*) Joe leaving the Chicago Tribune Building, 1983. (*Above*) Joe with his trademark fedora and iconic bullhorn. (*Below*) Joe being arrested in Denver, Colorado, on charges from Pensacola, Florida, June 1986.

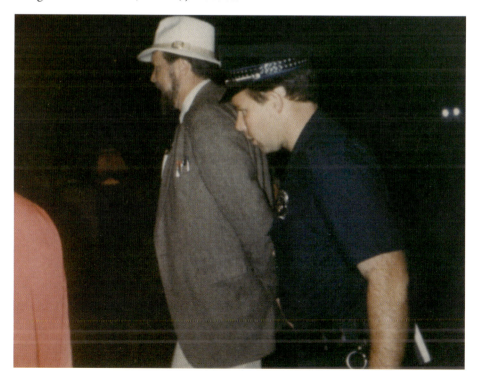

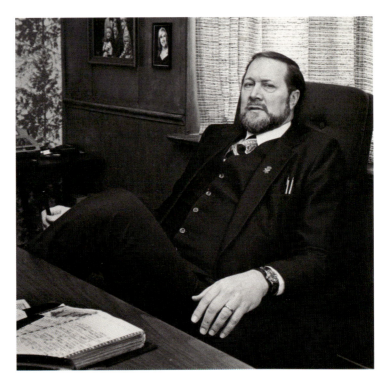

(*Above*) Joe at his desk in the first Pro-Life Action League office, 1980. (*Below*) Joe leading a protest in London, Ontario, Canada, February 1992.

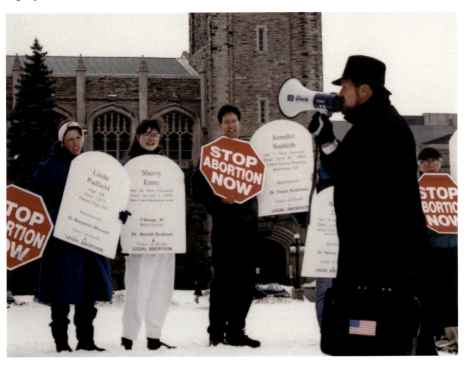

## CHAPTER 11

# The Abortionists

Immediately after the Supreme Court legalized abortion on demand in 1973, clinics began opening in all the major cities. Within days of the ruling, four clinics opened up on Chicago's Michigan Avenue, and a larger one opened at the corner of State and Randolph. These were in high-rise office buildings. Some clinics were in smaller freestanding buildings, like Concord Medical Center on State and Grand and the Midwest Population Center on Ohio Street. There were also freestanding clinics outside the Loop. Others popped up in a dozen suburbs.

When I called the clinic phone numbers and the referral agencies that advertised in the local papers, I often recognized the voice on the other end of the line. Helen and I knew each other reasonably well; she was the director of Illinois Citizens for the Medical Control of Abortion (later National Abortion Rights Action League of Illinois), and we'd debated live a number of times at local colleges and on the radio. When I published a letter in the paper, Helen would write a rebuttal. We had a lot of back and forth, and on this day, it was her voice on the line.

"Helen, how do you handle all these phones?" I'd ask. "You must be an octopus!"

"This isn't Helen," she'd say.

"Come on, Helen. I know your voice."

She'd hang up. Then I'd call the next number, and Helen would answer.

One of the clinics Helen referred women to was Albany, operated by a young woman named Suzanne. Some members of the IRLC board knew that Suzanne was Catholic, and I thought that maybe, with my background in theology, I could perhaps convince her to quit the abortion business.

Suzanne was twenty-six, energetic, and headstrong. She refused to meet with me and made it clear she wasn't about to give up her job as clinic director. She drove a red Volkswagen convertible, and when I saw her at Albany, I'd put an "Adoption Not Abortion" bumper sticker on it. She'd drive around with it for a few days until someone pointed it out, and she'd tear it off. Then when she was inside the clinic, I'd slap on a fresh one.

I called the city health inspector to find out whether Albany was operating with a valid license. They had nothing on file. I had a friend who worked at the City Health Department, and we went to Albany together on a busy day. He asked to see their license. They couldn't produce one, but they said they were getting one soon. That wasn't good enough, the health officer said. He ordered the patients to leave and the clinic to close for several days until it received its license.

Suzanne, in the meanwhile, decided to go skydiving. Her main parachute didn't open, and something went wrong with her reserve. I saw the obituary. I felt sorry for her—she was young, and she never got the chance to get out of the abortion business. The obituary included the arrangements for a funeral Mass at St. Tarcissus on West Ardmore Avenue in Chicago.

Growing up, nearly everyone I knew, regardless of their religious affiliation, believed that abortion was wrong. But by the early '70s, a number of sects had weakened their rhetoric. The Catholic Church remained committed to the truth, but after *Roe*, some commentators, and even some theologians, began suggesting that the Church no longer viewed involvement in abortion as a serious sin—the sort of sin that, in the past, could preclude a funeral Mass or interment in a Catholic cemetery. Concerned, I called St. Tarcissus and spoke with the pastor.

The pastor checked with the Chancery, which replied that, according to canon law, St. Tarcissus couldn't have a funeral Mass. Suzanne's funeral was conducted at the funeral home with a bishop from the Old Roman Catholic Church, a dissenting splinter sect, presiding.

I called Suzanne's mother to express my condolences and my hope that Suzanne had reconciled with God before the end. She told me another part of the sad story: Her husband, Suzanne's father, had passed away only five months earlier. Our conversation was suddenly interrupted when one of Suzanne's sisters grabbed the phone, cursed me out for interfering, threatened to sue me, and hung up.

A few days later, I overheard my assistant on the phone spelling my last name very slowly. When she hung up, I asked who was on the line—it was a law firm representing Suzanne's family. They were threatening to sue me for harassment. I asked an attorney friend how concerned I should be, and he told me they had no real ground for a lawsuit.

That was the end of the matter from a legal standpoint, but the story made it into the papers and was picked up by the Associated Press. "The pastor at St. Tarcissus Church," the story read, "said he was told of the woman's abortion activities by a man who phoned the church. 'The decision was not a result of pressure from pro-life groups,' said Fr. Leonard Felczak. 'She chose that herself.'"

The AP story didn't include my name, but in an angry letter to the *Chicago Tribune*, Helen did. We traded letters over the incident, and some members of the IRLC board were annoyed that our organization was made out to look callous. It turned out, however, that the archdiocese only intervened in the matter of the funeral. Despite the strict dictates of canon law, Suzanne is laid to rest just a few feet from her father's grave in the family plot at All Saints Cemetery in Des Plaines, Illinois.

Over the years, I lost touch with Helen until the phone rang one night in the early '80s. Ann answered it and handed it to me. There was that voice.

"Joe," she said, "it's Helen. This may sound strange, but I'd like your help." Her son, she said, was doing a school project on fetal development. "I can't think of anyone who'd be better to talk to and get pictures from than you, Joe. Could we meet?"

We invited Helen and her son over to give him some material for his presentation. Ann made cookies, and we sat by the fire with hot tea, going over some information on life in the womb and talking about the old days. Helen assured me that she'd left the abortion business long ago and no longer had anything to do with helping women get abortions. It was a pleasant visit, and I felt it a small triumph that one of the abortion advocates I'd sparred with so often had left the grisly industry.

Convincing someone to quit the business is an uphill battle. Occasionally, however, it's remarkably easy. One day early in my pro-life career, I went into a clinic on the second floor of a Chicago building. I asked the receptionist there if she liked her job.

"It pays well," she told me.

"Is that all?" I asked. "I think you should quit."

"What?"

"Think about it. You're helping this doctor destroy lives. What's the excuse—that they aren't really human? That you needed the money? You can find a different job. That's all—think it over."

I went back downstairs to the sidewalk. One of our volunteers went up to make an appointment, a popular tactic for filling appointment schedules with "no-show" time.

"Is the doctor in?" she asked. But the receptionist, to her surprise, was packing up. "I don't know when he's coming back," she said, "but I don't care. I'm leaving this place!"

That, of course, is the exception—clinic workers preferred to call the police. Most just don't think—or don't want to think—about their role in taking an innocent life. My friend Bob Jonas also had a habit of taking clinic staff to lunch to ask them about their work. He didn't have much luck getting them to quit, but he got them to tell him what went on inside the clinics. He heard stories of fraud, unsanitary conditions, complete disregard for the women, and other sad stories.

Bob recorded some of these conversations, and he played the tapes for me. I put much of this information on my daily hotlines, first at the IRLC and later at the FFL, but I wanted to reach a wider audience. In the summer of 1978, I took a stack of this information to an investigative reporter, Pam Zekman from the *Chicago Sun-Times*.

I knew Pam from my days working with the city. Back then, it was my job to make Mayor Daley and Chicago city workers look good, and it was her job to make them look bad, so she was seldom interested in anything I had to share with her. This time it was different. She said she'd pitch the idea of an exposé on Chicago's abortion clinics to her editors. They were intrigued. Zekman and a team of journalists partnered with the Better Government Association and set out on a very thorough five-month investigation of Chicago's abortion industry. They sent covert informants to get jobs at local clinics and referral services, investigating from the inside.

On November 12, 1978, the front page of the *Sun-Times* ran the headline "Meet the Abortion Profiteers" with the subhead "Making a Killing in Michigan Av. Clinics." The series ran each day for three weeks and was later reprinted in a special issue. Zekman had warned me that she was not pro-life, and the introduction to the special reprint stated, "Our purpose was not to re-examine the morality of abortion—we favor legalization—but to determine whether women were receiving safe, competent care the Supreme Court had determined was their legal right. We found that in a startling number of cases they were not."

What they uncovered was far worse and more extensive than anyone had suspected. They did an exposé on Dr. Arnold Bickham, who had worked with T. R. M. Howard at Friendship Medical Center and took over the clinic when Howard died. Three years before *Roe*, Bickham had his Illinois medical license revoked for performing illegal abortions—some on women who weren't even pregnant. After *Roe*, he got his license back, and in addition to Friendship, he ran another clinic on Michigan Avenue near Water Tower Place and a third in Indianapolis. None of these clinics had valid licenses.

Zekman quoted Bickham as calling himself "the most notorious physician in the city," and the *Sun-Times* uncovered other incidents of his medical malpractice. One girl who'd undergone an abortion on one of Bickham's "Bargain Days" came back with her mother the following day with severe cramping. He refused to see her without an additional cash payment, since it wasn't a bargain day anymore. When they couldn't come up with the cash, Bickham called the police to escort them out. The girl's mother took her to an emergency room, where doctors found fetal remains in her uterus.

We knew that Bickham charged poor women cash for their abortions and then billed Medicaid as well. What we didn't know is that he'd earned more than three quarters of a million dollars from Medicaid, more than any other abortionist in the nation. Zekman also found that Bickham had a contract with a federal on-the-job training program, but instead of hiring and training unskilled workers, he hired experienced staff and had them lie about their experience on their applications.

As a result of the "Profiteers" series, Bickham lost his Indiana medical license. His Illinois license wasn't revoked, but his Chicago clinics were shuttered for failing to meet required standards. He was prosecuted for fraud over his job-training scheme and received a two-year prison sentence.[1]

One Sunday morning, years after the series ran, I gave a talk at the Moody Bible Institute on Chicago's Near North Side. A group stayed after for a discussion, and one of them asked why doctors become abortionists.

"The money's good," I said. "There was a doctor here in Chicago named Arnold Bickham who made seven hundred and fifty grand in one year."

At this, about five people nearly fell off their chairs.

"Our head usher upstairs is named Arnold Bickham," one of them said.

"You've got to look into this," I said. "Find out if he's done time in prison."

Moody member Donna Baer learned that it was the same Arnold Bickham. He'd become a Christian in prison and had vowed not to do any abortions after his release. But his resolve didn't last long. Donna discovered that he was performing abortions twice a week at a South Side clinic. I contacted the Moody leadership and told them that we'd picket their church unless Bickham was removed as an usher. They did, and we never had to hold that picket.

Two years later, Bickham killed eighteen-year-old Sylvia Moore. She was in her second trimester, but Bickham used a suction technique, which is only suitable for a first-trimester abortion. One of

---

1    Pamela Zekman and Pamela Warren, "Abortion Profiteers" (series), *Chicago Sun-Times*, November 12, 1987–December 3, 1979.

his instruments broke off inside Sylvia's uterus, but he apparently didn't notice. When Sylvia was unable to walk after the procedure, he accused her of being lazy, put her in a wheelchair, and sent her home. Sylvia's mother took her to an emergency room later that day, but by then the damage was too severe, and she died.

The medical examiner ruled the death a homicide, but Bickham wasn't charged. He merely lost his medical license, a decade after the "Profiteers" series made it clear that he should never have kept it in the first place. A year later, he was prosecuted for practicing medicine without a license. Bickham eventually reinvented himself and became a Chicago Public Schools principal, working in the same South Side neighborhood where he formerly killed children at his Friendship clinic.

Bickham was just one of several seedy physicians the *Sun-Times* exposed. Bob Jonas, the lunch-hour conversationalist, heard about two doctors, Ming Kow Hah and Ulrich Klopfer, who competed to see who could perform more abortions in a single day, and we passed the information on to Zekman. The *Sun-Times* did a story on them, running a disturbing illustration of a doctor with tally marks on his apron. One of them had given up on administering anesthetic, since waiting for it to take effect might make him lose the race. Dr. Hah lost his Illinois medical license.

The titles of the *Sun-Times* articles could have come directly from our newsletters. One, titled "Life on the Abortion Assembly Line: Grim, Grisly and Greedy," was written by a reporter who took a job with a phone-in abortion counseling service and found that operators were paid by the clinics for every abortion that came through their referrals. Another reporter took a job inside a clinic to write, "Abortion Mill Bosses Cut Corners on Care." For our sidewalk counselors, the facts the *Sun-Times* uncovered were a gold mine. The Profiteers series helped us develop the "Chicago Method" of sidewalk counseling, where we share information with women about malpractice claims against the provider they are about to visit.

Two weeks into the "Profiteers" series, I opened the *Sun-Times* to see the day's coverage. They had a story on the local pro-life movement, with a picture of the FFL activists at a sit-in we'd staged two months earlier at the Midwest Population Center on Ohio Street. One of the activists pictured was Pam Warren, a young woman who had come to my office a few months earlier.

"I've been volunteering at Illinois Right to Life," she said, "but all I'm doing there is answering phones and filing things. I told them I wanted to be more active, and they sent me here. Is this the right place?"

"Yes, ma'am," I told her. "This is where the action is."

Pam attended several of our meetings and joined in some late-night adventures. We still had the Dirty Dozen going, and she got dirty with the rest of us. Whenever anyone offered her a ride home, she always asked to be dropped off on Wabash Avenue by the Chicago River. She was with us for a number of weeks, then abruptly stopped coming. I'd seen a lot of people get involved and then drop out, but this case felt odd. She seemed to have so much zeal that I wouldn't have expected her to quit.

When I read the caption below the *Sun-Times*'s picture of the Friends for Life sit-in, I learned that Pam Warren was actually Pam *Warrick*, Zekman's writing partner in the "Profiteers" series. She'd been a plant. The *Sun-Times* offices were right next to the Wabash Bridge over the Chicago River.

The story covered our planning for sit-ins, with an explanation of our aims. "Our purpose," I was quoted, "is three-fold. Education, which we'll do by counseling people in the clinics waiting for abortions. Disruption—we will probably stop everybody from doing their jobs. And publicity. This is going to get attention. We'll call the papers and the television crews as soon as you're inside the clinics."

The article made it clear that we were risking arrest. "We are not conspiring here to break the law. We are conspiring to save lives."

The article also included an account of a meeting at the FFL offices one evening where the CTA maps and cans of spray paint were handed out. "Scheidler," it said,

> flicked a bit of dried black paint from under his finger-nails. "This is from our little crusade last night," he said. He explained how he and another Friend for Life had vandalized posters put up by abortion clinics and referral services at CTA elevated platforms. But the task, Scheidler said, was too great "for just the two of us. There are so many of these ads. We need your help."
>
> "This may be a big news story," said Scheidler. "If they send photographers out to get pictures of the ads, I don't want them to find any intact. We have to work fast."

Until then, the "Profiteers" series had focused on the abortionists, so a story on pro-life activism surprised us—especially to learn that we'd been infiltrated the same way the clinics and referral services had been. After being ousted from the IRLC for bringing them bad publicity with my activism, I was worried that this story might affect the FFL board the same way. I called the chairman, Tom Roeser, to get his take on the story.

"I just finished reading it," Tom said. "It's worth a million dollars in publicity. It shows we're actually doing things."

"Meet the Abortion Profiteers" was a popular series, and it generated a huge response from readers. The Letters to the Editor section of the *Sun-Times* was packed with comments about abortion. When the *Sun-Times* produced its special reprint of the series, we bought up hundreds of copies and sent them all over the country to show what had been uncovered in Chicago-area clinics and what our kind of activism had accomplished. We'd helped expose those who victimize women and kill their children for profit.

While they exposed the seedier clinics in the city, they also ran articles on the clinics they claimed offered clean, safe abortions. At the start of the series, the *Sun-Times* included a note to readers: "This newspaper has decided that it cannot determine safe and sanitary conditions at all the abortion counseling services and clinics which advertised in our classified pages. Thus we are ceasing publication of such advertising at this time." Pleased as we were with this development, it had the downside that our free pro-life ad was also dropped.

In 1982, an FBI agent came to the League office to see whether I'd ever heard of a group called "The Army of God." Dr. Hector Zevallos, an abortionist from Granite City, Illinois, and his wife, Rosalee Jean, were kidnapped by a group using that name. After Zevallos promised to get out of the industry, they let him go, but Zevallos returned to his practice almost immediately.

The agent wanted to know if I knew anyone who might have been behind such an attack. The idea of kidnapping an abortionist and making him promise to quit seemed ridiculous to me. Anyone with any experience in the pro-life cause would recognize that as a harebrained scheme. I thought it was a hoax designed to make pro-lifers look like radicals, and I told the agent as much.

The kidnapping, however, was real. It had been perpetrated by three men new to the pro-life cause: Don Benny Anderson and his two nephews. During the week that they had Dr. Zevallos and his wife detained, one nephew got a severe case of poison ivy. Zevallos wrote him a prescription for an ointment, and that was how the authorities began tracking the kidnappers. They matched tire tracks at the barn where the kidnappers had kept Zevallos and his wife to those left at the scene of a clinic arson in Florida. All three were arrested that fall and convicted early in 1983. Don Benny

Anderson got thirty years for kidnapping and another thirty for the fire bombings.

A few months later, in April 1983, I flew to New Orleans to picket the NAF convention being held there. When my flight arrived, it was nearly midnight. The airport was almost deserted. Another traveler asked if I was headed downtown, and we agreed to share a cab. On the way, he asked what I was doing in town.

"I'm going to the National Abortion Federation convention," I said.

"So am I," said my companion. "I'm Dr. George Tiller from Wichita, Kansas."

I didn't tell him my name—we just continued our conversation. He told me he was doing a presentation on using ultrasounds in abortions. He'd brought a film of an abortion he was going to show.

"You have to be sure you've got everything out," he said. "I don't understand why more of us don't use ultrasound. I'm going to be talking it up."

I remember thinking a film like the one Tiller had could be a powerful tool for pro-lifers. I wondered if I could somehow get a copy.

We got into town. Tiller was staying at a cheaper hotel some distance from the convention, and I was staying at the hotel where the conference was, so the cab dropped Tiller off first. Before he got out, he invited me to come see his clinic if I was ever in Wichita.

I'd arranged to share a room with Andy Scholberg from Minnesota, and I met him the next morning in the lobby. He had a badge on—he'd registered for the conference. Although the plan was to picket the convention, I decided to join him so we could monitor the presentations.

Some NAF members recognized Andy and me and tried to get us removed, but since we were registered and didn't cause any disturbances, security wouldn't touch us. We were able to attend all the talks. Bill Baird of *Eisenstadt v. Baird* recognized us, followed us, and sat near us every chance he got. The Pontchartrain Room hosted three talks: "Moral and Ethical Dilemmas," "Personhood," and "Religious Perspectives." They paid lip service to the idea that abortion might be wrong, but in the end, each session justified abortion.

Andy and I joined the picket at noon, then went back into the convention. In the exhibit hall, salesmen for suction machines and other abortion tools were peddling their wares. Andy and I had a picture taken at a table covered with curettes and cannulas. When word got around that two "antis" were at the convention, it upset a lot of people. The afternoon sessions included workshops called "Violence against Clinics" and "The Fetus Scandal," which was about the discovery the previous year of seventeen thousand dead babies in a California storage container.

The banquet speaker was Canadian abortionist Dr. Henry Morgentaler, who had opened Canada's first clinic in 1969 and was then running six clinics. Once while in Halifax to protest the opening of a new clinic, I learned that Morgantaler had purchased three houses in a row, then opened his clinic in the middle house. The other two were buffers to keep pro-lifers away. Andy and I got to the banquet and sat at the table right in front of the podium. His delivery was halting, which seemed odd for a polished public speaker. We figured we were making him nervous.

Near the end of the conference, Tiller was scheduled to give his ultrasound presentation. I was in the audience, but he flatly refused to start his presentation unless I left. He had by now discovered who I was. As the atmosphere in that room became more tense and hostile, I decided to leave. In a way, I was relieved that I wouldn't have to watch a baby being torn to pieces, but I still had every intention of getting a copy of Tiller's film.

The NAF convention in New Orleans was an educational three days for Andy and me. Being with abortionists almost the whole time, moving between the various lecture halls, looking at the displays along with the doctors and clinic workers, we simply became part of the group. At the cocktail party, with people laughing and socializing all around us, it was hard to believe that they were all involved in such evil.

Getting on the plane for my trip back to Chicago, I saw dozens of faces I recognized from the conference. That odd impression of camaraderie clearly wasn't reciprocated—I got a lot of icy stares.

A few months later, I took Dr. Tiller up on the offer to visit his clinic. Right to Life of Kansas was holding a convention in Topeka, and I was a guest speaker. At a break in the conference, some friends and I drove 150 miles to Wichita to join a protest at Tiller's clinic. When I went in to see Tiller, the press followed me with their cameras. The receptionist told me Tiller was gone for the day, and the staff started scurrying around to avoid the cameras. I did several interviews inside Tiller's clinic, then left. I'd accepted Dr. Tiller's invitation to visit his clinic. I'd seen the inside of another American Dachau.

In 2009, George Tiller was shot and killed. By that time, he'd earned a reputation as America's leading late-term abortionist. In 2013, the documentary *After Tiller* was released, profiling four late-term abortionists in America. I went to a showing at Chicago's Music Box Theater. A few of my pro-life friends have cameos in the film's footage of protests, but the only interviews are with the doctors and their patients. The film celebrates how dedicated and brave these four doctors are for continuing to perform third-trimester abortions in the wake of the Tiller killing. As the closing credits rolled, a woman in the audience cried out, "Abortion providers are heroes!"

I'd confronted abortionists in person for years, including some that were featured in the film. In the silence after her comment, I retorted, "They're murderers." That might have shocked some people, but later a woman came up to me in the lobby and thanked me for saying it.

One of the doctors profiled in *After Tiller* was Colorado abortionist Warren Hern, who literally wrote the book on late-term abortion: *Abortion Practice*. The forceps he designed bear his name. Hern forceps are specially designed to crush a baby's skull during a partial-birth abortion. Experienced abortionists advise beginners to perform at least one thousand first-trimester abortions before they attempt a second-trimester abortion. In a first-trimester procedure, the baby is torn apart and sucked into a jar, but for a larger fetus, the doctor needs to dismember the child and pull it out of the uterus piece by piece. In order to handle that kind of work, the abortionist needs to be desensitized to destroying a life. Some have become numb, but for others, the echo of guilt lingers.

One of Chicago's clinics was run for years by a survivor of the Holocaust, Dr. Jan Barton. We thought someone who lived through that genocide would have a respect for human life, but Barton was one of the most callous doctors I'd ever met. In the early '90s, we staged a series of protests at his Western Avenue clinic, picketing several days in a row. One day Dr. Barton came out and walked up to my assistant, Tim Murphy. In his thick Polish accent, he said, "Tell your boss Scheidler to stop having blitzkrieg at my clinic."

I put my answer on the hotline. It was meant for Barton, but it applies to any doctor still in business.

"Sorry, Jan. We'll call off the troops when you stop killing babies."

CHAPTER 12

# The Plank

"Mind if I join you?"

Henry Hyde had come out of the hotel and asked to join our picket line.

It was early 1974. The temperature was just above freezing. It was half snowing, half raining as I led a group of pro-lifers back and forth in the slush outside the suburban Chicago Marriott hotel where New York governor Nelson Rockefeller was being honored at a Republican event.

Four years earlier, Rockefeller's signature had granted any woman who could get to New York the right to an abortion. With so many women arriving from out of state, postabortion complications were severely underreported in New York, skewing the data on the safety of legal abortion. It was this inaccurate data that Justice Harry Blackmun cited in *Roe* as evidence that abortion posed no significant health risks to the woman. So when Rockefeller came to Chicago, we greeted him with a picket.

At the time, Henry Hyde was serving in the Illinois legislature, but he was launching a campaign for the US House of Representatives. Hyde had spoken at the Civic Center rally in 1972 that helped bring me into the pro-life movement. I was disappointed when he chose to attend the Rockefeller event, but I understood the political demands for party loyalty during an election bid. Nevertheless he'd seen us on the way in and decided to follow his conscience. In joining us, braving both the slush and the scorn from his fellow Republicans, Hyde showed he was a true pro-lifer.

Younger pro-lifers might think that the two parties' positions on abortion have always been the way they are today, but in the early days of the abortion battle, that wasn't the case. The majority of states that adopted the American Law Institute's abortion reform laws and three of the four that legalized abortion on demand before *Roe* were headed by GOP governors at the time. When the 1970 National Abortion Act was put forth to legalize abortion nationwide, Republican Bob Packwood of Oregon was its sponsor. Of the seven justices who gave us *Roe*, five were appointed by Republicans. The most vocal dissenter, Byron White, was a Democratic appointee.

Within weeks of the court's abortion rulings, lawmakers began drafting amendments designed to undo it. Blackmun himself had noted that his ruling would be void "if this suggestion of personhood is established," and a Human Life Amendment would not only reverse *Roe* but void all the state laws permitting abortion pre-*Roe*. Two versions of a states' rights amendment were put forward leaving the legality of abortion to individual states, but since they both recognized a legal right to abortion, neither, obviously, was pro-life. The two states' rights amendments were written by Republicans. The GOP was not the established pro-life party—yet.

The summer after we picketed Rockefeller, President Nixon resigned over the Watergate scandal, and his successor, Gerald Ford, appointed Rockefeller as his vice president. Ford had criticized the *Roe* decision as going too far, but he declined to endorse either the Human Life or the states' rights amendments. His wife, Betty, remained outspoken in her support of the ruling. "I feel very strongly," she told CBS's *60 Minutes*, "that it was the best thing in the world when the Supreme Court voted to legalize abortion and bring it out of the backwoods and put it in the hospitals where it belongs. It was a great, great decision."[1]

Early one Sunday morning in 1976, two years after Ford took office, I got a call. "Joe, it's Kathy Edwards. Remember me?"

I had met Kathy earlier that year when I attended a pro-life meeting in Washington, DC. The night before the meeting, a group of us went to see an exhibit of Civil War artifacts at the National Museum of Health and Medicine, which at that time was housed in the Walter Reed Army Medical Center. The bullet that killed Lincoln was on display, and other exhibits featured hundreds, maybe thousands, of amputated limbs of Civil War victims, many with bullets still embedded in their bones.

It was a somber exhibit, but when we entered one of the galleries, we heard beautiful music coming out of a small theater off to the side. We went in to see what was showing. It was a presentation on fetal development, with beautiful pictures taken in utero, of babies from the earliest stages to birth. That was where I met Kathy Edwards, an activist with Missouri Citizens for Life. As pro-lifers, fighting a new wave of national carnage, we were struck by the juxtaposition of the film's beauty with the display of America's bloody past.

Kathy was calling from Missouri. "The Republican Convention is about to start out here," she said. "Delegates are already arriving, and we need to get a pro-life plank in their platform. John Macke is here, and he suggested I call you. We need you out here. Today."

I understood Kathy's urgency, but I was a little surprised she'd called me. I wasn't a national leader in 1976, and I wasn't sure what she thought I could accomplish. But they were eager to do

---

1    Betty Ford, interview with Morley Safer, *60 Minutes*, CBS, July 21, 1975.

something, and if they thought I could help, I was happy to try. I went to an early Mass while Ann made flight arrangements, and by that afternoon I was in Kansas City.

This was the first presidential election after *Roe v. Wade*. Three weeks before Kathy's call, the Democratic Party wrapped up their convention, nominating Jimmy Carter of Georgia. Democratic delegates had approved a platform statement that rejected any effort to amend the Constitution with either a human life or a states' rights amendment.

A week later, Gerald Ford declared that he favored a states' rights amendment. With the incumbent lukewarm at best on right-to-life issues, getting a pro-life plank into the Republican platform might have seemed like a lost cause. But there had been some important developments leading up to the 1976 convention that we thought we might be able to capitalize on.

Amending the Constitution is one way to void a Supreme Court ruling, but another strategy is to bring the issue before the court again, giving it a chance to reverse itself. Unless the justices change their positions on an issue, such a change could only come about after retirements or deaths. At the time *Roe* was decided, only one of the justices, William Douglas, was over seventy years old. The dissenters were the two youngest members of the court. Justice Douglas, the judge who defined the "right to privacy," retired in 1975. Ford replaced him with John Paul Stevens.

A few months after the appointment, the court heard arguments in *Planned Parenthood v. Danforth*, regarding a Missouri law requiring married women to inform their husbands and minor girls to get parental consent when seeking abortions. Few thought the court would let the spousal notification stand, but how the court would rule regarding parental notification was less certain. A child can't even obtain an aspirin from a school nurse without parental approval, and most people recognize that allowing a doctor to perform nonemergency surgery on a minor without parental consent would violate not just the parents' rights but their responsibilities. Would the court concur?

On July 1, 1976, less than two weeks before the Democratic National Convention was set to kick off, the Supreme Court handed down its *Danforth* ruling. All six of the remaining pro-abortion justices voted to strike down the whole law. Justice Stevens, however, split his vote, siding with the majority regarding spousal notification but siding with Rehnquist and White in the dissent that argued in favor of parental consent.

If the timing had been different, the Democratic Party would perhaps have crafted a response to the abortion issue more reasonable than agreeing not to talk about it and hoping it would go away. As it was, since the Republican National Convention was five weeks after *Danforth*, the outrage over the court's abrogation of parental rights gave us an opportunity to push the right-to-life agenda.

The convention would be held at Kansas City's Kemper Arena, but the meetings to draft the party platform were held downtown at the Muehlebach Hotel, where most of the delegates were staying. Missouri was traditionally a very pro-life state, and it was a Missouri law that the high court had just struck down. This was a good setting for championing the pro-life cause.

The 1976 Republican National Convention turned out to be the last one for either party where delegates actually selected a nominee rather than just endorsing primary results. Ford's presidency was one of the most bizarre in American history. He hadn't even been on the ballot in 1972. He replaced Spiro Agnew as Richard Nixon's vice president when Agnew resigned in 1973 over a bribery scandal. Nixon's own resignation elevated Ford to the Oval Office, but his popularity plummeted when Ford granted Nixon a full pardon just days after taking the oath of office. In the 1976 primaries, former California governor Ronald Reagan gave Ford such a challenge that on the eve of the convention the nomination was still too close to call.

I had supported Reagan all through the primaries even though he didn't have a spotless pro-life record. While he was California's governor in the late '60s, a therapeutic abortion bill based on the American Law Institute model came to Reagan's desk. It didn't appear to allow abortion on demand, but it permitted abortion if the health of the mother, including her mental health, was threatened. The bill had broad support in the legislature, and Reagan feared a veto would be overridden and might even prompt the drafting of a more permissive bill, so he signed it. The mental health clause functioned in practice as a catchall exemption, and California saw a massive increase in the number of "therapeutic" abortions. After that debacle, Reagan became an outspoken critic of abortion and announced his support for a Human Life Amendment.

When Reagan came through Chicago during the 1976 primaries, I took a group of activists to meet him as he arrived at O'Hare airport. There were some media there, but the crowd was pretty small, so a few of us went around the terminal and told people a movie star was about to arrive. In those days, you could go right up to the gate to greet people getting off a plane, and a good-sized crowd gathered around the gate to greet Reagan as he came down the Jetway. Those of us with signs spread out through the group and stood on seats in the waiting area, so it looked like a large, well-coordinated Reagan rally. As I walked with him through the airport to his taxi, I said, "The next time you fly into Chicago, it'll be on Air Force One." My prediction was off by four years.

Those of us who gathered to work on the pro-life plank—Kathy Edwards, John Macke, Ray James, Tom Curtis, and some other dedicated activists who had answered the call—decided to call ourselves the Human Life Amendment Committee. We put on whatever Republican insignia and buttons we could come up with. John counted 107 delegates on the full platform committee who would be voting on the planks that would be submitted before the convention began. He determined that thirty-three of them were firmly pro-life, with nine others leaning our way. Since we were short of the number needed to get a full pro-life statement into the platform, our task was to convince enough of the other sixty-five delegates that such a plank would be good for the party.

As the delegates started filing into the hotel, we acted like a Republican welcoming committee. In a sense, that's what we were—after all, we *were* Republicans, we were a committee, and we were welcoming the delegates. We showed them around the hotel, sat with them in the lounge, and tried to impress on them how important the right-to-life issue was and that the Democrats had made a significant blunder coming down against grassroots efforts for a Human Life Amendment.

"Well of course abortion is an important issue," one delegate told Kathy, "but an amendment to outlaw it would never get passed."

"Maybe you're right," Kathy replied, "but telling the people the courts are the only ones who can change the Constitution makes a mockery of the words 'We the people.'"

We explained that the life issue could be a strong one to lure over some of these voters to the Republican side. Neither Republican candidate supported abortion as a right, and whether a delegate was inclined to support Ford's weak position or Reagan's stronger one, it was clear that both candidates opposed the court rulings.

Despite joining our picket two years earlier, Henry Hyde had won his seat in the US House in 1974. At that time, nearly half a million abortions each year were paid for by US taxpayers, and Hyde introduced an amendment to a Medicaid bill to ban federal abortion funding. The Hyde Amendment passed in the house, but just weeks before the convention, it was defeated in the Senate—which, thanks in part to the Watergate mess, had a huge Democratic majority.

We called Hyde and persuaded him to send a telegram to each of the 107 delegates on the platform committee. We also wanted to provide them with pro-life statements from each of the frontrunners. Finding Reagan's was easy—he'd gone on record that the Republican platform "must recognize once and for all that to perform an abortion is to take a human life." Since Ford's position was weak, we might have had a hard time finding a good quote from him. Providentially, however, the very day I arrived in Kansas City, Ford was in Philadelphia speaking at the Eucharistic Congress there. Ford, an Episcopalian, addressed the Catholic assembly, saying, "I share your deep apprehension about the increased irreverence for life."

That sounded sufficiently pro-life, so we printed both Ford's and Reagan's quotes on the kind of yellow paper that telegrams were printed on and stuffed them all into the delegates' mailboxes at the Muehlebach. Thanks to our Human Life Amendment Committee, each delegate was implored by Hyde and both presidential frontrunners to support a pro-life position. Regardless of which candidate they supported, delegates could argue that a pro-life plank would be consistent with their agenda.

Our next challenge was getting a committee to introduce such a plank. Platform statements on social issues were being drafted by the Human Rights and Responsibilities Subcommittee, which was chaired by Representative Silvio Conte of Massachusetts. Conte had a fair pro-life voting record but had never shown any leadership in the cause. He was a Ford delegate at the convention and was now a strong advocate of the Equal Rights Amendment. NOW activists were also lobbying the convention, and since the feminist movement had become radically pro-abortion, we didn't have any confidence that Conte could provide the kind of initiative it would take to introduce a pro-life plank. On the other hand, the vice-chairman, Charles Pickering of Mississippi, a Reagan supporter, was firmly pro-life.

John Macke was from DC, and he contacted a colleague there to see if there was some urgent business in the House of Representatives that might require Conte's presence. It turned out that there was, and Macke persuaded his colleague to call for a vote. Conte felt he had to leave the convention for a few days. In his absence, we floated the idea that if the Human Rights and Responsibilities chair couldn't be present for discussions about proposed planks, it would be best to choose a different chair. That worked too, and Pickering took over those duties.

The media reported that the change was engineered by the Reagan campaign, but it was primarily our small group that got it done, and the following text authored by Senator Jesse Helms was presented to the Human Rights and Responsibilities Subcommittee: "We protest the Supreme Court's intrusion into the family structure through its denial of the parents' obligation and right to guide their minor children. The Republican Party favors a continuance of the public dialogue on abortion and supports the efforts of those who seek enactment of a constitutional amendment to restore protection of the right to life for unborn children."[2] That was all in a day and a half's work in Kansas City. By Monday evening, I was headed back to Chicago, and on Wednesday, the subcommittee voted. We thought it was going to be a close vote, but under Pickering's leadership the subcommittee approved the plank thirteen to one. That Friday, it was resoundingly endorsed by the 107 delegates whose mailboxes we'd stuffed. One of the two major American political parties, the GOP, was now officially courting the pro-life vote.

It had been a good week.

---

2    Reproduced in Daniel K. Williams, *Defenders of the Unborn* (Oxford: Oxford University Press, 2016), 232.

## CHAPTER 13

# Nominations

When the 1976 Republican convention finally got under way, the question of which candidate it would select was answered quickly. Although the stronger pro-life candidate, Ronald Reagan, was passed over in favor of Gerald Ford, the convention still resulted in some strong pro-life victories.

Nelson Rockefeller had announced before the convention that he would not seek another term as vice president, so the big question in Kansas City was who Ford would select for his running mate. In a move that surprised political observers, Ford selected Bob Dole of Kansas. Of all the choices considered, none was as firm a supporter of the right to life as Dole. A month later, the Senate passed the Hyde Amendment.

Jimmy Carter claimed that he opposed abortion and that his view and Ford's were essentially the same, but his political party was clearly becoming the pro-abortion party. Pro-lifers began to picket Carter wherever he went, and when he came through Chicago after the convention, CBS anchorman Bill Curtis commented that abortion had become the number one issue of the campaign. If not for the efforts of our ragtag Human Life Amendment Committee at the Muehlebach, that might not have been the case.

Chicago is a traditional Democratic stronghold—the city hasn't elected a Republican mayor since the days of Al Capone. By the time I settled in Chicago in 1963, Mayor Richard J. Daley had already won three elections and cemented his reputation as an iron-fisted ruler. He went on to win three more and took great pride in delivering Chicago's vote to the Democrats' presidential candidate. There was a longstanding tradition of honoring the nominee with a torchlight parade. The 1976 parade would end at Chicago's Medinah Temple, where the Illinois Democratic Party was holding its convention.

We protested Carter twice that September day. The idea of a "personally opposed, but . . ." politician might be commonplace today, but in the mid-'70s, it was a comparatively new concept. He professed to be against abortion, but it was clear that he would follow the party line, and it was obvious where the Democrats were headed. We met in the afternoon at a mall in the south suburbs, where Pat Trueman started the "Life, Yes! Carter, No!" chant. In the evening, we gathered at the Medinah Temple, where pro-life guru Greg Morrow had parked a big flatbed truck. As the procession came around the corner, Carter, Mayor Daley, and the rest of the marchers were greeted by Greg dressed in a toga. Standing beside him on the truck bed were local activist Ron Compagna's two daughters. One held a basin while the other poured water over Greg's hands. A sign above them read: "Jimmy Carter; Pontius Pilate on the Abortion Issue."

Despite the efforts of pro-lifers, Carter defeated Ford. Carter never had a chance to make any Supreme Court nominations, but there was a key court case during his presidency that involved one of Carter's cabinet appointees. The day the Hyde Amendment was to go into effect, it was challenged by a woman on public aid, Cora McRae, who argued that her varicose veins required the government to pay for an abortion. She won her suit, and Medicaid paid to end her pregnancy. Since it was decided as a class action suit representing all women on public aid, McRae's case invalidated the Hyde Amendment, pending an appeal.

When Carter appointed Patricia Harris Secretary of the Department of Health, Education, and Welfare (later Health and Human Services), she defended the Hyde Amendment in federal appeals court and before the Supreme Court. McRae's lawyers, in addition to contending that the government had an obligation to provide abortions to the poor, challenged the Hyde Amendment on First Amendment grounds. They argued that it violated the establishment clause since it enforced Catholic values. While none of the justices bought that argument, the irony of asking for public funds for a procedure whose legalization hinged on a right to privacy was lost on some of them.

The court announced its decision in *Harris v. McRae* at the end of June 1980—another election year. The six remaining justices who had voted pro-abortion in *Roe v. Wade* split on the *Harris* ruling, with Chief Justice Burger and Justices Powell and Stewart joining Rehnquist and White in ruling that the Hyde Amendment "represents a legitimate congressional interest in protecting potential life." Justices Blackmun, Marshall, and Brennan were joined by Stevens in their dissents. After four years as a dead letter, the Hyde Amendment was now in effect.

High inflation, growing unemployment, and foreign policy embarrassments, most notably the Iran hostage crisis, left Carter with little chance of winning a second term. Some pundits thought that the 1980 election was in the bag, and with the high court's new pro-life ruling shoring up the social conservative vote, many thought the Republicans might retreat from the pro-life stand it took in 1976.

Instead, the 1980 Republican National Convention in Detroit adopted an even stronger pro-life plank, written by Phyllis Schlafly, who had also led a successful campaign to defeat the controversial Equal Rights Amendment. The 1980 plank supported the Hyde Amendment, the Human Life Amendment, and parental consent laws. "We affirm our support," it said, "of a constitutional amendment to restore protection of the right to life for unborn children. We also support the Congressional efforts to restrict the use of taxpayers' dollars for abortion." Further on, it reads, "We will work for the appointment of judges at all levels of the judiciary who respect traditional family values and the sanctity of innocent human life."[1] It was a great victory for the right-to-life movement—one that built on the work of our little ad-hoc committee of '76.

Reagan's momentum had been building throughout Carter's presidency, and he won by a landslide in 1980. On election night, Republicans won both the White House and the Senate. I was in Washington the night of the inauguration and attended the pro-life inaugural ball in the Indian Treaty Room of the Executive Office Building at the invitation of Ann Higgins, a Reagan staffer.

Five months into Reagan's first term, Justice Potter Stewart announced his retirement. We were thrilled—for a while. During his campaign, Reagan had committed to providing the high court with its first-ever female justice. Pro-lifers hoped he would nominate a strong supporter of the right to life, but in early July, we heard he was considering Sandra Day O'Connor for the post. On July 7, 1981, I summarized some of her credentials in my hotline message:

> Shortly after being elected to the Arizona Senate in 1970, O'Connor voted for liberalization of the Arizona abortion law. In 1973 she voted for passage of a senate bill to allow Planned Parenthood to give out contraceptives to minors without

---

1    "1980 GOP Abortion Plank," *CNN.com*, last modified 1996, http://edition.cnn.com/ALLPOLITICS/1996/conventions/san.diego/facts/abortion/1980.shtml.

parental knowledge or consent. In 1974 she voted against endorsing a Human Life Amendment. . . . If you have not yet done your duty as a pro-lifer, you may still have time to be part of what we hope will be the scuttling of this appointment. Send a telegram today to President Reagan, the White House, Washington, DC, telling him to stand by the Republican platform calling for court appointments only of people who respect human life.

That evening, Reagan wrote in his diary, "Called Judge O'Connor and told her she was my nominee for the Supreme Court. Already the flak is starting and from my own supporters. Right to Life say she is pro-abortion. She says abortion is personally repugnant to her. I think she'll make a good Justice."[2]

The next day, Reagan was on his way to Chicago, and we were determined to send him a message. We assembled a group of seventy demonstrators at O'Hare. This time we weren't greeting Reagan at the gate; we were going to meet him at the air force base at O'Hare with a message. Dick O'Connor from the *Chicago Tribune* art department made some signs for us, big square posters with solid block letters. Held aloft in a row, they read: LIFE, YES. O'CONNOR, NO. When I told Reagan in '76 that he'd return to Chicago on Air Force One, I never thought we'd be there to picket him.

When the Senate Judiciary Committee held hearings on O'Connor's nomination, Dr. Jack Willke testified against her, as did Dr. Carolyn Gerster, founder of Arizona Right to Life. They had no impact. The Judiciary Committee voted 17–0 to send her nomination on to the full Senate. When it came time for the vote, Jeremiah Denton, a hero from the Vietnam era and committed pro-lifer, voted with his fellow senators to confirm. Nobody voted against her

---

2    Reprinted in the *Washington Post*, May 2, 2007.

after that. I spoke with Senator Denton shortly after the vote, and he assured me that as long as Reagan was in office, she'd be a pro-life vote on the court.

We lost that battle, but we had made abortion part of the debate, and early in 1982, when Reagan had to fill a vacancy for surgeon general, he chose C. Everett Koop, who had produced a series of pro-life films called *Whatever Happened to the Human Race?* with Reverend Francis Shaeffer.

The next year, O'Connor heard her first abortion cases as a Supreme Court justice: *Planned Parenthood v. Ashcroft* and *City of Akron v. Akron Center for Reproductive Health.* The first case focused on a Missouri law that was written after the *Danforth* ruling. This time, by a five-to-four vote, a parental notification law was allowed to stand. O'Connor voted with the majority.

*Akron* focused on a city ordinance modeled after an Illinois law that we'd worked hard to get passed. After the Supreme Court's 1973 rulings voided abortion laws throughout the nation, state legislatures started writing their own abortion laws. The first section of Illinois House Bill 1851, passed in the spring of 1975, read in part, "The unborn child is a human being from the time of conception and is, therefore, a legal person . . . and is entitled to the right to life from conception under the laws and Constitution of this State." In the event that *Roe* were overturned, this bill would automatically outlaw abortion in Illinois. It banned all abortions after viability, except where the mother's life or health was endangered. The legislation was designed to address the *Doe* loophole that "health" could include economic and social wellbeing by defining health as an exclusively medical issue.

When HB 1851 reached Governor Dan Walker, he vetoed it. Overriding a gubernatorial veto in Illinois takes a three-fifths majority in each house of the General Assembly. We met that mark easily in the House. But the vote would be very close in the Senate. I went to Springfield with several other pro-lifers to lead the battle for a Senate override.

We needed thirty-six votes. By the end of a day of lobbying at the state capitol, we had thirty-four lined up. We got the thirty-fifth when a strong pro-lifer who had been in the legislature but was dying of cancer called a senator friend of his. As a final gift to his old friend, the senator agreed to support HB 1851.

We needed one more vote. Richard M. Daley, the future Chicago mayor, was serving in the Illinois Senate but was in Chicago on business. We called to let him know how close the vote was. He flew down to Springfield just in time. The Senate voted 36–15 to override Governor Walker's veto. HB 1851 became law. The young Rich Daley was the thirty-sixth vote, and for a while, Illinois had the strictest abortion law in the nation.

The Akron, Ohio, city council included many provisions of HB 1851 in their own city ordinance. Their Supreme Court case against the Akron Center for Reproductive Health would be another close fight. Those of us who had lobbied for HB 1851 were eager to help the Akron effort and try to gather support from notable figures.

Reverend Jesse Jackson was based in Chicago, but he'd gained a reputation as a national leader, and we hoped Jackson would lend his support to the passage of the Akron ordinance. In 1977, Jackson had published in *Right to Life News*. "It takes three to make a baby: a man, a woman, and the Holy Spirit," he wrote. "Human beings cannot give or create life by themselves, it is really a gift from God. Therefore, one does not have the right to take away (through abortion) that which he does not have the ability to give."[3]

Jackson had also published an open letter to the US Congress supporting the Hyde Amendment. Tom Roeser and I went to see him at his People United to Save Humanity office on Chicago's South

---

3    Reverend Jesse Jackson, *National Right to Life News*, January 1977.

Side. At first, he tried to be noncommittal, but we reminded him of his earlier pro-life statements. Eventually, he said that we could use his name in publicizing support for the Akron ordinance. We immediately sent telegrams to Akron news outlets announcing Reverend Jackson's support for the ordinance. It passed, but it was immediately challenged in federal court by a local abortion clinic, and some of its strongest provisions were struck down. The city appealed the decision, and in the fall of 1982, the Supreme Court heard the case.

Reagan's solicitor general submitted an amicus brief asking the court to overturn *Roe*—Reagan was serious about trying to get *Roe* reversed. But in 1983, the city of Akron was defeated in a 6–3 ruling. Justice Stevens had joined Rehnquist and White in their support of parental consent in *Danforth* but now joined the pro-abortion side of the court. O'Connor had not just joined with Rehnquist and White in support of the Akron law but authored their dissenting opinion.

O'Connor had earlier criticized Blackmun's invention of a trimester system in his *Roe* opinion, where he had tried to establish the middle phase as the boundary between free access to abortion and the state's right to regulate it. "The *Roe* framework is clearly on a collision course with itself," she wrote. "As the medical risks of various abortion procedures decrease, the point at which the State may regulate for reasons of maternal health is moved further forward to actual childbirth. As medical science becomes better able to provide for the separate existence of the fetus, the point of viability is moved further back toward conception."

O'Connor also addressed the ridiculous terminology that the court had used in *Roe*, saying, "potential life is no less potential in the first weeks of pregnancy than it is at viability or afterward." She quoted an earlier Supreme Court opinion that "when convinced of former error, this court has never felt constrained to follow precedent." Justice O'Connor appeared to be predicting that *Roe* would indeed be overturned someday and that she'd be one of the justices to do it.

Though the court's majority ruling in Akron was a disappointment, pro-lifers were pleased to find that O'Connor was on our side, at least for now. If she held firm, only two more judges were needed to shift the court to a pro-life majority. The prediction Reagan had made in his diary, that O'Connor would make a good justice, might have been accurate. Perhaps we'd been hasty in greeting Air Force One with anti-O'Connor signs. In my *Action News*, the Pro-Life Action League's monthly newsletter, I described how glad we were that our earlier concerns were apparently unfounded. "We only hope," I wrote, "that the president will have the opportunity to make at least two more appointments that turn out as well as this one did."

But that was while O'Connor was serving under the Reagan administration. Things could change.

## Chapter 14

# The Machine

"People are always picking on my husband!"

I was on the phone with Eleanor "Sis" Daley, wife of Mayor Richard J. Daley, talking about Illinois Masonic Hospital.

"Well, you can see why, can't you? They're going to be doing abortions there—late-term abortions. You were the one who said you'd rather have a baby on your lap than on your conscience."

Very early in my pro-life career, even before I started full-time with the IRLC, I learned that the North Side hospital performed late-term abortions. I met with administrators to discuss it, and I assured them that we'd picket the hospital if they continued. They didn't change their policy, and we kept our word. We staged many large pickets with hundreds of protesters. We even had doctors and nurses at the hospital come out and join our protests on their lunch breaks and days off.

Illinois Masonic had received a large grant from Chicago businessman W. Clement Stone to build a new wing. In the fall of 1973, they planned a reception to celebrate breaking ground for the Stone Pavilion, which would house the new abortion facilities. Mayor Daley was invited to the ceremony, and since I'd worked for him a few years earlier, I tried to reach him to convince him to turn down the invitation. When I couldn't make any headway through the mayor's office, I decided to call Sis Daley.

"Think what a powerful message it'd send if he refused to dedicate the abortion center," I told her. But Sis said the mayor's schedule was his business, and she didn't involve herself in those decisions. Plans went ahead for the mayor's appearance—and for our picket.

The IRLC organized a large demonstration at the Stone Pavilion dedication. We produced more than a hundred signs, cutting out neat white letters and pasting them on black poster board. The reception was in a large tent on the lot where the Stone Pavilion would eventually stand, and we marched along the front of the hospital and past the tent. Nobody went into that event without seeing our public display of opposition to the hospital's abortion policy.

During the picket, I noticed a television camera set up on an elevated train platform overlooking the tent. It looked as though the camera angle captured the dedication but not our picket. I paid the train fare and went up to talk to the cameraman. He was from the local NBC affiliate, and he confirmed my suspicion—the angle was deliberate.

As a journalist, I'd been taught what I later taught my students: Conflict *is* news. "We're an important part of this story," I told the cameraman. "We're protesting this dedication because abortions will be done in the Stone Pavilion. A whole floor for nothing but abortions."

"Well," he mumbled, "I was told to cover the dedication, not a protest." He refused to move his camera or widen his angle to include our picket.

It isn't always that way with cameramen—in fact, I've found that while editors and reporters are generally hostile, cameramen are often the most supportive members of the media. I've always worked to ensure our demonstrations are visually compelling. Reporters and editors who oppose our message are sometimes predisposed to edit us out, but cameramen and photographers are drawn to the spectacle of a well-coordinated protest. Occasionally I've helped them set up a shot. Once while picketing a State Street clinic, I had more signs than people, and I convinced the cameraman to do a close-up during my interview. Each picketer would switch signs off-camera as they circled behind me, making it appear that our group was twice as large as it was.

While we couldn't stop abortions at Illinois Masonic, we had better luck with Cook County Hospital. Thirty-five hundred abortions were performed there each year, costing Cook County taxpayers $1.5 million per annum.

Rich Freeman and I went to see County Board president George Dunne, a Catholic. Dunne was an expansive, handsome man, and when we walked into his office he asked, "What's your problem, boys?" We told him we were concerned about abortions performed at Cook County Hospital. "Abortions at Cook County?" he said. "We'll put a stop to that."

Ending taxpayer-funded abortions at Cook County required a vote by the Cook County Board. Dunne launched an investigation and hosted public hearings, and I recruited several pro-lifers to testify against publicly funded abortion. In 1977, after the federal courts invalidated the Hyde Amendment, Illinois and several other states passed their own laws to prevent state governments from funding abortions. Governor Jim Thompson vetoed the Illinois bill, but pro-lifers lobbied hard and won an override. After the Supreme Court's 1980 ruling in *Harris* upheld the Hyde Amendment, Dunne was able to convince the Cook County Board that if state and federal governments didn't have to pay for abortions, neither did a county government. There were no more taxpayer-funded abortions at Cook County while Dunne was board president.

*Chicago Magazine* did a story on our efforts with Cook County Hospital. They quoted a NARAL leader who said of me, "If you cannot admire that guy for his views or style, you've got to give him credit for his perseverance." My "view" is simply that human life is sacred—but he did get one thing right: This kind of work takes perseverance.[1]

Much of our early activist work focused on getting the courts to recognize that the unborn had some legal rights. We saw an opportunity in the 1975 case of Melvin Morgan, who shot his eight-and-a-half-month pregnant girlfriend during a domestic dispute. She had locked him out of her apartment and was talking with him through the door when he fired at her. She survived, but the child died, and Morgan was indicted on charges of aggravated battery and attempted murder of the girlfriend.

When we learned about this case, Pat Trueman, Tom Roeser, and I went to see State's Attorney Bernard Carey and convinced him to charge Morgan with murder for killing the unborn child. We thought this case could set a precedent that an unborn victim has a right to life, but in the end, Morgan's attorney got him off on the charges by arguing that since he'd fired through the door, there was no way for the girlfriend to positively identify him.

In 1990, George Dunne announced that he would not seek another term as Cook County board president. Richard Phelan announced his candidacy and made a campaign promise to return abortions to Cook County Hospital. The new mayor, Richard M. Daley, supported this move, along with Attorney General Neil Hartigan, who was seeking the governorship at the time. All these men were Catholic—Phelan was a former seminarian—and their pro-abortion allegiance came as a shock to many Catholics.

---

1 Alfredo Lanier, "Abortion War at Cook County Hospital," *Chicago Magazine*, March 1981, 150.

In March 1992, Phelan started to act on his campaign promise. He sent a memo to Hospital Director Ruth Rothstein instructing her to plan to reestablish a Voluntary Interruption of Pregnancy ward. That June, he issued an executive order to open the ward. My pastor at Queen of All Saints, Father Charles Cronin, had known Phelan for years and wrote him, asking him to reconsider his position or resign.

But Phelan didn't resign. His executive order was set to take effect at the end of July. The Pro-Life Action League and other pro-life groups, along with four expectant fathers, filed a lawsuit challenging the order. Phelan called a meeting of the Cook County Board to rubber-stamp his order, purposely convening it when several pro-life members of the board were out of town. Surprised, the absentees filed suit to challenge the vote, and we won a temporary restraining order, but ultimately the courts upheld Phelan's plan to bring abortions back to Cook County.

We held massive demonstrations and all-night prayer vigils in front of the hospital during these court battles, and we appealed to Joseph Cardinal Bernardin. The *Sun-Times* printed a front-page story in which Bernardin said he was appalled that someone who professed to be a Catholic would take such action, but the cardinal stopped short of excommunicating Phelan or advising his pastor to refuse him communion. The day abortions resumed at Cook County, I wrote to the cardinal. I pointed out that according to canon law, anyone who procures or assists in procuring an abortion incurs a *latae sententia* (automatic) excommunication. Now that Phelan's actions had claimed their first victims, Phelan had excommunicated himself.

The cardinal responded. "As regards the question of excommunication," he wrote, "I am aware of the canonical interpretations that would argue that President Phelan has incurred this penalty *latae sententia*. There are, however, other equally respectable canonists who would argue that the conditions required to incur this penalty have not been met. In light of this disagreement, I have decided not to take a public position on this matter." By then, more than a hundred babies had died as a result of Phelan's order. I wondered what other conditions the cardinal had in mind.

A year earlier, in 1991, I had attended an event in Rapid City, South Dakota, where I sat at a table with Bishop Charles Chaput. I asked him what he would do if he had any prominent pro-abortion Catholics in his diocese. "I'd excommunicate them like *that*," he said, snapping his fingers with such a hearty crack that several people looked over. I wish we'd had his kind of resolve in the Archdiocese of Chicago.

The week after abortions resumed at Cook County Hospital, I organized a picket at Hospital Director Ruth Rothstein's Gold Coast home. As we were gathering, the Chicago police arrived and cited an ordinance saying we couldn't picket a single residence. But nothing in the ordinance prevented us from marching around the block. We jogged around most of the block, then took tiny, slow steps in front of Rothstein's house. Our group was large enough that there was a constant presence in front of her home.

On the one-year anniversary of the reinstatement of abortion at Cook County, we held a memorial service there for the 1,560 babies killed there that year. Against the notion that taxpayer-funded abortions were good for the poor, Cardinal Bernardin provided a statement that was read by his director of the Respect Life office, Father Roger Coughlin: "This is a tragedy for the poor and a callous attempt to eliminate the less fortunate from our midst rather than give them the support and care they need."[2]

---

2    "Archdiocese of Chicago Statement of Cardinal Joseph Bernardin, Archbishop of Chicago Re: Taxpayer-Funded Abortions at Cook County Hospital," Office of Communications, Respect Life office, September 16, 1993.

Good as this statement was, it cast the issue only in terms of social justice and ignored the fact that specific individuals were responsible for the tragedy. We were disappointed that the cardinal declined to make a public statement regarding Phelan's self-excommunication.

In 1994, Phelan left the Cook County Board presidency to campaign for the governorship. I made a point of attending every one of his appearances. At one breakfast, I arrived early enough for a spot right in front of the podium. He recognized me and dodged the abortion issue. Pro-lifers opposed him vigorously throughout his campaign. He failed to win the nomination.

When Phelan stepped down, Joe Morris, a strong pro-lifer, made a bid for the Cook County Board presidency. But Morris was a Republican, and no Republican had won that post since the '60s. The election went to Democrat John Stroger, who, though a Catholic and originally a supporter of George Dunne's move to end abortions at Cook County hospital, refused to rescind Phelan's order. In fact, he oversaw a 50 percent increase in the number of abortions performed at Cook County.

Despite this record, the Chicago Catholic Lawyers' Guild decided to recognize Stroger as their "Catholic Man of the Year" in 1996. The guild had recognized some true pro-life heroes in the past. Dennis Horan and Henry Hyde had both received the award. Richard J. Daley won it before *Roe* was decided, and his son won it in the days when his votes helped secure pro-life overrides in the Illinois General Assembly. I heard about Stroger's receiving the award the morning of the event. I was flying back to Chicago from Washington, DC, and the lawyer beside me said she was flying in to attend the annual Red Mass for lawyers and judges at Holy Name Cathedral. She was planning to attend the breakfast at the Four Seasons where Stroger would be honored.

As Lawyers' Guild members filed out of the church, I led a hastily recruited group of protesters across the street from Holy Name with graphic victim photos. We followed them into the Four Seasons, where I spoke with Stroger about his position.

"Look, I'm still pro-life," he explained. "But as a public official, I have an obligation to execute the law."

"That's the right word for what you're doing to the unborn," I replied. We were able to talk to most of the attendees before we were ejected. Many thanked us for staging the protest. We followed up with letters to the guild directors suggesting they be more judicious when choosing future recipients.

One of the strongest enemies of the pro-life cause in Illinois was Attorney General Lisa Madigan, daughter of the House Speaker, who consistently blocked the Illinois's parental notification law from taking effect. The law was passed in 1995, but it languished in limbo for over ten years. At that point, the Thomas More Society got involved, demanding that the Illinois Supreme Court issue the required judicial bypass rules. The court finally obliged in 2006, and Madigan had to request the federal court to lift an injunction against the law. The judge who granted the injunction was, coincidentally, the same one who presided over my racketeering trial, David Coar.

All of Illinois's neighbors—Indiana, Kentucky, Michigan, Wisconsin, and Missouri—had parental notice laws, so without one in Illinois, teens from nearby states routinely traveled to Illinois to get abortions without their parents' knowledge. Madigan's insistence on blocking the law thus undermined parental rights and responsibilities not just in Illinois but also in neighboring states. Court challenges to the law continued for several years, but it finally went into effect in 2013—*eighteen years* after it was signed.

In 2009, at the behest of Planned Parenthood and Family Planning Associates, the Chicago City Council tried to outlaw private conversations in front of abortion clinics. Acting on the notion that offering a woman information on abortion alternatives infringes on her free choice and constitutes harassment, the council considered a bubble zone ordinance. I first heard of this law when a reporter called to ask me what I thought of it. Hearings were scheduled for the very next day. We got a copy of the ordinance and saw that it might be interpreted to ban any protests within fifty feet of a health facility—a clear violation of the right to assembly that would never withstand a constitutional challenge.

Half a dozen of us attended the city council hearings, and learned that they'd changed the language of the ordinance. It now said that within fifty feet of an abortion clinic entrance, nobody could get closer than eight feet from another person unless explicitly invited. Several pro-life sidewalk counselors testified against the ordinance at the hearing. The council would vote a week later.

In 1996, Mayor Daley had scuttled a similar proposed ordinance, saying, "We don't need that kind of thing here." The city council got the message, and it never came up for a vote. But this time was different. There was clearly broad support for a bubble zone ordinance, and only a mayoral veto could prevent it.

We had to act fast. I recorded a robo-call to send out to all our members asking them to call the mayor's office. The mayor's usual answering service got overloaded, so his office set up a recorded message instructing callers to press a button to leave a message either in favor of or against the law. Within a day, the "against" mailbox was full.

Even the American Civil Liberties Union (ACLU) weighed in on our side on this one, since the ordinance was such an obvious violation of freedom of speech. But this time, Daley had firmly allied himself with Planned Parenthood and the abortion clinics. He ignored our pleas, and the ACLU, and signed the ordinance. The same man who had voted repeatedly for pro-life bills in the '70s and '80s now blocked our efforts to get crucial information to women just minutes away from making a tragic decision.

The Chicago police couldn't seem to understand what the bubble zone ordinance meant. They threatened to arrest any pro-lifer who

came within fifty feet of a clinic. We called the city attorney for clar-
ification and faxed a letter explaining the law to every police station
near a clinic. Our sidewalk counselors continue to save lives, though
some have been harassed or even arrested under the Chicago ordinance, despite the 2014 *McCullen v. Coakley* Supreme Court ruling
that recognizes sidewalk counseling as protected speech under the
First Amendment.

The political machines that operate in Chicago, Cook County,
and Illinois have presented many challenges to the defenders of
the unborn. With so much of that machinery in the hands of the
predominantly pro-abortion party, it's been hard to find politicians
here who will stand up for the right to life. Chicago is by no means
unique—similar struggles play out continually across the nation.
Pro-lifers appreciate and recognize politicians who steadfastly
uphold the right to life, and we keep calling out those who don't.
It's a hard battle wherever you are, but it's one we have to fight. Our
future depends on it.

## CHAPTER 15

# The Tribunals

"The First Amendment is not an issue in this case," said US Solicitor General Ted Olson. "The issue here is the use of force."

"There is always a First Amendment implication in a protest case," replied Justice Anthony Kennedy.[1]

I was at the Supreme Court again. It was December 2002, and we were appealing the verdict in *NOW v. Scheidler* that found me and other pro-lifers guilty of violating federal extortion and racketeering laws.

At one point in the oral arguments, Justice Stephen Breyer brought up the lunch counter demonstrations of the early 1960s. Though RICO, the federal racketeering law, wasn't enacted until 1970, Breyer asked whether civil rights activists could have been sued for racketeering had the law been on the books at that time.

"Martin Luther King didn't tell his followers to go into the Woolworth's and bash people around and forcibly prevent the white people from getting service," answered NOW attorney Fay Clayton.

---

1    Trial transcripts and records of conversations come from Scheidler personal archives. Official trial transcripts are available as public record.

"No, but just obstructing," Justice Antonin Scalia chimed in. "You've used the term 'violence' several times. As your argument to the jury indicated, it was enough if they obstructed the entrance and failed to part like the Red Sea if somebody wanted to go in. . . . You told the jury that you could find an offense here under the Hobbs Act by the mere blockade. It wasn't smacking people around. It was not letting people in."

Justice Ruth Bader Ginsburg spoke next. "How about Carrie Nation? You could concede, I take it, based on your arguments, that if RICO had been around then—and the Hobbs Act—that she would have been in violation."

"I would, your honor," Clayton answered.

I leaned over to Tom Brejcha and said, "Tom, I think we've just won this case."

"All we need is five," he answered.

During our 1998 trial, Judge David Coar allowed Clayton to tell the jury that nonviolent protests that disrupted business at abortion clinics amounted to extortion and that even attending and speaking at conventions was part of the racketeering scheme. With the laws defined that broadly, it was clear to Tom and me that there was little chance of winning in Coar's courtroom. Victory could only come through the appeal process.

NOW's case named two abortion clinics as plaintiffs. Clayton persuaded the jury that our protests had cost these two clinics $85,926.92. Judge Coar granted NOW's request for an injunction barring us from staging sit-ins or clinic blockades. NOW initiated their suit in 1986, but the Freedom of Access to Clinic Entrances (FACE) Act had passed in 1994, so by the time the verdict came down in 1998, the government had already given Clayton much of what she wanted. We knew that an injunction could be interpreted to cover simple picketing, prayer vigils, or even sidewalk counseling. I could be cited for contempt of court for simply praying outside a clinic. We had to fight it.

The RICO statute included triple damages, so we were actually on the hook for $257,780.76. The appeal process cannot be used as a way to put off paying settlements, so in order to file an appeal, we had to come up with more than a quarter of a million dollars—fast. Since it was a class action suit, with NOW claiming to represent every other abortion clinic in the country, the monetary damages could have been much worse. But Clayton had neglected to submit requests for the financial costs for all those other clinics, and when she finally got around to it, Judge Coar turned her down. If he hadn't, the judgment would have been more than a hundred million dollars.

Even so, coming up with a quarter million was going to be tough. And that was just to file the appeal—not to pay for any of the court costs or the plaintiffs' legal fees. It would have been convenient to have a pro-life philanthropist put up the full amount, and we considered approaching our top donors, but we figured that nobody would be willing to commit such large sums to what promised to be a long battle.

Immediately after the verdict came down, we received a flood of letters and calls from supporters. The overwhelming generosity and outpouring of support from the loyal Pro-Life Action League family was uplifting and encouraging. We had to make a sacrifice worthy of that support. I was speaking in Baltimore when I got the idea of putting our house up for the appeal bond. When I got home, I started talking with Ann about our prospects of raising enough for the bond.

"Joe," she said, "I think the house is the only answer."

"I was thinking the same thing, but I was afraid that'd be asking too much. We'll win this together, or we'll be homeless together."

As we worked on our appeal, we got amicus briefs from a wide array of groups that stage protests or employ civil disobedience, ranging from Dr. Martin Luther King Jr.'s Southern Christian Leadership Conference to the People for the Ethical Treatment of Animals (a group of New Jersey furriers had filed a RICO suit against some animal rights activists, and PETA was eager to see us win). We secured several others, but all of these briefs were rejected by the Seventh Circuit Court of Appeals Judge Diane Wood, a former NOW member who had clerked for Justice Blackmun. She should have recused herself, but she didn't, and we lost again at the first round of appeals.

We appealed again. The Supreme Court agreed to hear our case, but they rejected our claim that the injunction trampled on our First Amendment rights. We thought the whole case would have to rest on the definitions of extortion and racketeering, so during the oral arguments, it was a welcome surprise when the justices started framing it as a First Amendment case.

On February 26, 2003, the Supreme Court handed down their ruling. I attended the 7:30 Mass that morning at Queen of All Saints. The psalm response that day was "O Lord, great peace have they who love Your law." Right after I got home, I got a call from Tom Brejcha. All along he'd been saying, "We only need five," but we did much better than that. We got *eight*—Justice John Paul Stevens was the lone dissenter.

Despite their allegations of a dozen or so violent acts by anybody connected with abortion protests from coast to coast, all of which they blamed on us, Clayton and her friends never proved that we committed or threatened any violent action against any clinic, their clients, or their employees nor did they prove that anybody obtained any property in violation of the federal extortion law. Regardless of what Judges Coar and Wood had ruled, the Supreme Court held that NOW was not entitled to change the definition of extortion to deny us our First Amendment right to protest. We had won. It looked like we were not going to be homeless after all.

There is a massive March for Life in Washington, DC, every year on or near the January 22 anniversary of *Roe* and *Doe*. Nellie Gray founded the march in 1974, and after Carter's statements about his personal opposition to abortion, she invited him to attend, but he never did. When Reagan took office, though, he began holding meetings with Nellie and other national pro-life leaders the morning of the march. At first, only the more reserved pro-lifers, such as those from the NRLC, were invited to his annual meetings.

In 1983, Reagan published a short book called *Abortion and the Conscience of the Nation*. In it, he discussed the Supreme Court's 1973 error and his administration's support for efforts to correct it, including support for a Human Life Bill, which, unlike an amendment to the Constitution, would be much easier to pass. Reagan encouraged pro-lifers to continue working toward a pro-life society both through the political process and through our protests and sidewalk counseling. He included a line that has been my philosophy of pro-life work: "Prayer and action are needed to uphold the sanctity of human life."[2] After that, he started inviting activists to his annual meetings, including me.

When I walked into the Oval Office on January 22, 1984, there were only a few seats left, and I took one in the middle of the table, in easy reach of a large jar of Reagan's famous jelly beans. The pro-life representatives were all there, and we went over a twelve-point agenda we planned to present to the president. One of the points I was to bring up was getting a strong pro-life statement into the State of the Union address, which Reagan would deliver two days later.

The door flew open, and in walked this dynamic, charismatic man. He greeted us all and took his seat—right across from me. I never got to present my agenda item because it became moot almost immediately—Reagan covered it in his opening remarks.

As the meeting concluded, Surgeon General C. Everett Koop shook my hand. "Keep up the good work, Joe," he said.

"You too, C. Everett."

---

2    Ronald Reagan, *Abortion and the Conscience of the Nation* (Nashville: Thomas Nelson, 1984), 36.

After the March for Life later that day, ten of us went into the Supreme Court building and started reciting the rosary in the vestibule of the courtroom. A woman in uniform came over and told us to leave.

"But we're praying for the court," I told her. "That they'll make just decisions."

"You're not allowed to do that here," she said. Reluctantly we left.

Two days later, Reagan delivered his State of the Union address, in which he said:

> America was founded by people who believed that God was their rock of safety. He is ours. I recognize we must be cautious in claiming that God is on our side, but I think it's all right to keep asking if we're on His side. During our first three years, we have joined bipartisan efforts to restore protection of the law to unborn children. Now, I know this issue is very controversial. But unless and until it can be proven that an unborn child is not a living human being, can we justify assuming without proof that it isn't? No one has yet offered such proof. Indeed, all the evidence is to the contrary. We should rise above bitterness and reproach, and if Americans could come together in a spirit of understanding and helping, then we could find positive solutions to the tragedy of abortion.

The comments about the humanity of the unborn were exactly what we had wanted to hear.

The day after the address, Chief Justice Burger was in Chicago to speak at an event at the Hyatt Regency. We had two dozen pickets out front, and I went into the reception hall hoping to confront Burger about the children who had died as a result of the 1973 rulings. But as I approached him, two security guards grabbed me and started escorting me out. I had to make my comments at full volume instead of in the conversational tone I would have preferred. Justice

Burger looked over at me with a look that suggested empathy for what I was saying, but he shrugged his shoulders as I was led out. I had a clear conviction that he was an unhappy man.

Six weeks later, I learned that Harry Blackmun was to be an honored guest at the Harvard Law Society's black tie event at the Drake Hotel. A year earlier, Marjorie Montgomery, the leading pro-lifer in Kentucky, had confronted Blackmun at a Louisville event. "How do you sleep at night," she asked, "with sixteen million babies crying in the background, all the babies you've killed through abortion? It's murder, but we're praying for you." Marjorie was promptly invited to leave, but later that year, I attended a Kentucky Right to Life Association convention in Owensboro and presented Marjorie with a "That Took Guts" Award. Instead of a plaque, I opted for a boxing trophy—it seemed to fit. Now we wanted to show Blackmun that same fighting spirit when he came to Chicago.

We staged a picket at the Drake Hotel with a dozen signs that read, "Blackmun's Decision Kills a Baby Every 20 Seconds," "Impeach Blackmun for Abortion Ruling," and "Blackmun: No Justice for the Unborn." Peter Krump came to the picket with a drum, keeping a dirgelike rhythm as we marched.

During the picket, a sympathetic guest came out of the hotel and handed us five tickets. Since it was a formal event, only the best dressed among us could use the tickets. I had a habit of leading demonstrations in a three-piece suit—a white one with a white hat in summer, all black in winter. I took one of the tickets and handed the others to Debbie Trulson, Andy Scholberg, Mary Ellen Biell, and Mary Kwilozs, and we went into the Drake.

We went into the ballroom where Blackmun would be speaking. There was a smaller VIP area where the justice was greeting guests at a cocktail party. We saw that the people going into that area had different tickets than ours, but we also noticed that Blackmun's granddaughter was there and that she was about eight months pregnant. Debbie Trulson was at about the same stage of pregnancy. She had the same hair color as Blackmun's granddaughter and was even wearing a similar dress. Debbie decided to march right into the reception room, and we followed, with Andy and me escorting the other women. Nobody checked our tickets. We figured they thought we were all with Blackmun's granddaughter.

We got into the reception line. Debbie was the first to greet Blackmun. "How does it feel," she asked, "to be responsible for the deaths of seventeen million unborn children, just like the one I'm carrying?" She was immediately told by security to leave the reception, but the rest of us stayed. When I got to Blackmun, I asked if he was aware of the picket outside and if he understood what we were trying to tell him. He nodded.

Andy was next. He said, "I just want you to know that I believe abortion is murder."

"Well," shrugged Blackmun, "it's all right to disagree." Then he looked up at the rest of us and decided he'd shaken enough hands. That was the end of the cocktail party.

We filed into the ballroom where we took seats in front of the podium. Blackmun devoted his speech to reminiscences about his childhood in Illinois and his time at Harvard Law School. He didn't say anything about *Roe* or *Doe*, but at one point during his speech, he declared, "There are no absolutes." He seemed absolutely sure about that.

As the spring of 1984 rolled toward summer, the presidential primaries began warming up. Walter "Fritz" Mondale, Carter's vice president, quickly became the Democratic frontrunner and announced New York Congresswoman Geraldine Ferraro as his running mate. She was the first woman to appear on a major party's ticket. Feminists nationwide were thrilled with the choice, but the reality was that the economy had recovered during Reagan's first term. He was very popular. It would take more than gender politics to defeat him.

Ferraro claimed to be a devout Catholic, but in 1982, she wrote the introduction to a congressional briefing held by Catholics for a Free Choice, a group with virtually no adherence to Catholic teaching, saying in part that "the Catholic position on abortion is not mono-lithic, and there can be a range of personal and political responses to the issue."[3] Like Carter, Ferraro adopted the "personally opposed, but . . ." stance, though unlike Carter, Ferraro tried to argue that this stand was consistent with her professed religion. Her blurring of her position on abortion confused the issues for both Congress and the American public, and we wouldn't let her get away with it.

I was determined that any press coverage Ferraro got would high-light her anti-life position. Working with activists across the county, our operations were so well coordinated that the Ferraro camp accused Reagan's campaign of organizing it. When it became clear that the Pro-Life Action League was coordinating the campaign, we were invited onto several talk shows.

I flew out to New Jersey to protest her first public appearance after the convention, and NOW reported the League to the Federal Elections Commission and to the IRS for violating rules about tax exemption and political activities. The Federal Elections Commission assessed us a mere seventy-five-dollar fine for paying for my "politi-cal" trip to New Jersey. But when an IRS agent came to my office and spent several days poring over our records, he praised my assistant, Barbara Menes, for keeping our accounts in such good order and gave us some tips on ways to take advantage of our 501(c)(3) status. In the end, NOW actually did us a favor.

Reagan won another landslide that November, with Mondale only capturing his home state of Minnesota and the District of Columbia.

---

3    Frances Kissling, "How a Good Catholic Girl from Queens Took On Her Church," *Alternet*, March 28, 2011, http://www.alternet.org/story/150395/gerry_ferraro's_other_legacy%3A_how_a_good_catholic_girl_from_queens_took_on_her_church.

Unseating an incumbent is tough under any circumstances, especially during an economic boom, but we still campaigned hard for Reagan's 1984 reelection. Abortion on demand had been the law of the land for just over a decade, and throughout our history, the American public's attention span for social movements hasn't lasted much longer than that. Reconstruction, the Progressive Era, and the civil rights movement only swelled for about a dozen years. Even the abolition movement only lasted about that long: The 1850 passage of the Fugitive Slave Act inflamed passions on a broad national level, and with the announcement of the Emancipation Proclamation in 1862, the national fervor waned again.

I was determined that the pro-life movement would not drop off the front page. My professional life has been as a publicist. While studying for the priesthood, I felt called to publicize the Gospel. I taught college students how to use publicity. When I started pro-life work, I publicized the facts about the humanity of the unborn child and the danger of abortion to women. Soon, I started publicizing activism itself. When I was working on my manual for direct action, *CLOSED*, I was trying to come up with enough ideas to subtitle it "101 Ways to Stop Abortion." In the end, my list totaled ninety-eight—chapter 99 is called "Write the Next Chapter Yourself."

The fight to keep the abortion issue under national scrutiny has led to some unusual moments. When we protested the pro-abortion Supreme Court justices, we carried signs calling for their impeachment. Though Congress wouldn't heed our suggestion, I considered staging a symbolic impeachment trial. The idea quickly expanded to include a whole host of defendants, and Paul Brown looked through a US atlas to find any cities or towns in America named after Nuremberg, Germany, so we could host our own atrocities trial. He found only one, a little town in northeastern Pennsylvania.

Late in 1984, *Newsweek* interviewed me for a cover story on abortion, and I mentioned the Nuremberg trial idea to the reporter.

When the story ran in January 1985, it read, "Scheidler is shameless in his pursuit of publicity—one possible gimmick is a mock trial of Supreme Court Justice Harry Blackmun, to be held, if he has his way, in a Pennsylvania town named Nuremberg." Once the national press had announced that we were planning a Nuremberg trial, other reporters started calling for details. I decided we had to take it from concept to reality.

Nuremberg, Pennsylvania, is a tiny hamlet with just a few hundred residents, and its only meeting place is a small American Legion hall. As a Legion member, I hoped to rent the hall and flew out to Nuremberg wearing my Legion cap, but the head of the Legion Post, Tom Makara, said he couldn't rent us the hall. He said the folks in Nuremberg were afraid we'd attract counterprotesters and that riots would break out in their town. He even brought up a concern shared by some residents about us inciting motorcycle gangs to raid their sleepy village.

The pastor at Sacred Heart Church in Nuremberg, Father Martin Gaiardo, was much more supportive. He allowed us to stage opening and closing remarks in his parish church. The original Nuremberg trial in Germany opened in October 1945. Nuremberg II opened exactly forty years later in October 1985. We started with a brief introduction and prayer in the town of Nuremberg and then processed into nearby Hazelton to hold the actual trial in a Holiday Inn ballroom. We had a massive grim reaper effigy with "abortion" across the front and a bus festooned with pro-life banners.

Our defendants included the heads of NARAL, NOW, Planned Parenthood, the NAF, and the Religious Coalition for Abortion Rights (RCAR); the doctors who perform abortions; the media and celebrities who promote abortion; the politicians who vote for abortion; and the churches, for not taking a strong stand against abortion. We used cardboard busts to represent each of these groups and had them affixed to chairs in our defendants' dock. On each chair was a basket, and the audience came up and wrote specific names to put in each basket.

We had a three-judge panel that included pro-life lawyer John Jakubczyk, a special advisor to Senator Jesse Helms named Earl Appleby, and a law student named Marcelle Richards. We called witnesses. A professor from St. Louis University, Dr. William Brennan, compared the Nazi Holocaust to the abortion holocaust. Robin Woodrow of WEBA, a postabortion healing ministry, testified to the trauma of abortion to women. Our witnesses also included abortion survivors: one was a little boy, Josh, whose mother had been pregnant with twins. The abortionist didn't realize this, and when his twin was aborted, his mother immediately felt regret. When she learned that she was still pregnant with Josh, she carried him to term. He'd been injured—part of his arm and head were scarred—and he wore a little T-shirt that read, "I survived the abortion holocaust."

Media from all across Pennsylvania had covered the planning stages of the trial, and the Associated Press and United Press International wire services picked up the story. Among the reporters was a film crew from Finland. The same crew had also covered an activist convention we held in Appleton, Wisconsin, earlier that year, and when we saw them in Pennsylvania, we were impressed at how interested the Finns seemed to be in the American pro-life movement. The director, Victoria Schultz, told us that Helsinki Films was going all across America documenting a variety of social protest movements.

Helsinki Films released *Holy Terror* the following year. It opened with news footage of clinic bombings, then cut to a scene of my testimony before the congressional subcommittee about abortion clinic violence. The film wasn't about an array of movements: It focused entirely on pro-life activism and tried to make the case that those of us who organized the clinic protests also organized the arsons and bombings.

It turned out that Helsinki Films was a front and that Schultz had been hired by NOW. *Holy Terror* was released within weeks of filing the *NOW v. Scheidler* suit, timed perfectly to coincide with their allegations of our violent nationwide conspiracy to put the abortion industry out of business.

The Appleton convention and Nuremberg trial were featured in the film, along with coverage of clinic protests and blockades around the country and a massive sit-in in St. Louis. For the Nuremberg scenes, they added German beer hall music. Though their intention was to mock our mock trial, the effect made it seem like we'd been able to hire a live band for our procession from Nuremberg to Hazelton, and then back to Nuremberg.

At the conclusion of the trial, John Jakubczyk declared, "This court finds the decision of Justice Blackmun very deficient. The medical evidence is overwhelming that the human being begins his or her life at the moment of conception."

We processed back to Nuremberg, and I spoke from a Lourdes shrine at the Catholic parish at our closing ceremony:

> America has lost its way. It has abandoned God and God's law and in abandoning God it has abandoned Man. So our verdict must be that since we are all a part of a nation that condones abortion, all of America is guilty of this evil. We are guilty of doing little or nothing to rescue the innocent being led unjustly to their deaths. This trial can only adjourn with the resolution that it resume in the towns and cities where our children are slaughtered. We must go back to our hometowns—yours and mine—and seek out the abortion providers and reconvene one Nuremberg trial after another, all across America, until the message of the slaughter of our children is heard everywhere in the land.
>
> Go, then, from here to Nuremberg, Indiana, to Nuremberg, California, to Nuremberg, Iowa, to Nuremberg, New York.

Try those who conduct the American Holocaust. In trying the guilty, we will educate the unwary. In trying the guilty, we will give new value to the lives of the unborn victims. And in trying the guilty, we will begin to end the injustice.

In the end it will not be a trial in Nuremberg, Pennsylvania, nor a criminal court anywhere in the United States that judges their guilt. It will be the High Court of Heaven where the Just Judge will mete out a just sentence.

And we pray for those whose testimony we have heard defending the killing of little children under the law of abortion on demand. Our prayer will be then, and is even now, may God have mercy on their souls.

## Chapter 16

# Hail to the Chiefs

On November 5, 1985, one month after we held our mock trial in Nuremberg, I arrived at the US Supreme Court to listen to the arguments in two abortion cases: *Diamond v. Charles* from Illinois and *Thornburgh v. American College of Obstetricians and Gynecologists* from Pennsylvania.

The Reagan administration submitted an amicus brief asking the court to use these two cases to overturn *Roe v. Wade.* Pro-lifers across the country collected petitions to reverse *Roe*, and a coalition of pro-life leaders held a news conference at the National Press Club the day of oral arguments. Later we went to the court building and held a prayer service outside before delivering the thirty thousand petitions to the clerk and entering the courtroom.

In 1979, the Illinois legislature had passed a law with parental consent and informed consent requirements, and Pennsylvania modeled its law after Illinois's. Informed consent meant that abortion providers had to share information with women about fetal development and the risks of abortion to women. In both states, abortionists challenged the laws and obtained injunctions blocking them.

Inside the courtroom, Dennis Horan, one of my former bosses at the IRLC, was arguing for the Illinois law in *Diamond v. Charles*. Dr. Eugene Diamond, an IRLC member, had challenged the injunction. As a parent of teenage daughters, he believed his rights and obligations as a parent were undermined by the judge's order.

The Diamonds had fourteen children. Once after a lecture, a woman asked Dr. Diamond what made him an expert on teenagers. "Well, for one thing," he answered, "I have a nineteen-year-old, an eighteen-year-old . . ." and continued on down the list. He had five teenage daughters at the time.

There was a disturbing irony about how the courts interpreted the rights of pregnant minors. Rulings prior to *Roe* established that a pregnant minor is partially emancipated and empowered to make her own decisions regarding the pregnancy, such as whether to give the baby up for adoption. After *Roe*, these decisions were extended to include abortion. Thus in order to challenge the injunction against the Illinois parental consent law, Dr. Diamond used a different tactic. He got a judge to appoint him guardian ad litem for the class of unborn children in Illinois, then sued obstetrician Seymour Charles, one of the abortionists who had obtained the injunction. When the Supreme Court agreed to hear the case, Illinois Attorney General Neil Hartigan refused to argue it—which is why it was Dennis Horan, not Hartigan, who was arguing before the court that day.

The concentration of power in that courtroom is palpable. The notion of an American democracy responsive to the will of the people is pleasant and convenient fiction, but we really live in a nation governed by a panel of nine dictators—unelected but appointed for life—with the power to circumvent the democratic process. That day in the court, the power wielded by the justices struck me as downright scary.

The court announced their *Diamond* decision in April 1986, dismissing the case and sparing itself from having to address the question of whether the unborn could have legal guardians distinct from their mothers. They threw it out on the grounds that private citizens have no standing to challenge an injunction against a state law.

In *Thornburgh v. American College of Obstetrics and Gynecologists*, argued the same day, the plaintiff was the governor, Richard Thornburgh. That case was not thrown out, and Harry Blackmun wrote the majority opinion, which was released in 1986. In *Roe*, he had claimed that states could regulate abortion to protect maternal health at least after the first trimester—which was precisely what an informed consent law was designed to do. But now he claimed that no state law can be valid if it poses a "danger of deterring the exercise of that right." Informed consent laws were now unconstitutional.

"There are no absolutes," he'd said at the Drake Hotel. But for him, the right to an abortion had become absolute. He'd dissented in *Harris v. McRae*, arguing for continued federal funding of abortions, and now he was even contradicting his own ruling in *Roe* about a state's right to regulate abortion after the first trimester.

Even Chief Justice Warren Burger, Blackmun's longtime friend and the one who had assigned him the task of writing *Roe* and *Doe*, thought he'd gone too far. In his 1973 concurrence in *Roe*, Burger had written, "The Court today rejects any claim that the Constitution requires abortions on demand."

"I regretfully conclude," he wrote in his 1986 *Thornburgh* dissent, "that some of the concerns of the dissenting Justices in *Roe*, as well as the concerns I expressed in my separate opinion, have now been realized. . . . I agree we should re-examine *Roe*." Burger had announced his retirement before the *Thornburgh* ruling was made public, and by the time he left the court that fall, Reagan's next appointment, Antonin Scalia—a strict constructionist and a practicing Catholic—had been confirmed 98–0. Reagan elevated William Rehnquist, one of the original two *Roe* dissenters, to chief justice.

The next summer, Lewis Powell, another *Roe* vote, announced his retirement. Reagan nominated Robert Bork to replace him. We were thrilled—Bork was a strict constructionist, and his wife volunteered at a crisis pregnancy center. Bork certainly favored overturning *Roe*. But this was also during the height of the Iran-Contra Affair, and the Democrats were eager to seize a chance to oppose Reagan. Within an hour of the nomination, Senator Edward Kennedy delivered a speech on the Senate floor, saying that "Robert Bork's America is a land in which women would be forced into back-alley abortions."[1]

The Democrats had retaken the Senate that year, and Joe Biden of Delaware became chair of the Senate Judiciary Committee. The *Philadelphia Inquirer* asked Biden about his view on future court nominees. "Say the administration sends up Bork," Biden told them, "I'd have to vote for him."[2] He subsequently received a flood of complaints from feminist groups, and after Powell announced his retirement, Biden made public statements indicating that his thinking had changed. He was obviously withdrawing his endorsement of Bork, and his line of questioning during the hearings revealed that he was looking back even further than *Roe* to support his about-face.

During the confirmation hearings, Biden spent a huge amount of time grilling Bork on his critique of Justice Douglas's finding in *Griswold*, the 1965 birth control case, about the constitutional right to privacy, the same argument on which *Roe* rested. Biden's concern over *Griswold* was a smokescreen for his concern that Bork might vote to overturn *Roe*. The smear campaign against Bork worked, and

---

1    "Senator Edward M. 'Ted' Kennedy Senate Floor Speech Opposing Judge Robert Bork's Nomination to the U.S. Supreme Court," *C-SPAN,* July 22, 2015, http://www.c-span.org/video/?c4545562/senator-edward -m-ted-kennedy-senate-floor-speech-opposing-judge-robert-borks -nomination-us-supreme.

2    Larry Eichel, "Bork Hearings May Give Biden a Chance to Recover," *Philadelphia Inquirer*, November 16, 1985.

the Judiciary Committee voted 9–5 against him. Then the full Senate voted against him in a landslide, 42–58, defeating him so badly that the word *bork* is now used informally to describe obstruction through systematic defamation. Later in 1987, Reagan nominated Anthony Kennedy, who was confirmed 97–0.

The next year's presidential election saw Reagan's vice president, George H. W. Bush, running against the governor of Massachusetts, Michael Dukakis. We held an activist convention that summer at the Bismarck Hotel in Chicago, where pro-lifers from across the nation agreed to protest Dukakis at his campaign appearances.

Bush defeated Dukakis that November, and the next big abortion case, the first for both Scalia and Kennedy, came the following spring. We were confident of Scalia's vote, but Kennedy had been chosen in large part because his abortion views were unknown.

The case concerned a law written by a very dedicated pro-life activist I'd known for years: Sam Lee of Missouri Citizens for Life. In 1978, I invited Sam to Chicago to train volunteers for our first Chicago sit-ins. He split his time between activism in St. Louis and lobbying in Jefferson City, but he eventually switched to writing the legislation itself.

And it passed! The act he drafted began: "The General Assembly of this state finds that: (1) The life of each human being begins at conception; (2) Unborn children have protectable interest in life, health, and wellbeing"—words that directly contradicted Blackmun's *Roe* opinion. It went on to bar state-funded hospitals and clinics from providing abortions, required doctors to perform a viability test if the baby was more than twenty weeks old, and banned abortions after viability.

When the Eighth Circuit Court of Appeals struck down the law, the Missouri Attorney General, William Webster, appealed to the Supreme Court. George H. W. Bush's Justice Department filed an amicus brief requesting that the court use this case to reverse *Roe*. This was also a victory—in 1980, when Reagan chose Bush as his running mate, we were disappointed because Bush had declared opposition to a Human Life Amendment. But now he was demonstrating pro-life credentials in line with Reagan's.

The Pro-Life Action League spearheaded another petition drive. For *Thornburgh*, we'd collected more than thirty thousand signatures. This time the effort was even more intense. We called the nationwide effort "Speak Out America," and it brought in more than three *million* signatures. At the DC press conference, bundles of the pages of names asking the court to overturn *Roe* filled the tables. In July 1989, the decision came down. *Webster v. Reproductive Health Services* was also decided five to four—but this time the five voted pro-life!

Mostly, anyway. Trying to figure out the *Webster* case can make a lawyer dizzy. The nine justices authored seven different opinions: two majorities, three concurrences, and two that were part concurrence, part dissent. Rehnquist wrote the main majority opinion and argued that the line "life begins at conception" was not unconstitutional—it didn't carry any legal force and thus couldn't violate any rights. So there it was: not a Human Life Amendment but a human life bill, in a sense. No such law had made any headway at the federal level, but at the state level, it was allowed to stand, and it was written not by a politician but by a pro-life activist. As for the parts of the law that did have legal force, the key details were that the restrictions on state funding and facilities were upheld but that the ban on second-trimester abortions was struck down. Still, the court had dealt a severe blow to Blackmun's second-trimester guidelines. States now had the right to pass some real laws protecting the unborn.

But it wasn't a complete victory. The court could have reversed *Roe* but didn't. Rehnquist's opinion stated that *Roe* was still in force, but particularly with regard to later abortions, its ruling was "narrowed."

Scalia wrote a concurring opinion criticizing the decision to "narrow" *Roe* when the *Webster* case offered a perfectly reasonable opportunity to reverse it. Had Bork made it onto the court, he almost certainly would have sided with Scalia. Kennedy wasn't willing to go as far as Scalia but signed onto Rehnquist's opinion narrowing, but upholding, the constitutional right to abortion.

Since a pro-life law had been upheld, Blackmun authored one of the dissents. He was joined by the two fellow pro-abortion votes from *Roe*, Marshall and Brennan. Blackmun was incensed that his precious abortion decision was being reined in and one day might be reversed. "I fear for the future," he wrote. "The signs are evident and ominous. A chill wind blows."

O'Connor's concurrence seemed designed to shield Blackmun from that wind. She managed to steer *Roe* away from the collision course with itself that she'd written about in *Akron*, writing that she voted to uphold the Missouri law not based on the narrower interpretation of *Roe* Rehnquist cited but because—using the same argument she'd put forward in *Akron* and *Thornburgh*—she didn't regard the provisions as imposing an "undue burden" on the abortion-bound woman.

Hence the partial victory. Had O'Connor taken a firmer stand, *Roe* may have been overturned in 1989. I thought about Senator Denton's assurances after O'Connor's confirmation. As long as Reagan was in the White House, he said, O'Connor's vote would be pro-life. As soon as he was out, O'Connor began retreating.

With *Roe* hanging on the vote of a single justice, pro-abortion members of Congress started pushing for a federal FOCA. Reversing *Roe* wouldn't outlaw abortion throughout the country. Rather, it would return the issue to state legislatures. FOCA was designed to keep abortion legal under federal law in the event that the court overturned *Roe*.

One of FOCA's sponsors, Republican Senator Bob Packwood of Oregon, had been pro-abortion for decades. He was among the defendants we named at Nuremberg II. He'd proposed a National Abortion Act as far back as 1970, and though that effort fell flat, his new attempt never made it to a vote after pro-lifers voted in a provision that federal law couldn't supersede state parental consent laws. Since then, several state legislatures also introduced FOCA bills of their own, and pro-life lobbyists and activists around the country had been busy keeping those from passing. Each time a case that could challenge *Roe* comes before the high court, FOCA battles heat up nationwide.

George H. W. Bush had only one term, but in that time he placed two justices on the court. In 1990, William Brennan retired and was replaced with David Souter. Nobody really knew what to expect from Souter—after Bork, court nominees were very coy. Souter dodged the abortion issue in his confirmation hearing, and there wasn't much in his career to lead us to any conclusions.

The next year, Blackmun's staunchest pro-abortion ally, Thurgood Marshall, left the court. Marshall had famously argued the *Brown v. Board of Education* school desegregation case in the '50s and was the first black person to serve on the high court. It had been a tremendous disappointment that somebody so connected with advancing equal rights used his time on the court to repeatedly deny those rights to the unborn. His retirement was welcome news.

Bush wasn't about to let the court revert to being all white, and in 1990, he nominated Clarence Thomas to replace Marshall. The confirmation hearings centered on an allegation of sexual harassment made by attorney Anita Hill, who worked for Thomas at the Equal Employment Opportunity Commission in the early '80s. During Thomas's confirmation hearings, I attended a meeting with other pro-lifers in Northwestern Virginia, and after the meeting, several of us went to the Senate Office Building in Washington to observe the proceedings. Judge Thomas ultimately convinced the Senate to admit him to the court, with the final confirmation vote a narrow 52–48.

The court decided its next important abortion case in 1992, when abortionists challenged a Pennsylvania law regarding informed consent, parent and spousal notification, and a twenty-four-hour waiting period. Again, the Bush administration submitted a brief asking the court to use this new case, *Planned Parenthood v. Casey*, to reverse *Roe*. Four of the five restrictions on abortion were upheld, but the one that was struck down was the spousal notification law. Men still have absolutely no legal standing regarding their unborn children. And once again the court refused to overturn *Roe*.

If trying to figure out *Webster* can make a lawyer dizzy, trying to make sense of *Casey* would nauseate a judge. Unlike nearly every other decision, there is no majority opinion in this case. There are instead five opinions. Four are combinations of concurrences and dissents. Blackmun and Stevens, of course, concurred with striking parental notification but dissented on allowing all the other restrictions. Rehnquist, Scalia, White, and Thomas all concurred on upholding the four provisions but dissented on the decisions to uphold *Roe* and strike spousal consent. Nobody was surprised at the positions of those six justices. The other three—O'Connor, Kennedy, and Souter—decided the case. Their opinion, called the "plurality opinion," was written by O'Connor.

In his 1989 *Webster* dissent, Blackmun argued that it would be unfair to overturn *Roe* since "millions of women have ordered their lives around reproductive choice." In her 1992 *Casey* opinion, O'Connor wrote about the "costs of overruling *Roe* for people who have ordered their thinking and living around that case." But O'Connor isn't the only justice to blame for failing to overturn *Roe*. Kennedy and Souter, nominated by Reagan and Bush, were also in the plurality. These justices weren't going to help us reverse *Roe*. Indeed, in his *Casey* opinion, Blackmun praised the dissenters for their bravery, criticized the court's pro-life faction for their backwardness, and lamented, "I am 83 years old. I cannot remain on this court forever."

Blackmun was not the most pro-abortion jurist on the court when *Roe* was decided. That distinction belongs to William Brennan. But over the years, Blackmun's position became more extreme, and by 1992, he was the staunchest abortion supporter on the court. Now with the court arguably leaning pro-life, he was hinting at his retirement—and another presidential election was looming.

That year the Democrats nominated Arkansas Governor Bill Clinton to challenge President Bush. To join Clinton on the Democratic ticket, Al Gore had to abandon an impressive pro-life record. Representing Tennessee in the House and then the Senate, Gore had maintained a nearly 90 percent pro-life voting record. He consistently supported the Hyde Amendment, and in 1984, he wrote to a constituent, "It is my deep personal conviction that abortion is wrong. Let me assure you I share your belief that innocent life must be protected, and I have an open mind on how to further this goal."[3]

But that conviction wasn't deep enough to survive his vice-presidential bid. The Democrats held their convention in Madison Square Garden that year, and the Clinton-Gore camp planned a massive postconvention bus tour from New York to St. Louis. When they released the itinerary for their bus-o-rama, I contacted pro-lifers in every city where rallies were planned.

In Carlisle, Pennsylvania, pro-life demonstrators were kept away from the rally, but Dr. Chris Kalenborn and Joe McLaughlin sneaked graphic victim pictures into the crowd, positioning themselves between the candidates and the cameras. When Clinton rose to address the assembly, they held their signs up high. Some of the

---

3    Michael Kranish and Jill Zuckman, "Democrats Debate Abortion, Bush Senior Campaigns Bradley, Gore Dispute Consistency," *Boston Globe*, January 30, 2000, A30.

press corps waded through the crowd to ask them to lower their signs, even promising them interviews, which both Dr. Kalenborn and Joe refused.

We used the two-by-two-foot signs again, this time with letters on both sides, and sent sets to cities along the bus route. The first time this technique was used, Clinton's staffers didn't know what was on the other side, and a group of eight activists were invited onstage. As Joe Garrett, president of the University of Pittsburgh Collegians for Life barked out "Give me a *C*! Give me an *L*!" cheerleader-style, the crowd chanted back until CLINTON was lifted up, spelled out in large black letters on a white background.

Clinton's name only has seven letters, but there were eight signs. As the final *N* was held up, the last sign was also raised: an equals sign. When Joe yelled, "What does that spell?" everyone flipped their signs, which now spelled ABORTION!

The staffer who had invited them onstage was furious. He tried to have them arrested, but when the police were reminded that it was a public park and the activists had been invited onstage anyway, they allowed the activists to stay at the rally.

Those signs appeared at stops all along the bus-o-rama route, and we were even invited on stage once or twice more by staffers who hadn't heard what was on the other side. Eventually, Clinton's people brought out huge blue tarps on poles to try to block the "Clinton = Abortion" message. Abortion supporters also began showing up at tour stops. In Utica, Ohio, a woman held a sign reading, "I am the face of pro-choice America." An activist named J. R. Gulateri held up a picture of an abortion victim's severed head—the true face of pro-choice America—right behind her.

Tim Murphy and I drove down to Evansville, Indiana, to join the protests as Clinton's tour wound to its finale in St. Louis. There was a huge group of pro-lifers there. Tim and I got into the reception line and tried to speak with the candidates, but when we mentioned abortion, they just smiled and dismissed us.

After the demonstration, the protesters stacked their signs in the parkway along the street. A little girl about nine years old walked up and looked at the pictures.

"Isn't that sad?" I asked her.

"No," she answered. "That's a woman's right."

Her mother stood nearby, beaming. To this day, that's the only time I've ever heard a child dismiss the graphic evidence that abortion kills children.

When the bus-o-rama would arrive at its stops, supporters would join the motorcade and form a Democratic parade. Tim and I followed behind as they made their way to Vandalia, Illinois. Tim suggested we take a detour, speed ahead, and get our car into the procession. The plan was a success: We merged into the motorcade a few cars behind Clinton's bus and held our "Stop Abortion Now" signs, which were shaped like stop signs, out of the car windows. When we passed pro-lifers who lined the parade route, huge cheers went up. When we got into Vandalia, a secret service agent jumped in front of our car and ordered us to stop. There was no way to turn around, so we backed up past the crowds to more cheers.

The bus-o-rama ran exclusively through cities in the North, and I'd only contacted pro-life groups along its route. But when we got to St. Louis, we were thrilled to find that Pastor Ed Martin had brought a group up from Florida to join the protests. Mary Maschmeier from Missouri Citizens for Life, nine months pregnant, was able to get into the VIP section of the St. Louis rally and shake Clinton's hand. "You're killing babies, Bill," she told him. "Four thousand a day. You've got their blood on your hands." Clinton, visibly shaken, turned red as a secret service agent pulled Mary away.

Mary wasn't the only one to slip through the defenses. A week later, Clinton visited Chicago. At one appearance, while most pro-lifers were kept far from Clinton, Rene Marbach and her sister, Kathy Mangan, got tickets to the VIP area. They sneaked graphic signs in with a duffel bag. When Clinton arrived, they pulled out the signs, and a minor riot ensued. Rene recognized a number of Clinton supporters as escorts from a nearby abortion clinic.

That afternoon, while Clinton attended a fundraiser at the Conrad Hilton, more than a hundred protesters greeted him with the "Clinton = Abortion" signs and chants. "Pro-lifers are hounding Clinton at every whistle stop," I told the press, "to remind the American people of his support for abortion. Everywhere Clinton goes, he can count on us being there too."

It was strange to be so close to the campaign and then to see the media's coverage. As much as possible, they edited the pro-life protests out of campaign coverage. Perhaps they had learned from our work against the Mondale–Ferraro campaign that giving our efforts any attention could actually have an impact in an election. Like the Democrats who tried to hide from the abortion issue back in '76 by voting to keep the issue out of their convention, the media tried to hide Clinton's position. But Clinton and his supporters certainly saw our protests.

We chased Clinton around everywhere we could, but he beat Bush. As we anticipated, he immediately began pushing a pro-abortion agenda. The anniversary of *Roe* is right after inauguration day, and a number of presidents have used the anniversary to enact an abortion policy as a way to send a message about their social agenda. Ronald Reagan's Mexico City Policy closed a loophole in the Helms Amendment, the foreign-aid equivalent to the Hyde Amendment, that made it possible to use US tax dollars to finance abortions performed under foreign aid. On January 22, 1993, Bill Clinton rescinded the Mexico City Policy. Exactly eight years later, George W. Bush reestablished it. Eight years after that, Barack Obama rescinded it again.

Hounding Clinton hadn't kept him out of the White House, but we weren't about to let up. In 1993, Pope John Paul II celebrated World Youth Day in Denver. He planned to meet with Clinton there. We held enormous demonstrations there—not to protest the Pope but to picket Clinton everywhere he went. We also went out to abortionist Warren Hern's clinic in Boulder for a huge demonstration there. If you were an abortionist in the early '90s, you certainly didn't want Clinton visiting your town.

Clinton had his first opportunity to appoint a Supreme Court justice early in his presidency when Byron White, the dissenter who had called *Roe* an exercise of "raw judicial power," announced his retirement in March 1993. He was replaced by Ruth Bader Ginsburg. Now that a *Roe* opponent had been replaced with a *Roe* supporter, Blackmun finally felt it was safe to retire and left the following year. Clinton filled his vacancy with Justice Steven Breyer. Ginsburg and Breyer would be Clinton's only court appointments, replacing both the author of the *Roe* decision and its biggest critic.

When he retired in 1994, Blackmun had been the last of the original seven *Roe* votes left on the court. After William Brennan died in 1997, he was the last one still living. When Blackmun died in 1999, Gloria Steinem eulogized him, saying, "Justice Blackmun saved more women's lives than any other person in history."[4] Francis Cardinal George was less out of touch with reality, observing that Blackmun now knew when life begins.

Clinton's support for abortion was even worse than we'd feared. In 1994, he signed the FACE Act, and he vetoed the Partial Birth Abortion Ban in 1996.

The 1996 Democratic National Convention was held in Chicago. It was the first Chicago convention since the riots of '68, and we

---

4    "Remembering Supreme Court Justice Harry A. Blackmun," *Feminist Women's Health Center*, October 17, 2007, http://www.fwhc.org/abortion/blackmun.htm.

knew the whole country would be watching again. Clinton's challenger was Bob Dole, a solid pro-lifer. Activists and demonstrators with a whole array of issues are present at conventions, but our group was the largest at every venue.

Convention security was extremely tight. A few times we were forced away from areas where Clinton was scheduled to appear, but whenever that happened, we took up positions visible to his motorcade. By this time, we were using three-by-five-foot signs reinforced with foam board, and even from far off, our message to Clinton and the public was clear. But media coverage of our protests was more disappointing than ever. The abortion issue was almost completely cut from campaign coverage.

Clinton defeated Dole in 1996 for a second term. The Partial Birth Abortion Ban passed through Congress again. Over the years, the court's rulings had left *Roe* mostly intact, but the *Doe* decision, the one that specifically allowed late-term abortions, had been chipped away. If the ban were enacted, it stood a good chance of being upheld, even with two Clinton appointees on the court. Clinton vetoed the bill again. The override vote easily got the two-thirds majority it needed in the House of Representatives but missed the mark by a mere two votes in the Senate.

Though the federal law failed to pass, several state legislatures enacted partial birth abortion bans of their own. Nebraska's ban was challenged in court by late-term abortionist Leroy Carhart. The case, *Stenberg v. Carhart*, went to the Supreme Court, which struck down the ban in a 5–4 decision. Predictably, Clinton's appointees were pro-abortion votes. O'Connor, it turned out, was the tiebreaker vote.

Her betrayal was complete.

CHAPTER 17

# Have a Blast

"If I can't show the jury the inference that his sign has at the enterprise's conference," Fay Clayton told Judge David Coar, "then we can't begin to prove our case."

It was March 4, 1998, the first day of the *NOW v. Scheidler* trial. Two jurors arrived late. One never showed up at all. So the judge dismissed the others and allowed the lawyers to use the time to go over pretrial motions. I spent the time doing interviews in the lobby, and I never knew Clayton had blatantly admitted how flimsy her case was until I read the trial transcripts years later.

The sign in question was a photograph of seventeen activists standing by a big marquee at the first meeting of the Pro-Life Action Network (PLAN) in April 1985 at an Appleton, Wisconsin, motel. Its proper name was the Valley Christian Center, but the police had taken to calling it "the Good Samaritan Hotel." Reverends Jerry Horn and Norm Stone had purchased the building and turned it into a halfway house where police sent drunks or drug addicts they didn't want to lock up but couldn't release.

In 1983, the police presented Jerry and Norm with an award for outstanding community service. That same year the two decided to convert some of the space into a home for expectant mothers, to make it easier for them to choose life. But they wanted to do more: to go to clinics and offer women tangible alternatives to abortion. Jerry and Norm called me, and I invited them and their wives, Bonnie and Judi, to come to Chicago to learn about pro-life work. They were natural activists and immediately became deeply involved in the cause. The following spring, when I was looking for a location for a national activist convention, Jerry and Norm offered to host us at their "Good Samaritan Hotel" in Appleton.

This particular meeting was one of the central elements of NOW's case against us, in large part because it was the first meeting of PLAN. When I'd first settled on the name Pro-Life Action League in 1980, Ann's father Tom Crowley helped me incorporate it, and he was concerned about my use of the word *league*. "Might make you look like a communist outfit," he said. As it turned out, it wasn't the "league" part that gave NOW their opportunity to haul me into court: It was the "network." Their original allegation was that pro-life activism violated antitrust laws, but when NOW subpoenaed my files, newsletters, hotlines, and correspondence, they tracked down the dates and locations of all the activist meetings convened under the PLAN acronym. They decided to call PLAN a criminal enterprise in order to add the RICO charges to the case.

One of Clayton's favorite exhibits during the trial was an elaborate flowchart of PLAN and its "Leadership Council." PLAN was listed at the top. Under it were other organizations, including my Pro-Life Action League, Randall Terry's Operation Rescue, John Ryan's Pro-Life Direct Action League, and at the very bottom in the smallest type, Father Paul Marx's Human Life International, one of the oldest and largest pro-life groups in the country. In NOW's fantasy, I'd become my mentor's boss.

Another visual Clayton presented in court was a map of the United States with the dates and locations of all the PLAN conventions from the 1984 Fort Lauderdale meeting (before the PLAN name was used) to 1997. After Appleton in 1985, activists met in St. Louis, Atlanta, New York, Denver, Chicago, and elsewhere. On NOW's map, each site was indicated with a starburst—clearly meant to symbolize explosions, to suggest that our agenda included coordinating clinic bombings across the country. The map provided one of the few times that my lawyers' objections to a piece of evidence were sustained. Clayton had to change her blasts to dots before displaying the map to the jury.

The first day of the Appleton PLAN convention, Jerry Horn put a greeting on the marquee. He intended to spell out "Welcome Pro-Life Activists—Have a Ball." He was down to the last letters, but there were no more *L*s in the box. Jerry had something in the oven at the time—he also ran the kitchen—and he had no time to rearrange the whole marquee, so he grabbed an *S* and a *T*, switched the last two letters, and spelled out "Have a Blast."

During the convention, seventeen of us gathered at that marquee for a photo. Joan Andrews was in jail at the time, and some activists in the picture held up cafeteria trays with "Free Joan Andrews" written on them. Others held banners reading, "Jail the Baby Killers" and "Free Our Pro-Life POWs." That picture was the piece of evidence the lawyers were discussing on the first day of *NOW v. Scheidler*.

Our racketeering case was a double class action suit. NOW claimed that it directly represented all the women, NOW members or not, who'd ever visited an abortion clinic or would do so in the future, as well as all the thousands of clinics in the country. But they only had two clinics officially named as plaintiffs, both members of the Women's Health Organization, an interstate chain of clinics run by Susan Hill of North Carolina. She ran a dozen clinics. I'd protested at every one of them.

In the summer of 1979, I was picketing her Fort Wayne clinic, an old red brick house close to the sidewalk. About thirty of us were marching in front of the clinic when a car pulled up. Three men got out, one carrying a little black box. They entered the clinic, and a short while later, the staff and patients filed out to a park about a hundred yards away. Some time later, the three men came back out, got in their car, and drove off. The staff and patients filed back in.

As we continued marching back and forth, just feet from the building, a reporter approached me and asked about the bomb threat.

"What bomb threat? We didn't hear anything about a bomb threat."

"Why d'you think everyone left the building? That was the bomb squad that just left."

"Very interesting," I said. "Wouldn't a bomb have blown glass and brick right into our group? Why didn't they warn *us*? It tells you how much the abortion mentality has taken hold," I told him. "What if there *had* been a bomb? That bomb squad assumed we'd know when to leave to avoid the explosion. But we wouldn't have known."

There were several children marching with us, including my three sons. "Would they care if an explosion killed some of us? It'd serve us right, because *we're* the ones who are violent—even though it's the abortionists who are in there dismembering children." I gave that reporter an earful.

Two years later, I debated Susan Hill on ABC's *Nightline* with Ted Koppel. During the debate, Susan brought up that bomb scare at her Fort Wayne clinic, which gave me the opportunity to share our side of the story with a national audience and to show how ridiculous it is to think that all pro-lifers are terrorists.

But sometimes the bombs were real. Among his accolades as America's abortion pioneer, Bill Baird claimed that his Long Island clinic was the first target of anti-abortion terrorism in the United States. He used to display a photograph of his charred clinic at his talks. The NAF's extensive list of arsons and bombings at abortion clinics—which happens to list several instances where abortionists themselves were convicted of insurance fraud—cites a 1976 arson at a Planned Parenthood in Eugene, Oregon, as the first incident of anti-abortion violence. The perpetrator said it was retaliation for complications his girlfriend suffered from an IUD she had implanted at the clinic, yet they list it as *anti-abortion* violence.

NAF lists four arsons in 1977 after the Oregon arson. Three more arsons and four bombings occurred in 1978. Over the next three years, two clinics were set ablaze, but there were no bombings until 1982, when four more arsons occurred as well. There were two arsons and no bombings in 1983.

Then in 1984, there were *twenty-six* arsons and bombings. This sudden increase in violence repeats a pattern from other protest movements in US history. Of these twenty-six cases, ten were closed when the statute of limitations expired. The remaining sixteen were all solved. They were carried out by three different groups. Ken Shields and Tommy Spinks, working with Michael Bray, pled guilty to nine. Curtis Beseda was convicted for three and for one 1983 arson. Matt Goldsby and James Simmons were found guilty in four. Their patterns show that the six unsolved Texas arsons were probably related.

So it wasn't that dozens of pro-lifers suddenly started setting fires and planting bombs. But a handful of individuals, working alone or in small groups, managed to dramatically change the character of the abortion battle in the early 1980s. Most of these perpetrators were only loosely connected to a pro-life group or not even affiliated with one. With the exception of Mike Bray, they weren't leaders or regular protesters.

When Matt Goldsby and James Simmons bombed the Ladies Center in Pensacola, they reasoned that a sit-in closed a clinic for a day, only sparing the babies for twenty-four hours, but that destroying the whole facility could save them for good. One of the problems with this logic is that the women who had appointments at the Ladies Center could simply go somewhere else. Damaging or destroying a clinic may not have saved a single life.

As a pro-life activist, I had to decide how I would respond when clinics were bombed or burned. I'd had conversations with a few people who were so incensed over our nation's twisted morality that they thought they should attack clinics directly, but I always argued against that tactic and tried to talk them out of it. To dissuade others who wanted to go the vigilante route, I included a chapter in *CLOSED* called "Violence: Why It Won't Work." I pointed out that even though damage to property was far less serious than the violence that went on inside the clinics, it gave the real victimizers of women and children a chance to cast themselves as victims.

Matt Goldsby wrote me from prison, saying he hoped he didn't do too much damage to the cause. I wrote back that the cause was doing just fine and that he should focus on his own struggles while he was locked up. I felt sorry for these extremists. They were often singled out for especially harsh sentences. In addition to their natural opponents making them out to be monsters, the nation's pro-life leadership joined the condemnation. I thought they at least deserved to know that not everyone thought they were beyond hope.

When Don Benny Anderson, the Zevallos's kidnapper, was convicted, his wife and seven children were ostracized in their hometown. Some of his children refused to visit him in prison. I wrote to Don Benny's wife, Margaret, to let her know that she and her family were in my prayers. In June 1983, Andy Scholberg and I met Margaret and her twin daughters at a restaurant not far from the federal penitentiary in Oxford, Wisconsin, where her husband was incarcerated. We went together to visit him. We were given passes at the entrance, then led through an underground passage to a large recreation room. I'd only seen Don Benny's picture in the newspapers, so when he was brought in and I met him in person, I was struck by his resemblance to Paul Newman.

I thought it worthwhile to visit Don Benny. The Zevallos's kidnapping harmed the pro-life movement, making it difficult to argue our commitment to nonviolence, but one of the corporal works of mercy is to visit the imprisoned—not just the innocent incarcerated unjustly but the guilty ones too. I have seven children, and when I heard that some of his children were too embarrassed to visit him, I wanted to show him compassion.

Whenever I visited extremists, I found basically good people who wanted to save unborn children but who failed to consider that violence, even for a noble cause, is never justified.

St. Thomas Aquinas addresses the question of whether the ends justify the means—whether a bad action is permitted if undertaken for a noble cause. Aquinas explains that whether a particular action is moral depends on the goodness of the action's nature and the goodness of its end. The bombers only considered the end. But since bombing and arson have a real possibility of injuring or killing an innocent party, the action, by its nature, is *not* good. Having seen the student protest movement of the '60s lose support over violence, I vowed when I joined the pro-life movement never to advocate the use of violence.

Early in my activist career, I led a campaign to get the Catholic Church to pull out of a fundraising campaign called the Crusade of Mercy because Planned Parenthood was one of the groups funded. A *Chicago Magazine* story on this effort used a label Pat Buchanan had ascribed to me, "the Green Beret of the Pro-Life Movement." I felt proud to earn that title, because in many ways pro-life activism is a form of guerilla action. The media still refers to pro-life activism as "militant"—but it absolutely must be nonviolent.

My willingness to visit prisoners, to publish their addresses in my newsletter, and to encourage others to visit them made me a pariah in some pro-life circles. When *CLOSED* was released in the summer of 1985, I wanted to sell my books at the NRLC convention. However, because of my refusal to condemn the extremists wholesale, the NRLC refused to let me sell the books, so I carried around a box of copies at the conference to meet whatever the demand might be.

One of the speakers at the convention was Mother Teresa of Calcutta. I was late getting to her talk, and I came in by a side entrance near the front as she was being introduced. Mother Teresa was a tiny woman, and the podium was far too tall for her. The audience could only see the top of her head. I was carrying my box of books, so I walked over and set my case of books down behind the podium. "Here, Mother," I said, "try this." She stepped up on the box and started her speech as the audience applauded being able to see her. Since that speech, I've sold all the books she stood on, and with Saint Mother Teresa's canonization on September 4, 2016, a number of pro-lifers have a second-class relic of her in their bookcases.

While my compassion for the bombers and arsonists made me unwelcome in some pro-life circles, nobody in the movement ever suggested I was involved with the plots. Those accusations came from the pro-abortionists. When I met with Curtis Beseda at the La Tuna Federal Corrections Center in Anthony, Texas, I was surprised at how many security personnel were observing our conversation. I mentioned it to Curtis. "It's *you* they're keeping an eye on," he replied.

It was frustrating that we peaceful activists were being labeled bombers and arsonists. Partly as a way to laugh this off, a few of the attendees at the Appleton PLAN meeting put little firecrackers on their nametags. Those nametags made it into the abortionists' film, *Holy Terror*, and into our trial.

But the prize evidence in that trial was that marquee. When Fay Clayton talked to Judge Coar about "the inference that his sign has," she was referring to me and to "Have a Blast." But it was Jerry's sign—I had nothing to do with the wording. Nevertheless, the judge admitted the photograph along with Fay's inference that "Have a Blast" was a reference to bombing clinics.

Later in the trial, when Jerry was called to the stand, he was asked whether he'd had any idea that some people might think his marquee was a reference to violence. He said that Norm's wife, Judi, who was managing the motel, came to the kitchen to tell him that someone complained about the sign. "I told her she could change it if she wanted to," Jerry explained to the court, "but if she wanted me to, I was too busy baking potatoes and cooking steaks."

So the sign stayed for all to read.

## CHAPTER 18

# The House Hearings on Clinic Violence

With the increase in bombings and arson at clinics, the US House of Representatives Subcommittee on Civil and Constitutional Rights opened its 1985 session with hearings on these violent incidents. The subcommittee reached out to some well-known national pro-life leaders, but they all turned down the invitation. Finally, the subcommittee invited me.

I worried that if the hearings went ahead without a voice representing the pro-life position, they would simply serve as an opportunity for the pro-abortion faction to bash the pro-life movement and denounce us as fanatics, so I agreed to testify. The night before I appeared, I met with Earl Appleby and Michael Bray at Mike's Maryland home to prepare an opening statement. At the time, Mike was being investigated in connection with some clinic bombings on the East Coast, but he assured us that he was innocent. As it turned out, he wasn't. I had no idea that the night before I testified on clinic violence, I was hosted by one of the perpetrators.

The hearings were held in the Rayburn Building. When I walked into the hearing room, I found that NOW and NARAL had packed the audience. Aside from a handful of pro-lifers on the committee itself, Earl and I seemed to be the only ones in the room who didn't believe abortion was a fundamental human right.

There were five Democrats and three Republicans on the subcommittee. All adhered to their respective parties' positions. The subcommittee chair was California Democrat Don Edwards. He called the meeting to order:

> Today we are going to begin a series of hearings on abortion clinic violence. Our purpose is to consider whether, in specific instances, unlawful activities directed against abortion clinics have infringed constitutional rights of reproductive freedom.
>
> The purpose of these hearings is most emphatically not to debate the pros and cons of abortion. We take as our premise the holding of the Supreme Court, which has ruled that abortion in the earlier stages of pregnancy is a fundamental right.
>
> We have received reports about clinic entrances being blocked, clinics being invaded to disrupt activities, telephone threats, property damage, and so on. We strongly condemn all forms of violence that infringe the exercise of constitutional rights. The purpose of these hearings is to explore the scope and impact of this problem. We also want to ask whether the federal government, and particularly the Department of Justice, should be involved in investigating such violence under the civil rights laws.
>
> We will receive testimony in a later session from the Bureau of Alcohol, Tobacco, and Firearms regarding its investigation of the bombings and arsons. We applaud their successes to date and we urge them to continue their efforts until each of the bombings is solved.
>
> The hearing today focuses on other forms of violence— the harassment and intimidation of patients and staff—that

may be equally injurious in discouraging the exercise of full constitutional rights. I should make clear that we fully support the exercise of first amendment rights by abortion opponents. The allegations that we will be investigating today go far beyond legitimate first amendment protests.[1]

He went on to compare the rights of women to access abortion in the 1980s with the rights of blacks to sit at a lunch counter in the 1960s. It was clearly going to be an uphill battle. Edwards's opening statement had its share of inaccuracies that favored the opposition—that the Supreme Court had established a right to abortion only in the early stages of pregnancy, for example—but the mood became more hostile as the hearings proceeded.

Mary Bannecker, administrator of the Northeast Women's Center in Philadelphia, was the first witness. She began, as abortion advocates almost always do, by listing the other services her clinic offered, as though calling it an abortion clinic was unfair or biased. Despite the fact that Congressman Edwards said the day's hearings were for discussing "other forms of violence," not arsons or bombings, most of the abortion providers who testified offered nothing but accounts of fires, explosions, bomb threats, and vandalism.

When they got to the subject of the alleged pro-life harassment, one woman admitted that she'd walked untouched through a picket line, then told the committee: "I just could not believe that it was

---

1    This and other quotations from the hearings have been taken from the official government publication of the hearings.

United States Congress, House, Committee on the Judiciary, Subcommittee on Civil and Constitutional Rights, *Abortion Clinic Violence: Oversight Hearings Before the Subcommittee on Civil and Constitutional Rights of the Committee on the Judiciary, House of Representatives, Ninety-Ninth Congress, First and Second Session . . . March 6, 12, and April 3, 1985; and December 17, 1986* (Washington, DC: US Government Printing Office, 1987).

legal for them to be right out in front of the clinic where I was supposed to be allowed the right to choose to have an abortion. One
sign had a picture of dead babies in a garbage can from something
that happened years ago in Canada, not the United States, where
abortion is safe and legal."

During the abortion providers' testimony, Congresswoman Patricia Schroeder, a Democrat from Colorado, said,

> Several of you mentioned sidewalk counseling, and I would like
> to have a description of what that is about. I take it that what
> is happening is that they are stopping people coming into your
> clinics and demanding that they listen to them, which, I think
> again, is a little beyond speech. It's as if I decided that I don't
> like a certain church, I can go down and line people up around
> the church and stop everybody going in, saying "Do you know
> what you are doing?" And I think Americans don't have to go
> through that to do something that is perfectly legal. They can
> go into a church, if they want to, without being harassed.

Schroeder's metaphor is worth examining. In addition to presag-
ing the issue of bubble and buffer zones outside of clinics, Schroeder's statement used the example of going into a church. The 1994
FACE Act, signed nine years after the clinic violence hearings,
banned blockades outside clinics. But despite its name, Congress
added a second place where blockades were illegal: places of wor-
ship. That day at the hearings is perhaps the first time a member of
Congress publicly connected abortion clinics and churches. One
of FACE's strongest supporters in the House of Representatives was
Pat Schroeder.

The bill's official House sponsor, Congressman Charles Schumer,
a Democrat from New York, was also on the subcommittee on clinic
violence. He arrived late and hadn't delivered an opening statement.
He was the last member of the committee to offer any comments,

but he did ask the four abortion providers present, "How many of you have, either in clinics you run, clinics you are affiliated with, or clinics you've heard of, experienced violence? Just raise your hand. That is, arson, invasion of clinics, trespass, et cetera. Let the record show that all four have raised their hands."

Adding trespass to his list meant that a peaceful sit-in was now classified as violence, and the "et cetera" meant that anything they decided to label violence—whether now or later, including peaceful pickets—met that definition. Furthermore, since his question included incidents they had heard about, and we had all just listened to testimony alleging violent harassment, there was no option to *not* raise their hands.

"I, for one, respect the views of people on both sides, okay?" Schumer said. "I think those of us who are pro-choice often make the mistake of thinking we're morally superior to the people who aren't. We're not. It's not an issue for government to decide. That's all there is as far as I'm concerned."

But the government *had* decided it, and the committee had accepted that ruling as its premise. Now it was considering whether the right to abortion was so fundamental that it abrogated freedoms of expression.

Eventually, I got my turn. I had ten minutes to deliver an opening statement. I corrected Congressman Edwards's misstatements about the extent of the *Roe* decision and explained how our investigations contributed to the *Chicago Sun-Times*'s "Meet the Abortion Profiteers" series that exposed the dismal underside of Chicago's abortion industry and resulted in the closing of several clinics.

I told the committee that pro-lifers are deeply concerned not just with the children killed but with their mothers as well. I talked about the three thousand pregnancy help centers established throughout the nation. I explained why we conduct other forms of activism—picketing at hospitals, offices, and homes, the use of graphic images, sit-ins at clinics, all of it peaceful. I spoke about how effective sidewalk counseling is and how it has saved many women from postabortive grief.

I pointed out that the other side has its own transgressions. I testified to my own damaged eyesight, the result of an assault from a clinic guard. I described how my office had been vandalized so many times that my landlord refused to renew the lease. I mentioned telephoned death threats.

"As activists," I said, turning to the stated purpose of the hearings, "we caution the abortionists and those defending their lethal trade to cease their campaign to deny us our constitutional rights. Nonviolent direct action to end abortion is preferable to bombing abortion clinics, but if access to free speech, assembly, and redress of grievances is denied, the violence of abortion will be opposed by other means. Our methods are open and above board. Our abortion clinic sit-ins are within the law, in light of the defense of necessity."

I closed by quoting a letter I'd received just as I was leaving my office to attend the hearings. It was from a mother whose daughter Becky was just entering kindergarten. The mother had met me five years earlier in front of Park Medical Center in Chicago. She'd written to thank me for being there.

"There were forty abortions scheduled for that day," I told the committee. "Becky was the only one we saved. I wonder about the other thirty-nine who will never go to kindergarten, never learn to write, or never have their mother write a letter like this. That's what this battle is all about."

Then the interrogation started.

John Conyers of Michigan asked whether I had any concern for people after they are born, particularly those born into poverty.

"I have a very deep concern for all human beings," I answered. "But I don't believe you solve problems of hunger and poverty by killing people."

"What we are here about today is not to discuss your theories, but violations of the law, criminal violations of laws that are not being protected," Conyers replied. "And it seems to me that you have advocated that there are some violations of the law that you would support, apparently based on your notion of a higher law. And that is why we are here, I think, to try to draw the line a little bit more carefully on how we protect the first amendment, which I happen to be a great supporter of, but how we give everybody the right to be free from assault, intimidation, threats, harassment, and violence."

"I don't believe in any of those things," I assured him.

"Well, that's what we heard from the whole panel in front of you, and I thought you were in the room when they described, in rather graphic detail, not only verbal assaults, but physical assaults as well."

"I don't agree with those assaults," I answered. "I have a book . . . *CLOSED: 99 Ways to Stop Abortion*, and I don't advocate any kind of assaults at all."

"You mean you don't agree that you heard people describing assaults here for the last hour?"

"I said I don't agree with those assaults. I heard everything you heard. I tell my people, 'never touch anybody, never stop anybody, never stand in front of anybody.'"

"Are you aware that you can commit an assault verbally, without touching anybody?"

"Yes, I know that. I've been verbally assaulted many times by the abortionists."

"Well, I just wanted to establish that on record," he said, "because we've been spinning a lot of wheels acting like somebody has to get beaten up before they can be assaulted."

Patricia Schroeder was the next one to question me. "It's my understanding that you have advocated followers to go into clinics posing as patients, and then begin shouting slogans, locking arms to block off labs and procedure rooms," she said. "Now, do you think that's legal?"

"The shouting is not accurate, but the rest is pretty close. The sitters are trying to pray quietly, and a proper sit-in has a single spokesperson inside to tell why we are taking that action," I answered.

"You don't consider that conspiracy or trespass?" she asked.

"It's trespass if you think of an abortion clinic like a dentist's office," I answered. "But they are killing people inside those rooms. We'd like to get that point across. When we go in to save a human life—and I have the letter here from Becky's mom—"

"Now wait a minute," she said, cutting me off. "A Human Life Amendment has not passed—we're operating under a const—"

"Well, let's get a Human Life Amendment, then, out of this committee."

"—a constitutional decision that says it's legal to go into these clinics," Schroeder finished.

"It's still immoral," I said, meaning abortion.

"That's your decision."

"No," I replied, "that's God's decision. 'Thou shalt not kill' is not *my* decision."

"Well, the way I read this, the chapter headings in your book are kind of amazing," Schroeder went on. "'Taking Information from License Plates,' 'Using Private Detectives,' 'Pressure,' 'Graffiti,' 'Get the Dirt on Them,' 'Night Telephone Messages,' 'Use of Inflammatory Rhetoric,' 'How to Rattle Your Opponent,' 'Don't Let the Garbage Men Collect Garbage,' 'How to Deal with Goon Squads.' I mean, I could read all ninety-nine."

The book would not be out for a few more months, but she had a copy of the table of contents. If she *had* read all ninety-nine aloud, she'd have noticed chapter 81: "Violence, Why It Won't Work."

"It's clear you haven't read the book," I said. "It's actually very low-key." Some of the chapter titles she read may have sounded threatening to the committee, but these titles were written to draw readers into the book. "Inflammatory Rhetoric" was a reference to the pro-abortion claim that words like "baby" instead of "fetus" were inflammatory. But Schroeder wanted to give the impression that I advised activists to act like thugs.

She tried to bring the discussion back to the alleged assaults that the other panelists mentioned. I said that they had exaggerated and that my organization had a strict code against violence. But because yelling was now being characterized as assault, I said, "Sometimes when you are in a pitched conversation in front of a clinic there are some heated words. I don't condone that, but I don't think it is nearly as important as the fact that this woman is taking a child in there to have its arms and legs pulled off, be disemboweled, and have its brains sucked out."

"Sir," Schroeder replied, "I think one of the great tragedies is if you go back and look at the Supreme Court decision, it talks about the right to privacy, and we're not talking about one life, but two. The woman walking in there is a human being also. You are making a value judgment about women walking into these clinics who could be in life-threatening positions."

"You don't go into a freestanding abortion clinic in a life-threatening situation. You go to an emergency room," I replied. "You said there are two lives at stake here, two lives in the balance. But there aren't two lives at stake—we're talking about a woman deciding to take a life."

"But the woman still happens to be a human being. We still classify them that way. Women may not have equal rights in this country, but we are still classified as human beings."

"But her life is not at stake. Can't you understand the distinction?" I asked.

"Sir," she said, "I resent that very much. I want to tell you why, okay? I have two children, and I have lost two children, and it is not an easy thing for me to talk about."

"Then you should be pro-life."

"I am pro-life," she said.

"But you're defending the killing of children."

"Let me continue," she said. "I could be in a very threatening situation if I were pregnant again, and I resent you sitting there telling me that women take this decision lightly."

"I never said that," I replied.

"Well, you implied it."

"I'm not sure I did that either," I said. "But you are implying that it is a serious decision. Why is it so serious?"

"Because they are trying to deal with their situation, with the child's situation, and it's tough. Women are walking into those clinics under tremendous stress."

"Why?" I asked. I wasn't trying to be callous; I was trying to get Congresswoman Schroeder to admit that the stress, the anxiety, came in great part from the mother's knowledge that she was taking a life, doing something terrible.

Schroeder deflected. "You miscast the Supreme Court's decision, saying it allows abortion at any time," she said. "It does not."

"It certainly does."

"It says only in the first three months. That's a very different situation, sir."

"The Supreme Court has allowed abortion for the full term of pregnancy," I answered. "No state has been able to pass a law to protect the child in the third trimester."

"Sir, you are not a lawyer," she said.

"I may not be a lawyer," I said, "but I can read. I've read the decisions many times, and it is abortion on demand for the full term of pregnancy. Read it yourself and you'll see that."

"It's not 'abortion on demand,' sir, and I don't think anyone has interpreted it that way. I wish you could respect the fact that it is legal for women to get contraception, it is legal for women to go to these clinics. You have a right to express your opinion, and I respect that, but you don't have the right to break in, you don't have the right to intimidate, you don't have the right to verbally abuse them and call them 'murderers.' You don't have the right to take the law into your own hands. This is a government of laws, and not of men and women, and you're trying to turn that around because you say you are above the Constitution and above the law."

"Laws are for the people. The people are not for the laws," I answered. "When the laws are allowing the killing of innocent human beings, we will change those laws. But until we can, we will find ways to go around them."

"But sir, you are the one saying that. It is not the law saying that. You are the one redefining life. And I think that is something that all sorts of people, all sorts of religious groups, have been debating for thousands of years, and no one has come to a consensus as to exactly what does life mean, exactly when does it begin, and so forth. But you have decided, and therefore you were saying that all the laws and everything we have about it are irrelevant because of your position."

With that dressing down, Schroeder's time was up. The next questioner, Michael DeWine of Ohio, asked me to confirm that I wasn't involved in any of the incidents described earlier. I told him that was correct.

"The only thing I've heard you describe that you do that would be considered a violation of civil law would be trespassing—would that be a fair summary?" he asked.

"Yes. It would be trespass into an abortion clinic for the purpose of saving lives."

"All right. But you do not feel that you commit any assaults?"

"No, I would not touch anybody. Never have."

"All right, thank you. Thank you, Mr. Chairman." DeWine's few questions did help clarify my position about what laws pro-lifers could violate.

Then it was Charles Schumer's turn. He stated that he had several questions, first asking whether I condemned the acts of violence that were mentioned in the earlier testimony. It was a tough question, since so much nonviolent action had been labeled violence.

"I'm not sure I'm in a position to condemn them, since I'm not sure they're true," I said.

"Let's say they are true."

"I don't have the evidence."

"Let's say there was evidence, it was uncontrovertibly true that there had been an arson—an attempt to destroy a clinic. Would you condemn it?"

"I wouldn't condone it. But I wouldn't condemn it until they (the abortion providers) are willing to condemn their violence." This was exactly what I'd said in my opening statement.

"So you would not condemn it."

"That's right," I answered, "and I've said that many times."

"Well, I think that speaks for the value of your general testimony," he quipped. "In your exchange with Ms. Schroeder, you said that God said they are children. You and I are of different religions. My God does not say that. Are you telling me the United States of America should impose the view of your God on me and my family?"

"I believe in one God," I answered.

"So you believe your God has to be my God."

"I believe *our* God has to be the God that—"

"Let's say I don't believe in one God."

"Then you're wrong."

"I'm wrong? What should be done to make me believe in your God?"

"Well, maybe you need some education on the existence of God," I answered, "and the fact that in Scripture, God himself said: 'The Lord Your God is One God.'"

"Should I believe in Jesus Christ?" he asked.

"I think you should."

"Would you want to pass laws saying I should?"

"No."

"No. And now I want you to tell me the difference between passing laws as you advocate on *this* issue, because they are exactly the same. They are religious beliefs."

"You know, the Nazis had this nice little law that you could kill people, and you had to obey that law. They could have had hearings in Germany and anyone who tried to help Jews escape was a culprit and could be victimized or executed himself."

Schumer was Jewish, and in bringing up the Holocaust, I'd obviously touched a nerve. He sat up and started talking faster.

"You know why Nazism developed? Because there were people who said, 'I am right—you are wrong.' There was no one who said, 'We have a pluralistic government, and people can live here by their own beliefs in what they feel and what they do.'"

The crowd of abortion supporters began to applaud.

"Adolf Hitler did not think," Schumer went on, "that I had—no, I don't want any applause—"

"And you don't deserve any, either," I retorted.

"—because I consider this an important issue. Of course you think I don't deserve applause. You think a lot worse about me than that—"

"Because you are trying to—"

"No, no. Let me finish my point," he said. "What happened in Nazi Germany, what happens in Soviet Russia, is a group of people say, 'my laws must be your laws,' and there is no room for pluralism, no room for people to disagree.'"

This was coming from a member of a committee that was considering the issue of using civil rights laws to ban sidewalk counseling.

"That's what you are saying," he continued, "and as an American who believes in this country as deeply as anyone, I resent it."

"Well, I hope you do," I said.

"And then you say, 'It's okay for me to advocate illegal acts because my law is higher than your law.'"

"This country, for over a hundred years," I began, "protected its unborn."

"Did it ever call it murder? Was anyone ever executed?" Schumer asked.

"Oh, that's the important thing? To call it murder?"

"No, no, no. Well, you were saying what happened a hundred years ago—"

I said, "Gassing Jews was not called murder in Nazi Germany."

"So you're calling it 'murder'?"

"Yes, I am."

"Okay. The country never did."

"Well, we will," I said.

"Don't tell me what the country did or didn't do," he said.

"It outlawed it," I told him.

Ignoring this, Schumer changed the topic. "Let me ask you another question, sir. You said your organization does advocate trespassing, locking arms, trying to prevent abortions from occurring. Correct?"

"Yes."

"Now, if someone were to determine that this amounts to conspiracy to violate the law, would you willingly go to jail?"

"If they came up with some foolish notion like that—" I started. The idea of labeling pro-life civil disobedience as conspiracy seemed foolish to me at the time. It still does. For the NOW leadership in the room, though, Schumer was sketching out a strategy to shut down pro-life activism.

"No, it's not a foolish notion," Schumer continued. "It's our law right now, but you have such utter contempt for our law and our concept of America that you call it foolish. But let's say that it was law, that an organization got together and said, 'In different parts of the country, we're going to go in and trespass, and we're going to stop things illegally.' You admit that it's illegal, but you feel you're following a higher law, and I respect that."

"Thank you."

"I don't feel you should be doing what you're doing," he said, "but I respect that you think you're following a higher law. But let's say we found a hundred lawyers of all different ideologies, all different stripes, and they all said, 'This is illegal; in fact, it's a violation of certain criminal or civil statutes,' would you willingly pay the penalty under those statutes?"

"I have paid the penalty for my actions. I've been arrested five times."

"That's not the question," he said. "Would you willingly—"

"I've been in jail. I will willingly pay the penalty for my actions. We all will."

"Okay. Do you think what you are doing is criminal?"

"No."

"Why?"

"I think I've explained that," I said.

"You can't argue a higher law," he said, "because our criminal law does not allow each individual to decide or follow his or her higher law."

"Do you know that in every state in the union," I asked, "there is a common law defense of necessity that allows people to do things to try to save human lives?"

"No," he answered. "My knowledge—and I *am* an attorney—of the defense of necessity is quite different than yours. And once again—just like you interpreted the Supreme Court—you just twist it to interpret it the way you want, and then you go ahead and follow it."

"It has been applied."

"No. Not the way you're suggesting," he said. "It has never been applied in the way you have understood."

"It has been applied in trespass cases."

"Give me a court case that says you can go in and form a conspiracy, an organization, to go and invade and trespass other organizations because you don't agree with what they are doing. Give me a case."

"We have a Missouri case—"

"Cite one for me. Cite one." He was getting excited and wouldn't let me cite the case he was requesting.

"I resent your implication that I am making things up. We have three cases, and we will send them to you."

"I don't think you do," he said.

"Will you accept them if I send them?" I asked.

"If they say what you say, we'll accept them and put them into the record."

At that point, the chairman cut in and told Schumer his time was up. Immediately after the hearing, we forwarded to the committee the decisions in *St. Louis County v. Klocker* from Missouri, *Commonwealth v. Berrigan* and *Commonwealth v. Capitolo* from Pennsylvania, *City of Cleveland v. O'Malley* and *State v. Blasch* from Ohio, and *Fairfax v. Balch*. To their credit, the committee did introduce them into the record.

The hearing ended with Schumer making another objection to my referring to a higher law and saying that our "violence" was against human beings. But the issue of clinic violence was far from over.

NOW had their framework for a legal strategy to go after prolife activists: conspiracy. When the documentary *Holy Terror* was released the next year, it opened with news coverage of clinic bombings before cutting directly to my testimony at these hearings and my statement that I wouldn't condemn the bombings. They edited the footage down to Schroeder's claims that my book advocated violence, Schumer's speech about Nazism and the ensuing applause, and Conyers's assertion that I supported harassment. Just a month after the release of *Holy Terror*, NOW filed their suit against me and other activist leaders.

Thirteen years after these hearings, where Schumer had suggested a conspiracy trial of pro-life activists, when I was on trial for racketeering, NOW wanted to show that clip from *Holy Terror*, but my lawyers managed to convince Judge Coar that it wasn't an accurate representation of what had transpired that day, and Fay Clayton and her team were not allowed to introduce it.

But even without the film, NOW won their RICO case, and Judge Coar applied the triple damages mandated by the statute—not including the costs for NOW's legal fees, which they would have forced us to pay if we'd lost on appeal. But that was 1999. We would have multiple appeals and two more visits to the Supreme Court before it was all over.

In May 2009, eleven years after the RICO trial and after we'd won a reversal at the Supreme Court, I was invited to have dinner with a small group of pro-lifers from out of state. During the meal, I mentioned the film *Holy Terror*. None of them had seen it or even heard about it. I invited them to my office to watch it.

It had been a while since I had seen the video. During the opening scene, as footage of charred, bombed-out clinics appeared onscreen, I recalled visiting the site of a clinic bombing in Maryland several years earlier. The front porch had been blown to pieces, with shrapnel from the metal railing flung in all directions. It chilled me to think that a passerby could have been struck by that shrapnel. A pro-lifer's commitment to the intrinsic value of every life means just that—*every* life. Violence could never be the answer.

## CHAPTER 19

# Rescue Those Being Led to Slaughter

Early in 1986, I was invited to Binghamton, New York, to share my experiences in organizing pickets and protests. A young evangelical preacher who ran a crisis pregnancy center had started an activist group called Project Life. He wanted me to help organize his group and lead a picket. On Saturday morning, the group gathered at the top of a hill overlooking the clinic. I assumed we'd march down the road to the clinic, but they simply started marching back and forth where they were, nearly a block away.

"Why are you all the way up here?" I asked the leader.

"This is as close as they'll let us get," he answered.

"Who's 'they'?"

"The clinic."

I called out to the group, "Forward, march!" and led them down the hill.

As our group started marching back and forth in front of the clinic, the leader asked, "We can do this?"

"The sidewalk is public property," I answered. "We have a right to picket here."

That young preacher was Randall Terry. The next week, he and six others were arrested for holding a sit-in at that clinic. By the end of the year, Randy would have a new name for his group: Operation Rescue. Two years later, he coordinated a series of clinic blockades he called a "National Day of Rescue."

The National Days of Rescue that we coordinated in the early 1980s involved all kinds of activism, including pickets, prayer vigils, sit-ins, sidewalk counseling, and pro-life rallies. I organized events in Chicago but also reached out to other groups across the country to ensure that we all got some press on the same day. I wrote about one of our first events in my *Action News*, saying, "It is the hope of the League that these successful, highly visible, positive and effective National Days of Rescue will be adopted by other right-to-life groups across the country."

Randy would take the National Day of Rescue to a new dimension, but the plea I'd made in my newsletter eventually became a plaintiff's exhibit in my racketeering trial. NOW's attorney, Fay Clayton, claimed, "It shows the background of the conspiracy. We know of a hundred groups taking part in a rescue. It sets out the general guidelines of the kinds of groups he is recruiting for PLAN."

Fay's statement demonstrates a confusion about the term "rescue" in the pro-life movement. When we first used it, "rescue" meant *any* form of public activism—whether pro-lifers went specifically to clinics or just out in the public square, it was a rescue. By the end of the 1980s, it referred only to using human barricades to prevent the killing. Some of these human barricades were in clinic waiting rooms, sometimes in the hallways, and sometimes across the entrance to a building. They often involved arrests. When Clayton spoke of a "rescue," she was insinuating that I was somehow coordinating hundreds of clinic blockades as early as 1980. That just wasn't the case.

But one of the reasons *rescue* was such a significant term for activists is that the text of Proverb 24 resonates with those who recognize the evil of abortion. "If you faint in the day of adversity," it says, "your strength is small. Rescue those who are being taken away to death; hold back those who are stumbling to the slaughter." For pro-lifers, this line's instruction—save the unborn—is unmistakable, but it's combined with a second charge. We have responsibilities toward mothers and fathers clearly stumbling toward slaughter. We're called to try to rescue them too.

At the time when the Supreme Court enacted abortion on demand, the nation had become familiar with social protest. In the '60s, the sit-in became one of the most celebrated tools of the civil rights movement. As the Vietnam conflict accelerated, antiwar protesters staged sit-ins at the Pentagon and student demonstrators occupied buildings on college campuses. When *Roe* was decided, it was natural that some pro-life activists would see the sit-in as an appropriate protest strategy. But there is a fundamental difference between occupying a seat at a lunch counter and trying to save babies from abortion.

The pioneer of the pro-life sit-in was John Cavanaugh O'Keefe. In 1970, he applied for conscientious objector status in the Vietnam War and spent two years doing community service as a hospital orderly. He struck up a friendship with a nurse there, who one evening confided in him the horrible guilt she suffered over an abortion she'd had years earlier.

O'Keefe started doing research, and what he learned about the humanity of the unborn child and the brutality of the abortion procedures convinced him that his friend's guilt was the result of a grave evil. When *Roe* was announced, O'Keefe felt called to expose the evil of abortion and help save other women from the guilt his friend had experienced. He saw civil disobedience as an appropriate strategy.

In 1977, O'Keefe formed a group called the Pro-Life Nonviolent Action Project (PNAP). The group held sit-ins in Maryland and northern Virginia and, at trial, appealed to the "defense of necessity," a legal doctrine that exonerates a defendant of a lesser crime if the law in question had been broken to achieve a greater good. O'Keefe and his colleagues were acquitted of trespassing charges in Fairfax County, Virginia, on the grounds that they'd acted to save innocent human lives—a ruling that contradicted the Supreme Court's position that the lives of the unborn don't deserve protection.

O'Keefe composed a pamphlet explaining his sit-in initiative. It emphasized the importance of being completely nonviolent in order to reflect the helplessness of the child, the fact that halting abortions for a while gives women a last opportunity to reconsider, and how, by demonstrating a willingness to be arrested, activists who stage sit-ins draw public attention to the value of the lives destroyed by abortion. The pamphlet, *A Peaceful Presence*, quickly circulated around the nascent pro-life movement. In Cleveland, Mary O'Malley, Nancy Hackle, and Pat Perotti began organizing sit-ins. They called their group PEACE: People Expressing a Concern for Everyone.

Sam Lee, a student of theology and philosophy at St. Louis University, read O'Keefe's pamphlet and began leading sit-ins at clinics there, borrowing the PEACE name for his group. At first, the charges against sitters were simply dropped. Then, once they became more frequent and sufficiently large, the demonstrators were brought to trial and acquitted under the necessity defense.

In Chicago, local activists and I would go into clinics to talk to women in the waiting rooms, but we always left after the police were called. When I learned that the necessity defense had won in Maryland and St. Louis, I decided it was time to stage a Chicago sit-in.

On Saturday, March 11, 1978, a hundred demonstrators gathered at Concord Medical Center on Grand Avenue. Thirty entered the clinic while the rest marched out front or sat against the entrance to the building. Inside, some sat down along the walls in front of the doors to the procedure rooms. The clinic staff called the police. One of the women inside acted as a spokesperson for our group. She'd had an abortion at Concord a year earlier.

"I know from my personal experience," she told the women in the waiting room, "that this clinic will not tell you the truth about your baby and it will not tell you the truth about the real consequences of abortion—the tears, the anguish, the guilt, the loss you will feel when that baby is taken from your body. We are here to help you. Please, let us help you."

Just as the police showed up, reporters from the major newspapers, radio stations, and TV networks arrived. Each time a new arrestee was hauled out into the street, a cheer went up from the picketers outside. While this was going on, sidewalk counselors spoke with the women who had appointments at Concord that day. Two changed their minds and canceled their abortions. About twenty others turned away. While many may have come back another day or gone to a different clinic, it's possible that after witnessing so many people advocating for the lives of their children, some reconsidered and chose life.

Even though some pro-lifers disavowed sit-ins, the movement spread throughout the country. But while the necessity defense was permitted in districts in Virginia, Missouri, and a few other places, in more than twenty other states, judges refused to admit it, citing the *Roe* argument that unborn children lack legal personhood. Furthermore, the sentences for those convicted of trespassing were getting more severe.

Yet activists continued to stage sit-ins. For many, prevailing in court wasn't the main point. Their presence in the clinics could defend the unborn for as long as they were there. A stay of execution—if only for a few hours—was worth it.

Even if police hauled them away as soon as they arrived, or if clinic escorts ushered patients past the demonstrators, sit-ins were necessary. Activists arrested and roughed up in a sit-in experienced some personal suffering on behalf of the unborn. They believed in the redemptive aspect of their discomforts desperately needed by a nation that kills its posterity. Even if the courts weren't going to be persuaded that the unborn have a right to life, the witness of the sitters could convince the public, and some abortion-bound women, of its value.

At the 1984 NRLC convention in Kansas City, I contacted a reporter at the *Kansas City Star* to let him know pro-life activists would be staging a massive demonstration at a local clinic. When we arrived the next morning, the clinic was closed. I called the nearby Fox Hill clinic; it was closed. We called another one—closed. There were seven clinics in the Kansas City area, and we'd closed them all. A recorded message at the clinics directed patients to Truman Memorial Hospital. I sent word around our circle, and a hundred pro-lifers set out for Truman Memorial. I got there first and spoke to the security guard on duty for the hospital. I explained that we were planning to picket the hospital and offer prayers for the babies killed there.

The officer of the day (OD), as it turned out, was a born-again Christian. "Why don't you come in and have your prayer service here?" he asked. "You can use the waiting room—it's practically empty. Have your group come in through the lobby."

When the group arrived, I instructed them to come right in without letting on that I'd already spoken to the OD. After all, the original plan had been to stage a sit-in that day. When the OD came around smiling and showing people where the cafeteria and bathrooms were, I think most caught on that we weren't risking arrest. We held our prayer service, then went back to the NRLC convention.

That evening the lead story on every Kansas TV news program was the massive pro-life demonstrations in town. In the papers, the NRLC was hardly mentioned. We sensed some resentment from the convention organizers that our activism had stolen their coverage, but we knew that none of the speeches or displays could have shut down every clinic in the way we had. This event gave us a name for an effort we'd discussed in Fort Lauderdale earlier that year to get pro-lifers to commit to taking part in some form of activism at least once a year: picketing, counseling, joining a sit-in—some activity to bear witness to the value of unborn human life. We called it "the Kansas City Pledge."

Two weeks later, we held a "National Day of Blitzes." We'd been doing clinic blitzes in Chicago for years. The idea was to enter the waiting room, stuff pro-life literature into the magazines, talk with patients for as long as possible, then leave. In Chicago, we accomplished ten blitzes in one morning. There were similar blitzes in one hundred other cities with almost no arrests.

While we were looking for ways to get pro-lifers engaged in activism without risking arrest, abortion advocates were looking to get us arrested without our having broken any laws. In June 1984, Monica Migliorino and I were invited to speak to the Milwaukee Pro-Life Coalition. Afterward, we visited the Bread and Roses Women's Health Center on Wisconsin Avenue to do a blitz. The clinic was on an upper floor of its building, and we took the elevator to get there. When the elevator door opened, we found the entrance to the clinic was directly across the hall from us. A staffer recognized us and darted over, locked the door, and began shouting at us to leave. We took the elevator back down to street level. Two police officers met us on the sidewalk.

"Can you tell us how to get to Mader's?" I asked. Mader's is a famous old-world German restaurant in Milwaukee.

"Are you Joe Scheidler?" he asked. I was taken aback.

"Yes," I said. He handed us city citations for disorderly conduct and told us we had to come back to Milwaukee a week later for a hearing. Then he gave us directions to Mader's.

We duly appeared in court, and the charges were dismissed, but I was bothered by the precedent that pro-lifers could be subject to legal action simply for being pro-life. Pro-abortion activists were stepping up their own militancy, and with the law on their side, pro-lifers over the next few years would be served with injunctions, arrested, detained, and imprisoned all over the country.

The next month, in July '84, there were more than a hundred pro-life pickets organized across the country. August saw all-night prayer vigils at clinics nationwide. In the mid-1980s, after a decade of legal abortion claiming more than fifteen million victims, the idea of physically doing something about it began to appeal to more and more people. A generation too young to take to the streets in the '70s came of age during the flowering of our national tragedy and was eager to take a stand in defense of their unborn brothers and sisters.

Three months after my Milwaukee hearing, in September '84, I was arrested in Fargo, North Dakota. The charge was "emitting an illegal noise." I was leading a picket when the police informed me that they had a local ordinance against using a bullhorn. I set the bullhorn down. A young boy at the demonstration picked it up and pressed a button that produced the "illegal sound." I was happy to take the rap. In January 1986, I was invited to give a talk and lead a demonstration in Gainesville, Florida. I arrived the day of the space shuttle *Challenger* disaster, and as I got off the plane, the eerie, twisted plumes of smoke were still looming in the sky. The next day, when we were demonstrating, I was again told about a noise ordinance, so this time I asked to see it. The police said it was back at the station house and offered me a ride. The ordinance required a permit to use a bullhorn, so I filled out the forms and got my permit, and the police drove me back to the demonstration. Everyone there was surprised to see me return—they'd seen me leave in a squad car and assumed I'd been arrested.

So many pro-lifers were getting arrested at protests that I created a "Jailed for Life" award for any pro-lifer jailed for activism. The first of these was awarded in the spring of 1985 to Bob Rust of Greensburg, Indiana. Bob had been arrested for picketing an Indianapolis clinic and was sentenced to 160 hours of community service, picking up trash along highways on Wednesdays and Saturdays. Those days were selected precisely because they were the ones on which the local clinic performed abortions.

In the spring of 1986, we held our PLAN convention in St. Louis, where Sam Lee had been leading sit-ins for years. John Ryan joined Sam, and together they formed the Pro-Life Direct Action League. John had done hundreds of sit-ins and was already notorious for getting arrested: By the time I met him, he'd already been arrested four hundred times. John was one of the first activists to push for very large crowds with lots of arrests. It was at the St. Louis PLAN convention that we decided to stop using the term "sit-in" and call them "rescues." We planned five National Days of Rescue—clinic blockades on the same day nationwide—for the year ahead.

This was the first PLAN convention that Randall Terry attended. He'd just spent a month in jail in Binghamton for leading rescues there, and I gave him a Jailed for Life award.

The young preacher had come a long way.

CHAPTER 20

# Extradition

In 1985, Norm Stone and Jerry Horn began a public awareness campaign called Walk America for Life. They set out from Santa Monica, California, and as they headed east, they collected names on petitions demanding protection for the unborn. In May 1986, they finally got to Washington, DC, where they presented nearly three million signatures to President Reagan.

Along the route, Norm and Jerry joined a number of pro-life events. I met them in 1986 in Wilmington, Delaware, where the three of us appeared on a cable TV show hosted by a local pastor. A protest was planned for the next day at the Delaware Women's Health Organization (DWHO), one of Susan Hill's clinics. After the show, the host mentioned that the DWHO administrator had an Irish name, Cathy Conner, and that maybe she was Catholic. I was the only Catholic on the program. As a fellow Catholic, the host suggested, maybe I could talk her out of working there.

After our show, the four of us paid a visit to the clinic. It was on the second floor, and there was a "welcome" sign on the front door. As soon as we walked in, Ms. Conner said, "We're closed." No other staff was present, but there was a woman sitting in the waiting room.

I tried to tell Cathy about the fact that one day she would have to answer to God for the role she had in so many abortion deaths. While we were talking, the phone rang. Jerry answered it. "I'm sorry, the clinic is closed today," he said, and hung up.

Conner refused to engage in conversation, so I started looking at the waiting room to see which doors led to procedure rooms.

"What are you still doing here?" she asked.

"I'm casing the joint," I joked. I was kidding, but if one day local pro-lifers wanted to stage a rescue there, I'd be happy to share what I'd seen of the layout. "We're having a large protest out in front tomorrow."

"Well, I'll see you tomorrow, then. Now, please—get out!" We left the office and headed back down the stairs.

The next morning, when I arrived to lead the picket, I was greeted by a large police presence, including mounted police. Even if someone had planned a sit-in, there wouldn't be one that day. The police captain came over and handed me a warrant for my arrest for harassment and trespassing—no warrants for the three who had been with me at the clinic. I talked with the captain, who agreed to let me lead the protest march on the condition that I turned myself in afterward. So after the march, I walked a few blocks to the police station, where I was charged with trespassing and harassment and led to a cell. I spent several hours that afternoon waiting for bail. When I was released, I was told I'd have to return to Wilmington for trial.

Jerry and Norm posted my bail, and we walked across the street to St. Joseph Catholic Church, where I said a prayer of thanksgiving for my release. When we came out of the church, we heard sirens— the roof of the police station was on fire. I joked that we should get away before someone charged me with arson.

That afternoon, thirty of us drove over to Cathy Conner's home and picketed while she sat on her front porch with her arms folded.

A week later, I submitted an article to the *Wanderer*, a Catholic weekly, called "Thoughts from a Wilmington Jail."

What kind of justice will a pro-life activist get in Wilmington? That is anybody's guess. But whatever the verdict, the fact that the defenders of life are being judged at all is an outrage. An abortuary has no moral right to exist. It should be no crime to go into one in an effort to talk the abortionists into closing it down.

My few hours in the Wilmington jail were nothing compared to sentences served by heroes and heroines of the pro-life movement—people like John Ryan, Joe Wall, Joan Andrews, Fr. Ed Arentsen, Fr. Ed Markley, Randy Terry, Sam Lee, Rev. Jack O'Brien, Marjorie Reed, Christy Ann Collins, Teresa Lindley, Grace Gerl, Dan Scalf, and hundreds of other pro-lifers who have looked through prison bars for days and weeks and sometimes months and years because they stood up for truth. These are the saints of the movement, whose courage we admire and try to emulate.

Thoughts of these good people filled my mind in the Wilmington jail. I was proud of the good company I was in. Besides suffering with the saints of the movement, I was suffering with all the saints of every movement that stood for truth and justice in this country and elsewhere, in modern times and in ancient days. The list is endless. It includes our Savior, His Apostles, the prophets of old.

In a prison cell, we also identify very clearly with the unborn child, who is locked up in his mother's womb, awaiting a punishment much greater than ours.[1]

---

1   Joseph Scheidler, "Thoughts from a Wilmington Jail," *Wanderer Newspaper* (St. Paul, MN) 119, no. 20 (May 15, 1986).

The arrest was in April, and the trial was scheduled for early July. In the meantime, I was arrested again. In June 1986, I flew to Denver for the NRLC convention at the Marriott City Center. NOW was holding their convention just two blocks away at the Radisson Hotel that same week, so there were going to be some big demonstrations.

When I landed, I went straight to a studio for a radio show. Later, when I got to the Marriott, I registered at the desk, then turned around to see four police officers standing there.

"Are you Joe Scheidler?" one of them asked.

"That's me," I answered, as friendly as I could.

"You're under arrest."

"What? I just got here. The only thing I've done was a radio show. Was it that bad?"

"You're on the national crime computer for a warrant in Florida," he answered.

"What crime do they say I committed in Florida?"

"Burglary."

They handcuffed me and led me toward the door. Fortunately, I spotted Heather McCormick across the lobby. She was a young Australian pro-lifer I'd worked with on an Australian tour the year before. "Heather!" I called out. "Tell my lawyer, John Jakubczyk— he's here in the hotel—that I've been arrested."

During the ride to the station, I racked my brain trying to figure out what Florida burglary they could possibly think I'd committed. When we got to the station, they led me through a series of doors. I started counting as they locked behind me—fourteen in all. Finally, I was put in a holding tank. There were about thirty guys packed in there, several drunk, some banged up from fights. Of course, no one there was guilty—same story in any police holding tank anywhere.

There was a brand-new payphone in the cell, but all my money had been taken when they brought me in. I dialed zero to see if I could call Ann collect. It was about 2 AM in Chicago when I finally got through.

"Guess where I am," I said.

"In jail," she answered. "What'd you do?"

"I don't know. Burglary in Florida, they say. I can't figure it out. I've never burgled anything anywhere. I'm trying to get in touch with John Jakubczyk. I'll have him call you if I need bail money." I told her not to worry. But I knew she would—and so would I.

I'd barely finished the call when somebody shouted my name. I was taken to a cellblock and put in my own cell overlooking the prison parking lot. There was a little corridor that ran between the cellblock and the outside wall. I looked through the two blurry windows, feeling very cut off from the outside world.

There was a Bible in my cell on a little table beside a cot and a sink. I thought to myself that I'd been in a cell before, in the monastery. So I planned a routine of reading a few verses from the Bible, taking a rest, then doing some exercises to pass the time. I barely started into my routine when an officer unlocked the cell door and led me to a small room with a stool facing a Plexiglas window smeared with lipstick where women had tried to kiss their boyfriends. A reporter sat on the other side. I did the interview and was returned to my cell.

I picked up the Bible and started on the Gospel of St. John. But the officer came back. He led me out for another interview. Then another reporter arrived. Eventually, they quit locking my cell. When TV reporters showed up, I asked the officer, whom I'd gotten to know pretty well, if I could do the interviews on the other side of the Plexiglas, for a better picture. He agreed, and I asked the reporter to get him on film. We walked toward the camera together, and the officer seemed happy to get his fifteen seconds of fame. I did nineteen interviews that night and into the morning.

Late the next morning, John Jakubczyk came to see me with another lawyer, Charles Onofrio.

"So, John," I asked, "what's this burglary charge all about?"

"It's from Pensacola. You're charged with burglarizing a place called the Ladies Center."

"But I didn't steal anything."

"Some people went in and damaged some equipment," he said. "In Florida, that counts as burglary. And it's serious."

"I never went in that place," I said.

"They say you were on the porch, directing the break-in."

I'd been down in Pensacola in March for a demonstration at the Ladies Center. I flew in with John Ryan. We both agreed that we weren't going to risk arrest, because we didn't want to have to come back to Florida for trial. John was used to being arrested, but he had the advantage of protesting in places where prosecutors and judges were more sympathetic to the cause. Pensacola was different. Two of its three clinics had been bombed a year and a half earlier. The trial had been a media circus, and the bombers, Matt Goldsby and James Simmons, each got ten years. John and I didn't want to take our chances with the Pensacola courts.

During their trial, local activist John Burt protested outside the courthouse and drew a lot of media attention for publicly proclaiming that the bombers be exonerated because they were trying to save lives. I'd gone to Pensacola for the sentencing. I didn't agree that the necessity defense could justify bombing a clinic, but I was interested in these young people, and I wanted to discuss why they turned to bombs when the real solution to abortion is in counseling and working to change the culture. Matt Goldsby had written me a letter from jail expressing regret that his actions might have hurt the pro-life cause. I had written back that though I disagreed with his tactics, I admired his zeal. I wanted to meet him, but the judge barred him from seeing anyone but his lawyer.

John Burt and his wife, Linda, ran a halfway house for unwed mothers called Our Father's House, where John Ryan and I stayed when we visited in March 1986. The night before the protest, we drove by the Ladies Center, an old house with a long front porch and a shorter side porch. The women and girls waited for their abortions in the living room off the smaller porch. There were two doors along the front, one on each porch.

Back at Our Father's House, we held a short meeting to discuss the possibility of staging a rescue. John Ryan said that neither of us was willing to take part, but Joan Andrews said she was willing to go in. Joan was a veteran of sit-ins with John Cavanaugh O'Keefe and was accustomed to getting arrested. In fact, when O'Keefe and Harry Hand held their massive sit-in at Gaithersburg, Maryland, in 1984, there was only one arrest: Joan Andrews. The Gaithersburg clinic had been closed, but Joan got into the building and was arrested for trespassing. From there, she moved to St. Louis to join John Ryan and Sam Lee in their rescues and was arrested numerous times.

John Burt asked if I'd go into the waiting room to try to talk women out of having abortions while he, Joan, and others started the sit-in. I agreed but said that I'd leave as soon as I was asked, since I did not want to face trespassing charges in a state so far from Chicago. This was a month *before* my Wilmington arrest, so I really didn't consider it likely that I could be charged with trespassing for simply going into a building.

That night's meeting was very informal. It wasn't a real planning session, and John Ryan and I were unclear as to what would transpire the next day. But we were guests, and it was John Burt's event, so we didn't complain. I assumed we'd find out what we needed to know when we got to the clinic.

The next morning, several of us went to an early Mass and then returned to Our Father's House for a breakfast of bacon and eggs at a long dining room table. We ate at a leisurely pace, which was fine with me, since I still wasn't sure of our plans for the morning's activities.

The later we got to the clinic, the less likely it was that someone would go inside.

When we got to the clinic around eleven, there were sixty demonstrators outside and at least fifteen clinic personnel, guards, and escorts on the clinic grounds. Its doors were closed. They'd clearly taken precautions to ensure that no rescue could take place that day. The local pro-lifers and clinic staff seemed to know each other. There was a lot of conversation. The atmosphere was almost friendly. I was relieved to see that it was just going to be a picket.

As the pro-lifers marched and the pro-abortionists stood guard on the long porch, I walked up the steps of the side porch and tried the door to the waiting room. It was locked, and I was actually relieved that I couldn't get in. I turned toward the picket line and started a chant: "Life, yes! Abortion, no!"

Then I went back and joined the picket. In the meanwhile, John Burt, Joan Andrews, John's daughter and a friend went behind the clinic, came around the side, and waited. When someone came out the door that opened on the long porch, John, Joan, and the two girls all ran in front of the porch and rushed into the clinic through the open door.

Police arrived in minutes. Joan was arrested trying to pull the wires out of a suction machine. John Burt was arrested and later accused of assaulting clinic staff. The two girls with them were also arrested. A pro-life attorney at the protest, John Haring, tried to intervene with the police and was also arrested. He fought like a madman while being shoved into the squad car. Haring had been a POW in Vietnam and had been held in a tiger cage. He'd been severely claustrophobic ever since. He was one of the first released, but he stayed at the station to counsel John Burt and Joan Andrews, who were both held in custody. The two young women were released that afternoon.

John Ryan and I stayed in Pensacola for a couple of days, walked the white sandy beaches, and enjoyed some superb seafood before flying out from New Orleans. John Burt and Joan were still in jail.

What I didn't know was that after the protest, the clinic staff showed the police a picture of me on their porch and claimed I was behind the effort to get into the building. The Pensacola police looked for me for two days, then put out a warrant for my arrest. Somehow, some NOW members knew that I was on the national crime computer and, months later, notified the Denver police that I was coming to town for the NRLC convention. That was how I got arrested almost as soon as I arrived in Denver.

John Jakubczyk told me that Dr. Jack Willke offered to post a bond up to ten thousand dollars for my release. I've always appreciated that, but I didn't have to take him up on the offer. Jakubczyk and Onofrio got me out on my own recognizance. It took most of that Saturday, but by five that afternoon, I was released.

Those fourteen doors were unlocked one by one, and I walked outside to find 150 pro-lifers with hastily made signs and chanting, "Let Joe go!" Jack Ames had gone up and down the convention halls with his bullhorn, recruiting protesters to come to the jail. As I stepped outside, a loud cheer went up. It was a colorful welcome, but I hadn't slept or eaten in hours, so I thanked the crowd and headed back to the hotel.

They'd given me a meal in jail, but I didn't eat it. They let us out of our cells to sit around a large metal table where we could eat and talk about the crimes we didn't commit. I'll never forget the menu—tuna casserole and mashed potatoes—but there was another prisoner there who'd already wolfed down one meal and looked like he needed another, so I gave him mine. He was there on a murder charge.

For the time being, I wasn't allowed to leave Colorado. We had a host of activities planned for our Denver stay, including a rescue at Rocky Mountain Planned Parenthood and a picket of Warren

Hern's clinic in Boulder. At Rocky Mountain, a SWAT team came to drag rescuers away from the clinic. They were very aggressive, using pain compliance on protesters. When they came for one demonstrator, Dan Scalf, they broke his arm. You could hear the bone crack across the parking lot.

On our trip to Boulder to picket and pray at Hern's clinic, the Denver police followed our car. Each time we left one jurisdiction, police from the next jurisdiction were waiting to pick up the trail. They followed me all the way to Boulder and back to Denver. Detectives followed me on foot everywhere I went, even into the restaurant where I had lunch.

When we finally got back to Denver, I went before a judge. Jakubczyk and Onofrio had worked out a deal to allow me to return to Chicago on the understanding that I'd return to Denver later to be extradited to Florida to stand trial for burglary. When I got back to Chicago, I had to call Denver every day to see whether the extradition papers had come through.

In the meanwhile, I had to fly back to Delaware for my Wilmington trial. There were three judges who could have decided my case. The worst would have been the one that local pro-lifers nicknamed "the hanging judge." Of the other two, one was Catholic and the other Jewish. I was relieved when I was assigned to the Jewish judge. It might seem odd, but we'd learned that Catholic judges, in an effort to demonstrate their impartiality, usually doled out the harshest sentences to pro-lifers. I was found guilty on the trespassing charge but not harassment, and I had to pay a fifty-dollar fine plus seventy-five dollars in court costs.

At the end of the month, I called Denver, and Onofrio told me my extradition papers had come through and I had to be in Colorado the next day. Two bailiffs would accompany me on a flight to Pensacola.

"Couldn't we save Colorado some money and just have me fly directly to Florida?" I asked. Onofrio said he'd see if he could work it out with the judge. He called back to tell me I could, but that when I didn't show up in Denver they'd put out a warrant for my arrest. When I landed in Florida, I'd have to call Denver to have them cancel the warrant. So that saved me from going back to Denver to fly to Pensacola handcuffed in the middle seat between two bailiffs with a burglary charge hanging over me. That night I called a lawyer in Florida named Art Schimick. I'd never met him, but I knew his father. He agreed to take the case and said he'd meet me at the airport the next day.

I had no idea what was going to happen in Florida. Joan Andrews and John Burt were still in custody awaiting trials. I was told that if I were allowed to post bond, it would have to be in cash. I had no idea how much the bond might be, so I scraped together as much cash as I could from my own account and the League's and headed off to the airport with three thousand dollars in my wallet.

I was nervous carrying that much cash. I was nervous in general—it didn't help that the plane encountered turbulence the whole way. When I took out my wallet to recount the money, I pulled out a little pamphlet that I'd picked up in a church in San Antonio. It was called "Hail Mary." I read it there on the plane. It explained the prayer word for word and said that most of us rush through the line "Pray for us sinners, now and at the hour of our death." We all know we'll need prayers at our death, the pamphlet said, but we're also asking for prayers *now*. "You, dear reader," it continued, "may be in a situation where you need help *now*." How right they were—so I prayed, "Mary, I'm on my way to Pensacola, and I may be on my way to jail. Please, get me out of this mess."

When we landed, I was the last person off the plane. A young man approached me and asked, "Mr. Scheidler?"

"Yes?"

"I'm Art Schimick. I got you off."

"What?"

"I got you off, but you have to leave town right now, and do *not* talk to the press. I understand you have a talk to give in Houston tonight."

It was true. I hadn't canceled the Houston talk on the hope that my stay in Florida would be brief. I had a ticket for a later flight from Pensacola to Houston in my coat pocket.

"Well, there's a Delta flight leaving for Houston in a few minutes. If you can get on that plane, you're off the hook here. There's no time to explain everything right now. I've talked to your wife. Call her when you get to Houston—she'll tell you about it."

I walked to the counter and exchanged my ticket for the next flight. When I got to Houston, I called Ann and found out what happened. When I'd been in Pensacola for the sentencing of the Pensacola bombers, Matt's fiancée Kay Wiggins, and James's wife, Kathy, were also being sentenced for serving as lookouts and driving the getaway car. Each got five years' probation. They were free to go but had to pay one hundred dollars in court costs. Kathy had the money, but Kay didn't. Someone had recently given me a hundred-dollar bill. I still had it in my wallet, so I motioned Kay over to me and handed it to her.

After Matt went to prison, he and Kay broke up. Now she was dating a lawyer—Art Schimick. When he told her that he was representing me, she said, "Joe Scheidler? That's the guy who gave me the hundred-dollar bill! Get him off!"

Schimick knew that the local sheriff wouldn't want any more press about Pensacola and its problems with pro-lifers. So he alerted the media that I would be at the airport. Then he called the sheriff and told him about the impending media circus. The sheriff asked Schimick what he could do to avoid it, and they worked out a deal to drop the burglary charge against me on the condition that I catch a plane out of town and not return to Pensacola until after the sentencing of John Burt and Joan Andrews.

As I took my seat on that flight to Houston, I thought about my prayer on the previous flight. I'd always envied my brother Bob's strong devotion to the Blessed Mother. I'd always done the things that you're supposed to do to be close to Mary—say the rosary, meditate on her humility and her exaltation—but I never felt real closeness to the Mother of God. That day changed me. She'd heard my prayer directly, when I needed her most, and wrapped her mantle around me.

I'd written of my time in the Wilmington jail about how a prisoner can identify with the unborn child scheduled for termination. Now I felt the opposite sensation, feeling enclosed and protected by a Mother's love, a feeling every child should be able to enjoy. Ever since that day, I've felt a devotion to Mary that I never had before and a stronger conviction that my calling is to help make the womb a safe place for every baby.

If that was the purpose of the arrests, incarceration, trial, extradition—and the rescue—it was all worth it.

CHAPTER 21

# Go Forth and Teach

Chicago is known worldwide for the 1929 St. Valentine's Day Massacre, when seven mobsters were executed in a Lincoln Park garage allegedly on orders from Al Capone, who then seized control of Chicago's criminal underworld. But a far greater massacre was plotted in Chicago on St. Valentine's Day exactly forty years later, when a group of abortion advocates met at the Drake Hotel, just two miles south of the site of the notorious gangland slaying. They met to create NARAL. Millions would be massacred as a result of this 1969 meeting.

One of NARAL's founding members was Betty Friedan, author of *The Feminine Mystique*. In 1973, just months after the *Roe* decision was announced, Friedan met with Pope Paul VI, the author of *Humanae Vitae*, the 1968 encyclical that confirmed the Church's opposition to artificial birth control and correctly predicted the widespread moral decline ushered in by the contraceptive mentality. The pope congratulated Friedan on her work promoting women's rights, but after the meeting, Friedan told the press she'd challenged the Holy Father on the Church's position on abortion.

A year after I started working for the IRLC, I learned that Friedan was scheduled to speak at Mundelein College, where I'd taught and met Ann. I worried that she'd spin the pope's congratulations into an endorsement of abortion, so I went to her talk. I told the nuns I wasn't there to cause trouble. I just wanted to ensure that Friedan didn't use the forum to attack or ridicule the Church's moral teachings at a Catholic college. At that moment, Friedan came in and the nuns started greeting her, so I went up to her.

"I'll be in the front row during your talk," I told her. "If you say anything even remotely pro-abortion, I'll come up onstage and counter you." She ignored me and turned to the nuns. The stage wasn't very high, so if I had to make good on the promise, it wouldn't have been difficult.

I picked my seat in the front row. Friedan said some interesting things about the Church and the hierarchy, and not all of it was positive, but she did compliment Paul VI and never went near the subjects of abortion or contraception. That was a relief—I'd come on strong, but I didn't want to have to interrupt her.

College campuses were destined to become an important front in the abortion wars. As a legal, moral, ethical, scientific, and theological issue, it comes up in lecture halls all the time. But it's also true that many of those seeking abortions are students themselves. Before *Roe*, one of the best-known illegal abortion referral services was the Jane Collective, founded in 1969 by a University of Chicago student. So from my earliest days as an activist, I've worked to get the pro-life message out to college students.

About a month after Friedan's Mundelein talk, I visited another Catholic women's college. My assistant at the IRLC, Laura Canning, lived with her parents in north suburban Lake Forest, near the campus of Barat College, a Catholic women's college. Laura contacted the school and issued an invitation to the student body to attend a pro-life talk I would deliver at her house. Her family had a huge living room, and she'd set up chairs and ordered refreshments.

But nobody came. Finally, I went over to the campus and asked them to make an announcement about our presentation. It was after classes, and they allowed me to use the PA system in the academic building. I invited the students to come over to Laura's. I said that whatever their positions on abortion, I would answer their questions. I also mentioned the free food.

While I worked at Mundelein, it was often referred to as a girls' school. While I was on the PA at Barat, some students came down and sat on the stairs in front of the reception desk where I was speaking. "I know what you're thinking," I said into the PA. "I used to teach at a girls school, and—" That was it. The young women on the stairs started shouting me down. I'd called them girls, and now they refused to listen to anything I had to say. I went back to Laura's, and no one followed. It was just the two of us in that huge living room, with all that food.

That was an early lesson for me that the feminist rhetoric that helped lead to legal abortion had also cultivated a defensiveness among young women. If we wanted anyone to listen to us, we were going to have to be careful about the words we used.

Words matter. A college campus is one place where this should be most apparent. In 1982, a dozen activists and I attended the graduation ceremony at the Northwestern University Medical School. We had obtained a copy of their commencement program and had printed a version of our own. Both programs included the Hippocratic Oath, the pledge that medical students take, or at least used to take. Our version, true to the original, contained the line, "I will maintain the utmost respect for human life from the time of conception." Northwestern had cut the phrase, "from the time of conception." We put it back.

We handed out our programs to about a third of the graduates. When it came time to recite the oath, everyone proceeded in unison until they came to the amended line, at which point the recitation got garbled. Both graduates and attendees were curious why this happened and started looking at each other's copies. When they saw the two texts, they got the point, and we managed to make the subject of abortion a topic at that graduation.

Having done hundreds of talks and debates on college campuses, I have faced my own share of disruptions. Sometimes the opposition is very hostile, and sometimes it's surprisingly cordial, but in either case, I've managed at times to change some minds, or at least help those who support abortion as a right to better appreciate our perspective.

In the spring of 1990, I was scheduled to give a talk one evening in Fowler Hall, Purdue University's student union. A large sign had been set up in the lobby inviting pro-choice students to gather outside Fowler to protest my talk. It was a beautiful April day, so I decided to walk over to the lecture hall early. I ran into a few dozen protesters carrying picket signs. I introduced myself and invited them to attend my talk. I told them they'd have to leave their signs outside, but so would the pro-lifers.

There were about 150 students in the audience, and I said that despite our disagreements it was good we could be civil to each other. I related some of the stories of being interfered with and verbally attacked on other campuses. After my talk, I took some questions. Some of the opposition asked questions that revealed genuine interest. At the end of the evening, I received a standing ovation, and I noticed that some of the pro-abortion protesters were among those standing and applauding.

Among the incidents I recounted to those Purdue students was a trip I made to San Francisco 1985, just days after our Appleton PLAN convention. Energized by that meeting with an enthusiastic group of pro-lifers, I set out to deliver two talks in one day, the first at San Francisco State University and the second at Berkeley.

My aunt, Merle Pursley, lived in San Jose, and Ann and I stayed at her home. Aunt Merle wanted to hear my talk, so she drove us to the San Francisco State campus. The first sign that my talk was causing a stir was that police met us at the entrance to the campus and stayed close while we parked. When we got out of my aunt's Mercedes-Benz diesel, they walked with us through the campus to the performing arts building where I was to give my talk.

A crowd had gathered outside the performing arts building to protest. In the middle stood a massive eight-foot-tall papier-mâché pig. Its bearded face, a caricature of mine, wasn't exactly flattering. A sign around its neck read, "Joe Scheidler," and on the pig's other flank was another sign: "An American Hitler." It was mounted on a wheeled platform, and two students were pulling it around through the crowd.

When I got into the auditorium, it was nearly empty. The pro-abortion faction had torn down all the notices about my talk, and perhaps the hostilities outside the auditorium dissuaded interested students. Only a few professors, a handful of pro-life students, and my Aunt Merle listened to my forty-five-minute address. On my way out, the shouting resumed, and so did our police escort.

That evening, I gave a talk across town on the Berkeley campus. Someone had circulated flyers saying there would be people there with syringes of HIV-positive blood planning to stick people when they went in to attend the talk.

There was a large police presence on campus, most on motorcycles. Perhaps because of the syringe threat, the officers moved the protesters to either side of the entrance, then turned their motorcycles toward the building where I was speaking and kept their motors running. The idea was apparently to use their exhaust to keep the crowd away so nobody could follow through on the syringe threat. The venue was packed—the threat actually helped publicize the talk.

In 1984, while giving a talk on activism at the Camden County Right to Life convention in East Brunswick, New Jersey, I noticed a group of women in the front row furiously taking notes as I spoke. At the end of the talk, I got a standing ovation from everyone except the women in the front. Not long after, a colleague forwarded me a document from NOW. It was a report of the talk I'd given in outline form. It was so well done that I used that outline for the next several years whenever I gave a presentation on activism.

At one of my college talks, a group of pro-abortion feminists dressed in white robes doused themselves in red paint and laid down all around the podium while I spoke, each holding a cardboard gravestone that read, "Joe Scheidler Killed Me." When I spoke at the University of Florida in Gainesville in 1986, a small group of women sat in the front row as I spoke, holding up coat hangers and signs bearing "Keep Abortion Legal" and "My Body, My Choice." To my relief, they didn't shout their message, but at the end of the talk, they came up and dropped dozens of coat hangers on the floor around the podium.

"First time I've seen such mild-mannered pro-abortionists," I joked into the microphone. "You actually let me talk. Thanks—and thanks for the hangers."

Some time later, I learned that the coat hangers were supposed to have been woven into a wreath, but that it fell apart when they tried to give it to me. I found this out at a rescue in North Carolina led by Reverend Ed Martin—coincidentally, the same man who helped me get the speaking engagement in Gainesville. Some of the activists there started talking about how they came into the pro-life movement. "I was at the University of Florida, and I was a NOW activist," said a rescuer named Kathy Green. "Joe Scheidler came to give us a talk, and our group gave him a wreath of coat hangers. But while I was standing there holding a pro-choice sign, I couldn't help but think that he was making some sense. When I went home, I thought about it some more. Eventually, I decided I should be pro-life."

Probably the worst treatment I've ever had at a talk was in the spring of 1992 at Indiana University (IU) in Bloomington. Maybe one of the reasons the pro-abortion crowd was so hostile was that it was just weeks before the Supreme Court heard arguments in *Planned Parenthood v. Casey*, the first chance to reverse *Roe* since President Bush put Souter and Thomas on the court, replacing *Roe* votes Brennan and Marshall.

I spoke in a lecture room in Alumni Hall. It was laid out like a Greek theatre, with an elevated central area mostly surrounded by seats for the audience. About a hundred protesters crowded into the front and surrounded me. They screamed "Heil Hitler!" through the first half of my talk. I kept trying to speak, but they approached the podium to grab my notes. They stole a rare hardbound copy of Warren Hern's *Abortion Practice* right off the podium, then started spitting at me. Finally, one of them came up, jammed a finger down his throat, and vomited toward me. Vomit splashed all over the podium, but I jumped back and didn't get sprayed.

At the end of my talk, campus security—who stood by and watched all this—escorted me from the lecture hall to another room where I tried to do interviews with the press gathered there. The same group of angry students surrounded me and drowned out my efforts to talk with reporters. When I returned to Alumni Hall to take questions, the hecklers followed, shouting. Later that night I did interviews with the *Bloomington Voice* and *City News*. I stressed that the hecklers—despite their spit, vomit, and interference— hadn't prevented me from finishing my talk. A few months later, an IU student sent me a video tape of my talk, and the harassment looked worse than I remembered.

I wasn't surprised to find that my worst receptions were at secular colleges. The opposition at religious schools was far more cordial. My reception at public high schools was generally good. Sometimes a teacher or pro-life group coordinated these appearances, but over the years, I'd received calls from parents who were concerned that representatives from Planned Parenthood had been to their children's schools to advocate for birth control and promote the notion that abortion should be a guilt-free choice when contraception fails. I explained to them that these occasions offer an opportunity to invite a pro-life speaker, and I was frequently invited as a result.

Oddly, the most hostile crowd I faced when speaking at a high school was at a Catholic school. Colleen Kelly Mast, a teacher at Bishop MacNamara High in Kankakee, Illinois, invited me to address the student body in the gymnasium. I knew that some families had already withdrawn their children from the school due to concerns over heretical teachings and that more were considering it, so I felt I should take the opportunity to make sure the students there learned the Church's position on abortion.

The invitation incensed an English teacher there. He'd been teaching his classes that the pro-life position was unconstitutional. He taught at every grade level, and by the time I arrived at the gym, he had the students riled. Some started booing me even before I began, and after I started talking, more joined in. Finally, I stopped, expecting the booing to die away. It didn't. "I don't believe this is a Catholic school," I said. "You won't even allow a Catholic speaker to discuss the critical issue of abortion."

As I walked away from the microphone, the English teacher walked up and lowered it. "Mr. Scheidler is violating the Constitution!" he said. "All he talks about is life, but I'm talking about liberty and the pursuit of happiness!" The students cheered. Personally, I was glad he taught English and not Civics. The rights he mentioned are enumerated in the Declaration of Independence, not the Constitution. But his main error was failing to recognize that life was listed first because it is the most essential right. The rights to liberty and the pursuit of happiness can never outweigh the right to life.

## CHAPTER 22

# These Tactics of Yours

In 1982, NARAL board member Anne Gaylor, author of *Abortion Is a Blessing*, contacted the press to announce a fundraising campaign to pay for an abortion for a pregnant eleven-year-old Madison, Wisconsin, girl. Gaylor was further victimizing this poor child to use her as a poster child for the abortion rights movement, and I wasn't going to let her get away with it. I hired a private detective to find the girl and contacted the media telling them what we were doing.

He learned that the child was staying with her aunt in Chicago, in the Cabrini Green housing project. Several of us went to Cabrini and spoke with the girl's aunt. We never did meet the girl, but some weeks later, I talked with her mother, who told me the girl hadn't had the abortion.

The *New York Times* did a story on our use of a private detective. The story generated dozens of interviews, and while it may have made us look extreme to some, it generated discussion on how seriously pro-lifers take their mission to save the unborn. The *New York Times* is decidedly liberal-leaning and notoriously pro-abortion, and some people were shocked that I considered it a victory for them to do a story on us hiring a private eye to track down a pregnant child.

But I've always believed that the only bad press is no press. When pro-lifers say the media are the enemy, they forget that much of the information we receive comes through the media and that the media have helped keep the abortion issue alive for nearly five decades. We can take advantage of existing media, and we can produce our own.

When I left the IRLC and set up the FFL, I knew communication and education were key elements of our mission. We aired a Sunday morning radio show called *Back to Life*. I read the news, Father Charles Fiore spoke on abortion, and Tom Roeser discussed the political scene. Then we'd take phone calls. Guests on the show included Mother Teresa of Calcutta and Congressman Henry Hyde.

When we closed down *Back to Life*, we launched a TV program that aired on a local Christian station. We called it *Abortion: Exploding the Myths*. A good friend, Jerry Rose, ran a TV studio in the Chicago Lyric Opera House building, and he let us record our program there free of charge.

Local sportscaster Bill Berg was our MC. He was pro-life and very upbeat, and he kept the program moving. We covered the entire pro-life issue, showing pictures of fetal development and the results of abortion. We had several guests in our ninety-minute program. We borrowed six telephones from the phone company to use as props and had some young women pretending to answer calls and write down donations throughout the show. The night the program aired, we rented a bank of real telephones and had volunteers at the FFL office answering the real calls. We raised five thousand dollars and added two hundred new members.

*Exploding the Myths* aired on a Christian station, so we were reaching an audience that largely agreed with us. But there are many pro-lifers who oppose showing abortion victim photos, picketing doctors, and counseling at clinics. A show on a Christian station might convince some of these more conservative types of the value of activism, but it probably did not reach many abortion supporters.

And we have to reach that crowd. In my press releases, I always included my home phone number to make myself available for interviews. No matter how small a radio station might be or how late at night the program, I was always happy to have the airtime. A listener might be considering abortion, and presenting the case for the unborn could help save a life and save a mother or father from a lifetime of regret.

Early in 1984, I was contacted by Jane Chastain of American Portrait Films in California, who was working with Donald Smith on a film, *Conceived in Liberty*, about a young woman forced to have an abortion. The topic intrigued me. Abortion apologists stress that the issue is all about a woman's right to make her own choices, but anyone who has stood outside an abortion clinic for any length of time has seen pregnant women coerced into the clinic by boyfriends or parents.

I met the film crew outside the Michigan Avenue Medical Center in Chicago. They wanted to film the front of the building, but from enough of a distance that they wouldn't have to fuzz out the faces of the people going inside. We crossed over to Grant Park and filmed from there. As they filmed, I described one young woman I'd seen whose boyfriend had her in a hammerlock, twisting her arm painfully behind her back. But, I explained, most kinds of coercion are more subtle, like threatening to leave her if she chooses to have the baby.

Almost on cue, a couple came down Michigan Avenue to the clinic building. The young woman wore a red scarf, and she stopped in front of the revolving doors at 30 South Michigan. She hung back, but as we watched, the young man with her grabbed her by her scarf and pulled her into the revolving door. It was chilling.

This is why a key element of pro-life activism must always be outreach to women in trouble, women who think they have no options. Tangible, material help is essential. A crisis pregnancy center can be a nexus for a variety of crucial resources. If a woman needs a place to stay, those who see the value of the life she's nurturing will find her a place. Five chapters in *CLOSED* address things pro-lifers can do to help, including opening their own homes to pregnant women. Crisis counselors can help women find jobs. They can help provide women with the goods and services new mothers need—everything from prenatal care and counseling to diapers and bottles.

I'm happy to say that the Michigan Avenue Medical Center eventually closed down, as did several others in downtown Chicago. When they were in operation, we staged an annual parade the day before Mother's Day that visited about half a dozen clinics in downtown Chicago, three of which were on fashionable Michigan Avenue. Our theme was "Whatever Happened to Motherhood?" Marchers would place a single rose at the door of each clinic.

One year it rained on our procession. The march was led by a teenage boy carrying a white cross, flanked by two young girls carrying candles. Behind them four volunteers carried a white baby casket on a platform. A few dozen of us walked to the first clinic, said some prayers, and read a scripture passage. We fixed a rose to the clinic door, then moved on.

A reporter from the local CBS station, Mary Laney, came out with her cameraman to cover the procession. At the last clinic we visited, Arnold Bickham's Water Tower Clinic, Mary came up to me and complained that they weren't getting many visuals. She was right. We hadn't had any confrontations, and while we did go into one clinic to pray, we left as soon as we were ordered to leave. The cameraman had no chance to get any footage of us inside. As a news story, our protest didn't offer much. We were just a group of people walking in a light drizzle.

But I knew of a small park just a block east of Water Tower Place. I directed the procession over to the park, then hurried ahead and got to the park before the rest of the group arrived. It was still drizzling, and the place was deserted. The park had a metal carousel you could spin by hand, and I got it going as fast as I could. I went to the swing set and got all the swings moving. I pushed the little rocking horses on metal springs so they swung back and forth. It made for an eerie sight, all this playground equipment moving in the mist with nobody there. When Mary Laney and the cameraman came along, she saw the whole park in motion. She told her cameraman, "Get that!" He obliged, focusing on a lonely, empty swing swaying back and forth before panning back to capture the whole park.

"Where are our children?" I asked, standing at the park gate. "They've been killed by abortion. They should be playing here. There should be noise and laughter, but there is silence, and we only have their ghosts."

Then Mary asked something sincere and thoughtful. She almost whispered it. "Do you ever save any with these tactics of yours?"

While we were at the park, two women who'd been with our march were still at Bickham's clinic talking with a woman who had arrived there while we were putting the rose on the door. They'd dissuaded her from having the abortion and were making arrangements to help her. "We just saved one at that last clinic," I told Mary Laney. "Our counselors are there with her now."

That segment was their lead story on the evening news. They showed our march, the roses, the swings, and aired my comments about the dead children and the one we saved. It was powerful—this was good media coverage, and we hadn't planned it ahead of time.

While it's possible to reach women at clinics, when the abortion industry reaches out to recruit customers, pro-lifers need to do something to thwart their efforts. When clinics advertised on public transit, we set out to combat that initiative, and I based some chapters of *CLOSED* on our experiences. When the manual was finished, my editor sent the manuscript to a lawyer named Michael Woodruff to see whether any of the tactics included could get us sued. The first paragraph of the chapter "Remove Abortion Advertising" originally ended with the sentence, "It is imperative that pro-lifers do everything they can to counter such advertising, preferably by legal means."

The chapter went on to discuss how to contact the firm that owned the billboards or bus benches where the ads appeared, but Woodruff wrote back, "'Preferably by legal means' implies that the author would also advocate unlawful means if legal means fail to remove the clinic advertising."

Many activists were perfectly comfortable pulling down or painting over those ads, and Woodruff picked up on the implication that I had no problem with that. He was right. Regardless of what the courts have said or what ordinances local legislatures pass, an abortion clinic has no *moral* right to exist, and thus no moral right to advertise. Nevertheless, we followed Woodruff's advice and cut the phrase from that chapter.

The only part of the book that discussed illegal activity was the chapter on sit-ins, where I explained that the lawbreaking in question was excusable under the necessity defense. Still, we added a disclaimer at the front of the book that read, "Wherever there is any question regarding the legal right of any person potentially affected by anything stated or implied in this book, the reader should consult legal counsel."

In January of 1985, just before *CLOSED* went to press, our publisher decided to have an independent editor look over the final draft. When it came back in February, it was an absolute mess. The woman who did the editing had changed every "him" to "him/her," and the introduction had been rewritten in such a way that it totally missed my intent. As I went through the chapters, I found that some of my best examples of how to close down the abortion business had been scratched out.

There were some corrections where the original grammar or spelling had been improved, but for the most part, this editor had destroyed my book. Ann and I spent the next five nights working almost without sleep to get the book back as close as possible to its original form, to make it worthy of publication. We sent that version to the publisher, and when they sent back the proofs they'd done, it was the way we wanted it.

*CLOSED* was released in May 1985. The following year, NOW filed their lawsuit against me, trying to use the courts to silence opposition to abortion. In his letter, Michael Woodruff had written that he thought my position "philosophically inconsistent in condoning the elimination of pro-abortion advertising while complaining in another chapter when only the other side is presented." If anything, the federal lawsuit against pro-life activists proved my point that the abortion industry was adamant that only one side could be heard.

Eventually, I had to answer their charges in court. I've debated countless abortion supporters and always had answers for their arguments, but the court battle promised a different kind of debate entirely. The real issue—whether or not abortion was the deliberate taking of innocent life—was excluded from the arguments.

CHAPTER 23

# A Global Cause

Pro-life work has taken me all over the world. In 1985, one of my busier years, I logged enough miles to circle the globe ten times by plane and twice by car. While on a plane, I prefer to spend my time reading or watching the in-flight movie. When the passenger sitting next to me asks what I do for a living, I respond that I'm a writer, but if I'm asked what I write about, I have to confess that my issue is abortion and that I'm against it. The responses range anywhere from delight to abject horror.

On one flight, the woman next to me told me she was an attorney and asked what I did for a living. After I told her, she rang for a flight attendant.

"What can I get you?" the attendant asked.

"A different seat," she said. "I can't sit next to this man."

When the attendant told her all the seats were taken, I suggested she could stand. She replied with an icy stare. Finally, a friend of hers exchanged seats with her. Fortunately, the friend didn't ask about my job.

Such interactions aren't all bad, of course. Another time, I boarded a flight wearing a Life Rose, a small stick-on rose with the world "life" embroidered below it. It caught a flight attendant's attention. She told me that she and her husband were desperate to adopt, and she asked if she could talk to me about finding a mother who wanted to put her child up for adoption. She asked a standby attendant to take her place so we could sit and talk throughout the flight.

In 1985, Margaret Tighe, head of Right to Life Victoria, invited me on a two-week lecture tour of Australia and New Zealand in August, the dead of winter in the southern hemisphere. My hosts were also the Society for the Preservation of the Unborn Child (SPUC) and Christians for Life of Christchurch in New Zealand.

I started my stay in a cold, dark motel in Melbourne, but after a welcoming party in Margaret's cozy home with fireplaces in every room, I moved into Margaret's daughter's room. Her teenage daughter graciously moved to the pantry.

After a dozen TV and radio shows in Melbourne, I joined sixty demonstrators in front of a private retirement home that also served as an abortion clinic. Margaret and others went into the clinic and tried to talk to the women. Police removed dozens of protesters who had gone into the facility, but there were no arrests. SPUC's Father Eugene Ahern blessed the biological waste incinerator, and I gave a talk.

I visited Brisbane, Coolangata, and Sydney, holding press conferences, addressing activists, and picketing abortion clinics. We caused quite a stir on the Queensland-Victoria border. At the time, abortion was illegal in all but one territory, so the police were in a quandary as to how to keep us away from the clinics that were operating illegally.

Back in Melbourne, I joined a massive picket of Bert Wainer's clinic, where fifty protesters were confronted by a dozen guards, twenty police, and several television crews. The heroine of the picket was Heather McCormack who entered the clinic half a dozen times but escaped arrest.

In Adelaide, I went to the Queen Victoria Hospital with McCormack to speak to the hospital administrator and later to the Queen

Elizabeth hospital to do the same. Both hospitals did late-term abortions up to twenty-four weeks. After talks and interviews with media in Adelaide, we flew to Perth on the west coast of Australia for more protests and talks.

The two Beardsley brothers, Darryl and Warren, kept me from getting lost as I traversed in New Zealand. I spoke and protested in Christchurch and Auckland, always aware that while abortion was outlawed in all but one Australian territory, and in all of New Zealand, the law was simply not enforced, and thus those who fought abortion were the ones treated as criminals, not the ones who did the abortions.

In the spring of 1987, I got a call from Notre Dame law professor Dr. Charles Rice. The Republic of Ireland was considering ratifying the Single European Act (SEA), and he wanted my help. I wondered what I could do, as I had very little knowledge of the SEA.

The concern over the SEA was that ten of the eleven countries that had already ratified it had legal abortion. Only Belgium didn't, but they were only a few years away from adopting it.

Once a nation adopts legal abortion, it's almost impossible to vote it out. Ratifying the SEA, which required economic cooperation on a number of issues, including health care, could become a gateway for legalized abortion in Ireland. An Irish pro-life group invited Dr. Rice to help impress on the Irish clergy and the population at large the dangers of ratifying the SEA. But he had other commitments and asked me to go in his place.

There was no way I could replace Dr. Rice, but I promised I'd give it the old college try. I flew to Dublin that May and stayed at the home of Youth Defense founders Una and Seamus Nic Mhatúna. During my stay, I traveled all over Ireland with Mike O'Connor and spent several nights at his home. I did dozens of radio shows, often from tiny unofficial stations with studios hidden in the upper room of a hardware store or in the back of a bakery or a pharmacist's basement. The night before I left, I visited the ruins of a Cistercian abbey with Mike's wife and two children.

By the end of the trip, I probably knew as much about the SEA as any member of the Irish Parliament. In a way, the trip was a failure in that the Irish Parliament ratified the SEA. On the other hand, the predicted legalization of abortion did not follow, so our efforts to publicize the need to keep abortion out of Ireland helped, for the time being.

When Ireland won its independence from Britain after the First World War, the more heavily Protestant areas in the northern part of the island, where English settlers or their descendants lived, remained part of Great Britain. Off and on again for the rest of the twentieth century, Catholics in Northern Ireland waged a guerilla war against foreign—and Protestant—control.

When the British Parliament legalized abortion through twenty-eight weeks gestation, a clause in the Abortion Act of 1967 exempted Northern Ireland. In the late 1990s, another legal initiative pushed to extend the act to the island. The pro-lifer who did the most to keep abortion out of Northern Ireland was Bernadette Smyth, the tireless and dedicated activist who founded Precious Life in 1997. In 1999, she invited me and other American pro-lifers to come to Belfast and help with her campaign.

Pastor Ed Martin, Joan Appleton, Mark Bomchill, and I flew into Dublin to join Youth Defense rallies before renting a car and driving north to Belfast. By this time, I'd been officially declared a racketeer, and those venturing to push abortion in Northern Ireland tried to make an issue out of a Chicago "gangster" coming to train Irish pro-lifers.

When we arrived, the press gave the Americans a lot of attention. Some Youth Defense members thought we were upstaging them when they were protesting at the office of Bertie Ahern, the Taoiseach (Irish prime minister) at the time. They asked me to make myself scarce, so I walked across the street to a pub. I struck up a conversation with some men at the bar, and we got along just fine. As the demonstration ended, the bartender looked out the window.

"Looks like they're leaving, Bertie," he said. "You can go back to your office now."

Back in Dublin, we spent the night at a bed-and-breakfast. There we met a stately elderly woman named Margaret Mary Doyle Dane, who was visiting a friend at the bed-and-breakfast. She started talking with us and asked if I was Catholic.

"Of course," I said. I asked her if she knew of a nearby church.

"I'm going to Mass right now," she said. "Why don't you come with me?"

So Ed and I went along. Ed didn't have the heart to tell her he was Protestant. He stood, sat, and knelt on cue and even made the sign of the cross. But after Mass, Margaret Mary Doyle Dane asked Ed why he hadn't gone to communion.

Ed paused. Then an answer came to him. "I haven't been to confession."

The next day, we headed back to Belfast, where we were to meet Bernadette Smyth at the Europa Hotel. She was waiting in the lobby with some friends, and when we came in, she rushed over. "I recognize you from the cover of your book," she said. "I was so impressed when I read it that I wanted to meet you."

She took us to the restaurant off the lobby, and we shared a lively conversation. I had an interview scheduled at the BBC, but I still had my bags with me, so Pastor Ed stayed behind and watched my bags in the restaurant while Bernie took me over to the studio. On the way, she told me that the Europa Hotel, where we had just eaten, is known as the most bombed hotel in the world. In the course of the Irish Troubles, it had been bombed more than a dozen times.

While I was doing the BBC interview, some reporters came into the Europa. "Where's this Joe Scheidler?" one asked. Pastor Ed told them I was at the BBC but would be back soon.

"Who are you?" they asked.

"I'm the Reverend Ed Martin," he answered.

"You're Protestant."

"That's right."

"This Catholic Scheidler's got a Protestant minister to watch his bags for him? Who is this guy?"

That's the way Ed told it, anyway. It might even be true.

A few years later, I returned to Ireland. Bernadette's campaign to defeat the Abortion Act didn't end there. Though no clinics opened in Northern Ireland, referral agencies arranging for Irish women to have their abortions in Britain were still active. There were once fourteen such agencies, but thanks to Bernadette and Precious Life, they were down to one.

Precious Life had arranged for me to give an address, and the event was an impressive one. Onstage with me were representatives of all the political parties, people who would never have shared a stage in the past, all united in the cause of life. Bernadette had done her job well.

After my talk, Ed Martin and I got a tour of Northern Ireland from a pro-lifer named Ned. We passed through a forest where St. Patrick was said to have spent so long preaching that his walking stick took root and became a living tree. We drove past abandoned huts and other ruins and came out at an amazing collection of volcanic crystals, huge hexagonal rocks jutting out into the Irish Sea. They call it the Giant's Causeway, named for the legends about giants using them as stepping-stones to pass between Ireland and Scotland.

But the weather was miserably cold and rainy. "I'd love to sit by a fire and have some Irish stew," I told Ned.

"I know just the place," he said. Minutes later, we were all in a cozy pub sitting beside a coal-burning stove enjoying a delicious Irish stew. The next day, I flew back to Chicago. About a week later, I got a phone call from Bernie Smyth. Ned had been carrying a large banner honoring the Blessed Virgin during a procession on the feast of the Immaculate Conception when he collapsed from a heart attack and died. A day or two later, I got a postcard from Ned, with a drawing of a beautiful castle on it. He wrote to say that he'd really enjoyed spending the day with Ed and me. He'd told his friends how proud he was to have taken the American pro-lifers on a tour of Ireland.

Every so often when I see pictures of Ireland, particularly pictures of ruins, I think of Ned and remember a story he told me on our tour about a day in his youth.

"There were about six of us," he told us. "We went into this old castle. It was hardly a ruins at all—it was in real good shape. We all had torches, and we snuck in and went looking around. Then we noticed one of our group was missing. We started looking around for him. We were all scared. We couldn't imagine what had happened to him—then he jumped out and spooked us. All of us dropped our torches and ran out as fast as we could. In a short time, the castle was gone. We'd burned it down."

What are the odds? There I was, the American pro-lifer accused of racketeering, under suspicion of encouraging burnings and bombings, just taking a short vacation in the Irish countryside with a nice elderly gentleman—and he turns out to be an arsonist!

On a trip to France in 1990, I met with Dr. Jérôme Lejeune, who discovered the extra chromosome that accounts for Down syndrome. He hoped for a cure for the condition, but he was horrified when his method started being used to abort babies likely to be born with Down syndrome. He became an outspoken pro-lifer.

Ann and I had dinner with Dr. Lejeune and his wife, Birthe, in their fifteenth-century home on the Rue Galande in Paris. He told us about his teenage years during the Nazi occupation of France. Our discussion was so engaging that Madame Lejeune let the dessert burn. During our visit, Dr. Lejeune spent a half hour on the phone with a reporter from the United States, about testimony he had given in a trial in Tennessee that involved the custody of frozen embryos. It was an exciting evening. As we were leaving the apartment, Dr. Lejeune described a notorious sword fight that had taken place on the stairway of his building four centuries earlier.

During our stay in Paris, we met with several pro-life activists. Ann was conversant in French, and she was invited to return the following October for a conference. At the conference, she met Patrick Bray, an activist from Tours, whose occupation was teaching English. Bray was excited about *CLOSED* and offered to translate it into French. Years later, on a pilgrimage to Lourdes, we walked into a book store and discovered *CLOSED, 99 façons de faire cesser l'avortement*. In 2011, my son Eric traveled to Belgium for a March for Life in Brussels, where he met a local pro-life activist who proudly pulled a French copy of *CLOSED* off his shelf.

I spent New Year's Eve 1992 in Moscow, Russia. With me was Bill Grutzmacher of the Chicago Nativity Scene Committee, who once complained to me that it'd be easier to put up a crèche in Red Square than in Chicago's Daley Plaza. My main interest was meeting with as many Russian pro-lifers as possible, to see what we had in common and find out how we could help each other.

Dr. Igor Ivanovich Guzov, the founder of the Russian group Support for Motherhood Association, met me at Sheremetyevo Airport and took me to a New Year's Eve party at the home of Serge Markus, a Moscow pro-life leader. My hotel, the Moskva, was a fifteen-minute walk from the only active Roman Catholic church in Moscow, St. Louis of France on Lubyaka Street. There were three daily Masses, one in Latin and two in Russian. I attended daily Mass within the shadow of the KGB headquarters.

I visited the Kremlin, where President George Bush was signing the Strategic Arms Reduction Treaty with then Russian president Boris Yeltsin. Later I took a train to Zagorsk, seventy miles from Moscow, to visit the monastery city.

I asked Dr. Guzov to write a column for my *Action News*, and he presented the work his Support for Motherhood Association was doing and their outreach to various pro-life groups in other countries. I invited him to the United States to speak to activists in Chicago.

In September 1995, Father Paul Marx of Human Life International invited me to accompany him on a trip to South Africa. Our four-man team included Reverend Johnny Hunter, an African American pro-life activist, and Brian Clowes, Father Marx's right-hand man. Our goal was to help defeat an abortion bill that had just been introduced into the South African parliament by a hostile government. Although South Africans opposed the bill 99.7 to 0.3 percent, the parliament was determined to pass it. The bill had draconian penalties for anyone who tried to thwart it, including doctors who would face long jail terms if they refused to refer for abortions.

Our host, Dr. Claude Newbury, met us in Cape Town and drove us to a convent of Visitation Nuns in Johannesburg who cared for the elderly and infants dying of AIDS. This was our home during our visit to Cape Town. We all gave talks and visited colleges and seminaries throughout South Africa.

Later, while staying with Dr. Newbury in Johannesburg, we debated a group of NOW members before nearly a thousand university students in Soweto, the vast majority of whom were pro-life. We did radio shows from underground studios whose owners were hiding from the authorities. We painted a fifty-foot sign on a graffiti wall with four-foot red letters that called abortion murder, and we included a phone number callers could use to voice their support for pro-life legislation.

It was obvious that South Africa was suffering. Crime was soaring. High walls, barbed wire, and locked gates spoke of fear and concern. Buildings sat empty, monuments tumbled, poverty abounded—but the pro-life message still resonated in people's hearts.

One thing was perfectly clear to me as I traveled the globe. The battle to maintain respect for human life is worldwide, and pro-lifers everywhere are members of a universal family.

## CHAPTER 24

# Sacrilege

Lawrence Lader, organizer of the fateful meeting at Chicago's Drake Hotel that produced NARAL, hosted a lunch in September 1966 with Reverend Howard Moody of the Judson Memorial Church in Greenwich Village and two other New York ministers to found the Clergy Consultation Service (CCS). The CCS was a network of clerics willing to counsel women on the theological and moral dimensions of abortion. In reality, it functioned as a referral service for illegal abortions. "As clergy," Moody explained in his 1973 book *Abortion Counseling and Social Change*, "we were bound to follow a higher moral law."

Lader wanted the group to operate in the open to prompt public debate on legalizing abortion. If religious leaders found abortion morally acceptable, he reasoned, it would be easier to do away with legal restrictions. He got the CCS featured prominently in Jane Brody's 1968 *New York Times* article "Abortion: Once a Whispered Problem, Now a Public Debate."

The same year the CCS started in New York, a similar group formed in Chicago: the Illinois Citizens for the Medical Control of Abortion. Its offices were in the First Unitarian Church in

Hyde Park. Don Shaw, an Episcopal minister, headed the organization, and later Reverend E. Spencer Parsons, dean of the Rockefeller Chapel at the University of Chicago, took over its leadership.

In 1967, the CCS teamed up with Planned Parenthood to produce a film, *Each Child Loved*, to advocate for legal abortion. CBS's *60 Minutes* aired the film in 1972. In it, a young woman goes to see her pastor, who assures her that having her child killed is the moral thing to do. God wants her to be happy, after all. After her abortion, she feels peace and contentment with her decision, while "Amazing Grace" plays in the background. It was a heavenly grace, the CCS implied, to be able to have an abortion. *Each Child Loved* was the first film I saw that used religion to justify abortion.[1]

The same year *Each Child Loved* was produced, the Jane Collective established itself at the University of Chicago to help women get legal abortions. Reverend E. Spencer Parsons worked closely with them. When New York legalized abortion with no residency requirement in 1970, the CCS chapters began specializing in interstate commerce. Local chapters arranged travel and accommodations for women to obtain legal abortions in New York. At the same time, the Janes, despite having no surgical training, started doing abortions themselves for women who couldn't afford to travel.

After *Roe*, the Janes disbanded, but Parsons remained active and helped found the Religious Coalition for Abortion Rights (RCAR). One of his motivations for creating RCAR was the US Conference of Catholic Bishops's strong condemnation of *Roe v. Wade*.

In May 1974, I invited Reverend Don Shaw to lunch. Shaw directed the Midwest Population Center, a clinic near the Chicago

---

1    *Each Child Loved*, an Airline Production televised on *60 Minutes*, CBS, May 14, 1972.

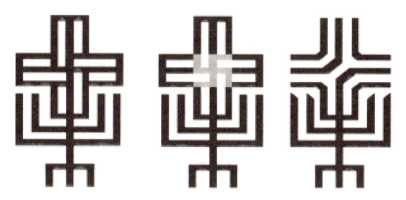

RCAR logos. Their initial logo is at the left. We highlighted the central swastika in red during our 1985 "Nuremburg Tribunal." Shortly afterward, they redesigned their graphic to the one on the right.

Gold Coast that specialized in vasectomies before *Roe* and abortions after the ruling. I'd met with abortionists who acknowledged that abortion ends a human life but justified their role by rationalizing that at least the abortion was a safe one. Shaw, however, viewed his role as an act of charity. He saw abortion as a *gift*. I also invited Reverend Parsons to lunch, and I got a similar impression—for him, the right to choose was practically a religious rite.

On the sixth anniversary of *Roe v. Wade*, RCAR hosted an Interfaith Celebration for Choice at a Lutheran church in downtown Chicago. "What do we celebrate in a woman's right to choose?" the leader asked the congregation. They delivered the response as one: "We celebrate her individual relationship to God."

"What do we express in celebrating her right to choose?"

"The hope that every child will one day be conceived in trust and love, and be nurtured as a uniquely wanted being."

In 1983, Dr. Marjorie Maguire, a Catholic theologian and a member of Catholics for a Free Choice, said that personhood begins when the mother "accepts the pregnancy." The remark was delivered at the NAF conference in New Orleans. Maguire

delivered her theory of personhood to a room full of abortionists in the business of rationalizing late-term abortions, especially
those in cases where amniocentesis indicated birth defects. In many
of those cases, the mother initially approved the pregnancy, only to
change her mind after the amniocentesis. In Maguire's theory, personhood was a condition that could be conferred *and withdrawn*
at the mother's whim.

In 1978, the Chicago Association of Catholic Priests decided to
confer a Humanitarian Award on Dr. Quentin Young, the Chairman of Medicine at Cook County Hospital. They honored him for
his promotion of quality medical services to the poor and neglected.
We'd already talked to Board President George Dunne about halting taxpayer-funded abortions at Cook County, but at that time, he
wasn't having much luck changing the hospital's policy—it would
take two more years to accomplish that. Quentin Young was one of
those opposing Dunne's efforts.

I'd debated Young on Warner Saunders's television program
*Common Ground*, where he vigorously defended taxpayer-funded
abortions. Pro-lifers were disappointed that an association of priests
would confer a humanitarian award on a staunch abortion advocate.
We knew they weren't honoring him for his position on abortion,
but we ultimately decided to picket the event, which was held at the
archdiocesan minor seminary in Niles, Illinois.

That February night was bitterly cold, and people arriving faced
seventy-five protesters lining both sides of the seminary driveway. I
had a bullhorn with a shoulder strap and a microphone attached to
the bell by a long cord. We brought a portable cassette player, and I
used the bullhorn to amplify a recording of the Mass of the Dead as
the guests arrived: "Requiem aeternam dona eis Domine"—"eternal
rest grant unto them, O Lord."

After all the guests arrived, Father Charles Fiore and I went in
to talk to the Association of Catholic Priests leaders. We explained

to the organizers that, since they were honoring an abortion advocate, we should get equal time to explain that their honoree opposed
Church teaching. They refused. I still had my bullhorn over my
shoulder, and while we were talking, I accidentally hit the button
on the microphone, which caused a loud feedback squeal. The organizers must have thought I was threatening to disrupt their event,
because they immediately changed their minds and agreed to give
Father Fiore two minutes on the dais.

Father Fiore's talk was a very thorough explanation of why an
abortion supporter should never receive a humanitarian award from
a group of Catholic priests. When he finished, one of the leaders of
the association invited us to a side room for coffee. He thanked us
for pointing out the importance of looking into a potential honoree's abortion positions beforehand.

In January 1982, I learned that RCAR was planning a religious
service at the New York Avenue Presbyterian Church in Washington, DC. I made a banner that read, "sacrilege" in large red letters.
The morning of the event, several pro-lifers from Chicago flying out
to DC for the March for Life made plans on the plane to disrupt
the service. There were nine of us all together. Rich Freeman would
sneak my banner in under his coat. I'd meet him and Greg Morrow
at a side aisle, enter the sanctuary, and unfurl the banner. The others
would infiltrate the crowd and stand in support of the pro-life cause
when we reached the sanctuary. We knew we'd be risking arrest.

Rich, Greg, and I got to the church just as the ceremony began.
We joined the congregation. As we went in, we noticed bundles of
green and white balloons tied to coat racks at the back of the church.

The pastor, Arthur McKay, opened the service. "Rejoice," he proclaimed, "for you are called to freedom. You are called to sanctify
life. You are called to decision. Rejoice in the freedom to transcend
ourselves through our ethical choices. Rejoice, for you are called to
translate your beliefs into deeds and actions."

We were planning to wait for Episcopal Bishop Brook Mosely's sermon to go into the sanctuary with our banner. But after Pastor McKay spoke, the B'nai B'rith Women, the YWCA, and Catholics for a Free Choice all presented "evidence" from scripture to show that God is pro-abortion. Goldie Kweller of the Women's League for Conservative Judaism quoted Genesis from the pulpit: "Let us make mankind in our image, in our likeness, so that they may rule over the fish in the sea and the birds in the sky, over the livestock and all the wild animals, and over all the creatures that move along the ground." When she said that we also have dominion over children, suggesting that the right to abortion was conferred in Genesis, I knew I couldn't sit through any more of this blasphemy.

I signaled Greg and Rich, and we took out the banner, walked into the sanctuary, and unfurled it. A woman in the sanctuary leapt up and tried to grab the sign, but we were all six foot four, and it was too high for her to reach. She jumped repeatedly, but she couldn't touch it. Several others in the sanctuary joined her effort. They couldn't reach it either.

"This is not a house of God," I said, and put on my hat. "But to make this a religious ceremony, we'll recite the Lord's Prayer."

We started the Our Father and walked down the aisle with the banner. Dr. John Hackett and his wife, Mary Anne, stood and joined our prayer, as did Rosie Stokes, Jack Ames, and the other pro-lifers scattered throughout the crowd. Their presence subdued the congregation, and nobody else tried to grab for the banner until we reached the back of the church. Someone finally caught it, and we lost the tug-of-war. We were right next to the green and white balloons, so we untied them. As they ascended to the rafters, we left the church, where we ran into some police coming up the steps. "Hurry!" I said. "It's chaos in there!" We slipped around the corner and rushed over to join the opening ceremonies of the March for Life.

NBC and some cable affiliates had some cameras at the RCAR service, and that night, the only coverage of the "Rejoice for Choice" ceremony was our "sacrilege" banner. Our plan had worked. We'd snatched their media coverage. Some of those interviewed complained that our disruption was "shameful," but later I answered that critique in my newsletter. "The 'Chicago Nine,'" I wrote, "entered the New York Avenue Presbyterian Church in the spirit of Christ entering the temple to drive out those who were desecrating it."

Two weeks later, workers from a storage supply company arrived at a California pathology lab to repossess a container that the lab was using to store aborted babies. The lab's check had bounced, and the workers opened the container before hauling it away. Inside, they found the bodies of aborted infants, some as old as thirty weeks. At first, news reports said that about five hundred bodies had been found. Within weeks, the estimate was in the thousands. The supply company turned the container over to the LA County medical examiner. The final count was 16,431. Two hundred were older than twenty weeks.

Pro-life groups asked permission of the medical examiner's office to hold a burial service for the children, but the ACLU and the Feminist Women's Health Center filed a lawsuit to block the service. Pat Boone recorded a song called "Sixteen Thousand Faces" that played at a memorial service for the children in May 1985. Finally, that October, they were buried at the Odd Fellows Cemetery outside Los Angeles.

Early in 1983, I learned that Auxiliary Bishop George Wirz of the Diocese of Madison, Wisconsin, was going to honor the new Wisconsin governor, Anthony Earl, at a Mass at St. Raphael's Cathedral. Earl had all the earmarks of a good practicing Catholic, but during his campaign, he'd promised NOW that he would support state funding of abortion in Wisconsin. Two years later, the Supreme Court upheld the Hyde Amendment, cutting off federal funding for abortion, and pro-abortion factions pushed to secure funding at the state level.

Father Charles Fiore was from Madison. He organized a large picket at St. Raphael's with the help of Albin Rhomberg of Catholics Concerned for Life, who placed full-page ads in papers throughout the state. "Persons of goodwill," they read, "who wish to protect the lives of our prenatal brothers and sisters are urged to express their indignation at Tony Earl's pro-prenatal-killing policies."

Rich Freeman and I made a banner that read, "Bishop Backs Baby Butchers." We drove up to the protest to find that Albin's ad brought out nearly a hundred protesters holding graphic images of aborted babies and signs that read, "Sacrilege in the Cathedral." Before the Mass, we chanted, "Life Yes, Earl No" as people filed into the church, but we didn't protest during the Mass.

Afterward, Governor Earl came out of the cathedral with his wife and two daughters. "We're sorry to have to do this," Father Fiore said. "We know it's embarrassing, but abortion is such a critical issue that after the stance you took in the campaign, we had to have a presence here."

"I understand," Earl said.

It's unsettling to protest at a church. As a Catholic, I can't help but remember the dire consequences of Martin Luther's 1517 protest at All Saints Church in Wittenberg that launched the Reformation. The mainline religions that resulted from his departure from the Church—Lutherans, Methodists, Presbyterians, Episcopalians, and most of their offshoots—almost all officially permit abortion. We pray that our protests at churches don't drive pro-lifers away from our cause. But sometimes it has to be done.

Why are so many pro-life leaders Catholic? It's not a coincidence. Catholics, I think, are more accustomed to believing in something they cannot see. During the Reformation, the Real Presence of Christ in the Eucharist was disputed. Most strains of Protestantism rejected the Divine Presence in the communion host. Catholicism didn't and never has. It takes a far greater leap of faith to trust that what appears to be a mere wafer contains the Divine nature than it does to trust that a human embryo has a human nature, and so Catholics are less disposed to disregard centuries of teaching on the sanctity of unborn human life.

Catholics also revere the mother of Jesus more than most Protestants do. One of the first prayers Catholics learn is the Hail Mary, which names as blessed "the fruit of thy womb, Jesus." Jesus' human body acquired its divine nature at his conception. The Incarnation, rightly, is not celebrated at Christmas but nine months earlier, on March 25, the Feast of the Annunciation. During the Middle Ages, the Annunciation was a more solemn feast than Christmas.

This isn't to say that the pro-life movement is, or should be, a purely Catholic one. Many non-Catholics of varying faith traditions respect the sanctity of life. And there are secular and even atheist pro-life organizations.

But in general, the commitment to upholding the sanctity of life correlates to a basic acceptance of Divine authority. Catholics accept that the authors of the Holy Scriptures were divinely inspired and that the Church, established directly by Jesus, has the authority to *proclaim* its meaning but not to *change* it. Evangelical Christians also believe in a divinely inspired Scripture that is not open to modification.

The sanctity of unborn human life is proclaimed throughout the Bible, and it's not for men to decide that verses like Jeremiah 1:5—"Before I formed you in the womb, I knew you"—are irrelevant. But many Protestant denominations follow a tradition where a congregational majority determines the content of the moral law. In the United States, the first of the main religious denominations to proclaim that abortion was an individual right was the Unitarian Universalists in 1963.

In 1984, I spoke to a Unitarian Universalist congregation in Chicago. I knew very little about that denomination at the time, though I knew that the name "Unitarian" indicated a rejection of the Trinity, and I knew Bill Baird was a Unitarian. In our debates, I'd learned that his god was basically indifferent to what people did.

It was Sunday. I went to an early Mass and then to the restaurant where the Universalists met. I asked the person who had arranged for my talk at what point in the service I should speak. He told me, "You *are* the service." It seemed to me that simply inviting in a guest speaker—no prayers, no hymns—was a poor excuse for a liturgy.

I set up my slide projector and screen and showed both pictures of fetal development and graphic pictures of babies killed by abortion. During the question period, a young man asked, "Do you ever eat hamburgers?"

"Yes, I do," I answered. "In fact, I'm going to have one for lunch in a little while."

"Then you're not pro-life. A cow has to be killed for you to have a burger."

"There's a great deal of difference between a cow and a person," I replied. "A human being lasts for eternity. A cow's existence has an end. Plus, God gave us dominion over the animals."

He wasn't impressed. The next question came from a young woman. "How do you know there *is* a god? Has he ever spoken to you?"

"Yes," I answered. "Through the scriptures." She was equally unimpressed.

It was a deeply negative experience. I'd gone hoping to explain why a tiny single-celled human being is of more importance than the whole universe, but there was simply no common ground for a meaningful discussion. I was a poor "service."

Even more discouraging was when the mother of a Catholic seminarian came to see me about the moral theology her son was being taught in the seminary. He said his class had been assigned a book by Father John Dedek, entitled *Human Life: Some Moral Issues*. Father Dedek wrote, "Taking lethal action against what is only probably (and therefore doubtfully) a human person does not necessarily represent conditional intent to murder. I would judge that the only sufficient reason would be to save the life of the mother, or, what I would think equivalent, her mental sanity. To be concrete, I would think that such circumstances as rape or even grave socioeconomic conditions could justify an abortion."

Of later-term abortions, Dedek wrote, "As the likelihood increases that the conceptus is in fact an innocent person with full human rights, the reason for attacking it would have to be more serious. Only very serious reasons, such as grave danger to the physical or mental health of the mother, or some very serious physical or mental deformity of the child could justify an abortion during that time, since there is increasing probability that the fetus is by that time significantly and fully human."[2] None of this, of course, was consistent with the Church's teaching on the sanctity of human life.

At the time, Father Dedek served as pastor of St. Julian Eymard Parish in Elk Grove Village, Illinois. I went with a friend to talk with him about his book.

We met in the sacristy. Father Dedek asked us to call him "Sam," a nickname he'd earned in the seminary for his resemblance to Humphrey Bogart's character Sam Spade in *The Maltese Falcon*. He stood very frankly behind what he'd written, and our conversation turned into an argument. A bell rang. Father Sam said, "You'll have to excuse me. It's time for me to hear confessions." On our way out of the church, I mentioned to my friend that I'd forgotten we were talking to a Catholic priest—it felt more like a conversation with an abortionist. My friend had the same feeling. Clergy who accept a pro-abortion theology preach a gospel of convenience and disposability, a gospel without Christ's wounds.

---

2      John Dedek, *Human Life: Some Moral Issues* (New York: Sheed & Ward, 1972), 88.

In Scripture, Jesus is known by his wounds. In Luke 24:39, Jesus identifies Himself by His wounds: "See my hands and my feet, that it is I myself." And he instructed his followers to "take up your cross and follow me." He never said it would be easy. A problem pregnancy may indeed be a problem, but it is not a catastrophe. If Christ was known by his wounds, then to be Christlike, we must also bear wounds. Clergy who counsel women that they can have their children, their "problems," simply aborted are not shepherding their flocks—they are misleading them.

Unfortunately, pro-life activists have had to picket at many churches over the years. In January 1991, I joined a picket in front of the Cathedral of the Blessed Sacrament in Sacramento, California. Pro-abortion politician Pete Wilson had just won the governor's race there and was to be honored by Bishop Francis Quinn in a special ceremony that was replacing the time usually set aside for Sunday Mass. During his campaign, Wilson had pledged to appoint a pro-abortionist to fill the state senate seat he was vacating.

When Albin Rhomberg alerted me to this planned ceremony, we began the usual protocol of letters and phone calls, trying to block the event. When I called the Chancery and spoke with a Monsignor, he told me he was also unhappy at having the cathedral used to honor a pro-abortion politician. He had tried to block the event but had been overruled.

The night before the protest, I flew to Sacramento. I stayed with Dr. Jack Hockel and his wife, Judie. That night, we stayed up late painting a banner with "sacrilege" in large red letters, and the next morning, we drove to the cathedral, where we got four "golden tickets," which put us just across the aisle from the governor. While a group picketed in front of the cathedral, we took our places inside.

Police soon arrested all of the picketers outside, holding them in a police van. Apparently, the police were waiting to see if there would be more arrests before pulling away. At the point in the ceremony where prayers were offered for governor-elect Wilson, I stood up and said, "Let us pray that Governor Wilson recant his pro-abortion position, which has rendered this ceremony a sacrilege." Then I reached into my coat and pulled out the banner. I handed the corner to Judie Hockel and we started unfurling it.

Security descended on us from all sides. They yanked the banner out of our hands and dragged me from the pew. They left Judie alone, but I was hauled to the police van where a cheer went up from the prisoners inside.

When the ceremony ended, I noticed through the small window in the back of the van that Bishop Quinn was coming toward us. It made me glad that he would want to talk to us, and I prepared to greet him. But then some of my fellow prisoners shouted "Judas!" and he turned away.

We were taken to the station and booked. We considered our protest a success, since we'd brought the abortion controversy into the ceremony. When I got back to Chicago and discussed the arrest with my lawyer, he advised me to sue the state of California for violating my rights to attend a service in a Catholic cathedral. I took his advice. Two and a half years later, I had to go back to Sacramento for a deposition. In the end, the court recognized that arresting me for disrupting a prayer service violated my civil rights, and I won a thousand-dollar settlement.

*Roe* had been decided by three Presbyterians, two Episcopalians, a Methodist, and a Catholic. When that Catholic, Justice William Brennan, died in July 1997, his funeral was held at the Cathedral of St. Matthew in Washington, DC. I met with a group of activists in DC the weekend before the funeral, and we went to the noon Mass at St. Matthew's. Afterward, several of us went to the sacristy to talk with the celebrant.

"You're aware that Justice Brennan's funeral is going to be held here in a few days?" I asked.

"Yes, I know," he said, "and I think it's probably a violation of Church law. Justice Brennan almost certainly excommunicated himself with that abortion decision. But I can't do anything about it."

"Well, we can," Jack Ames replied.

I was leaving for Ireland in a couple of days and couldn't be in Washington for the funeral, but I helped Jack plan the protest. He could only get a small group together, and the police kept them nearly two blocks from the Cathedral. Not many attending the funeral were aware of the protest, but we believed a picket was still appropriate. Brennan, after all, was more than just another justice who signed on to Blackmun's opinion. In some ways, he was the mastermind. It was Brennan who'd written in the birth control case that whether or not to *bear* a child was central to the right to privacy. In the conference after oral arguments in *Doe v. Bolton*, Blackmun originally declared that the Georgia law at issue seemed perfectly constitutional, but Brennan bullied him into changing his vote and striking down the law, allowing for abortion on demand throughout the full term of pregnancy.

It wasn't so much Brennan's funeral that Jack's group was picketing two blocks from St. Matthew's—it was those who allowed the ceremony to take place there. I don't like the idea of picketing a funeral. While I have no problem picketing a church that is honoring an abortion pusher, a funeral should be respected, regardless of whose funeral it is. But in the case of a public figure with no evidence of a recant, there is a scandal issue. The man on the street might assume that abortion isn't a major issue if the author of a national pro-abortion ruling can be honored with a Catholic funeral. We prayed that Justice Brennan made his peace with God, but we still had to hold the picket.

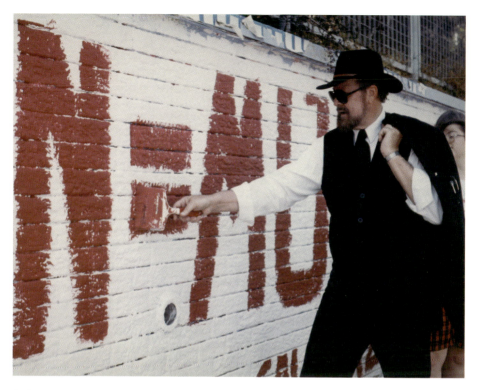

(*Above*) Painting a pro-life sign on an official graffiti wall in Cape Town, South Africa, 1995. (*Below*) Truth in media picket urging the New York Times to tell the truth about abortion.

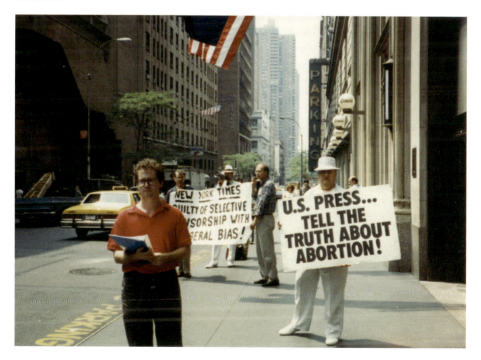

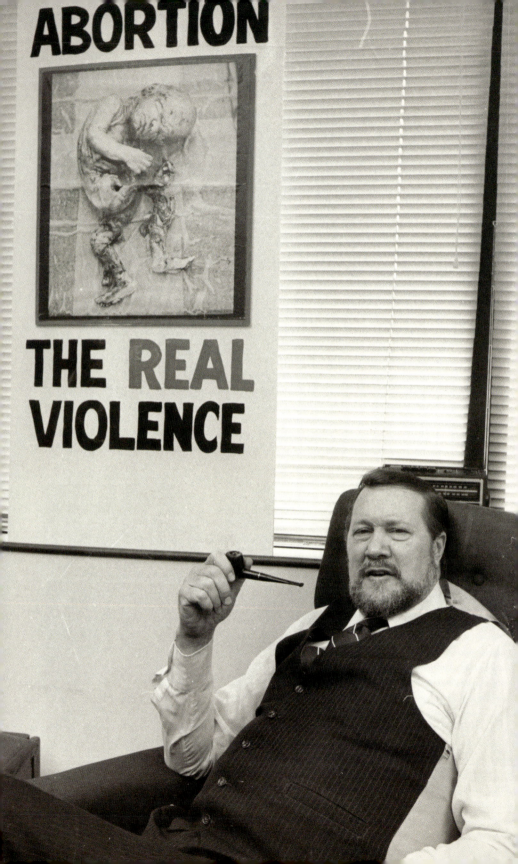

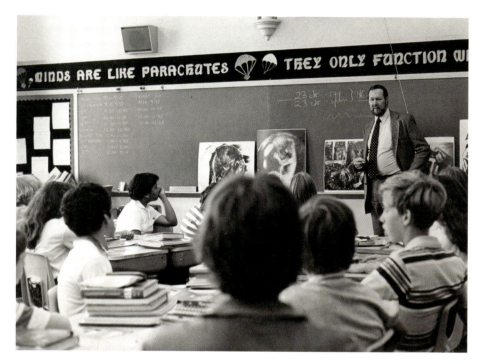

(*Opposite*) Joe in his League office, 1984. (*Above*) Educating students on life issues. (*Below left*) Joe recording his daily hotline message. (*Below right*) Tim Murphy in "lock & block" rescue at Park Medical Center with Joe and other activists.

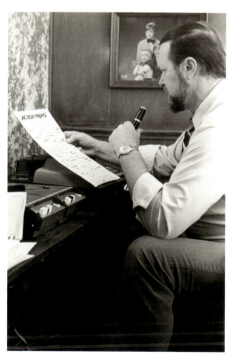

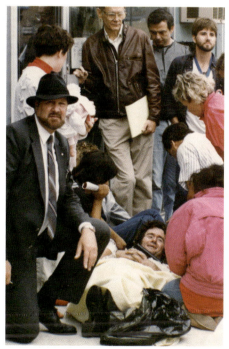

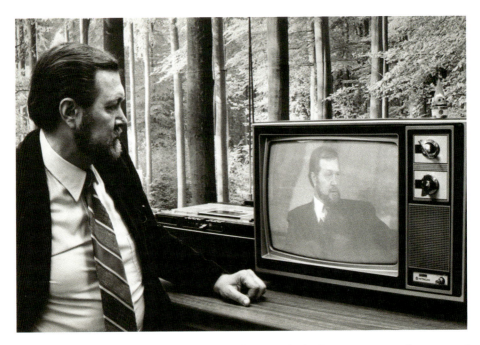

(*Above*) Joe watches an interview of himself on TV. (*Below*) Joe paints a garbage can of doll parts for dramatic impact in protests, 1981.

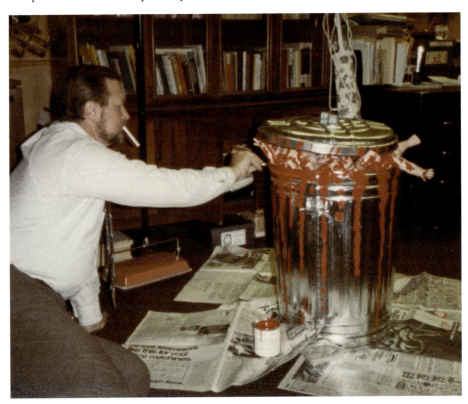

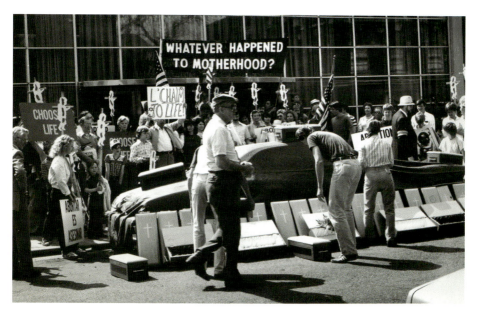

(*Above*) Mother's Day march, May 1982. (*Below*) Protest of Faye Wattleton at CBS TV in Chicago.

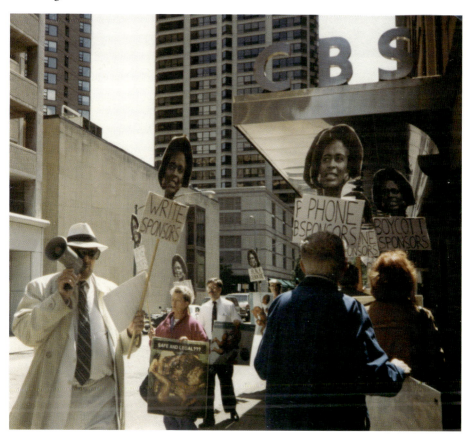

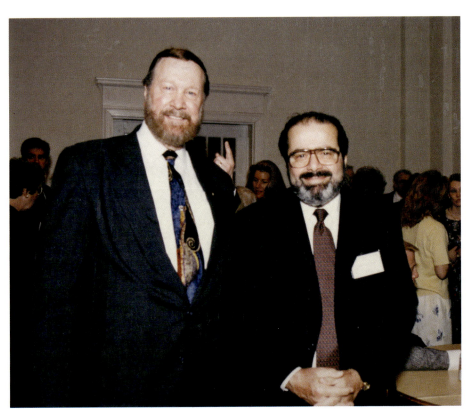

(*Above*) Joe with Justice Antonin Scalia. (*Below*) Joe with Justice Harry Blackmun.

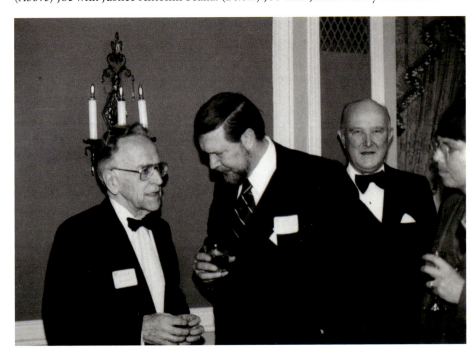

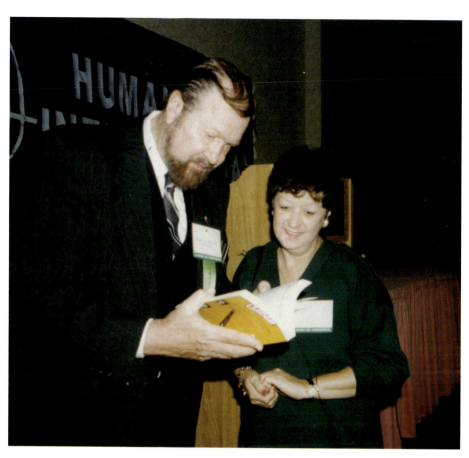

(*Above*) Joe with Norma McCorvey (*Roe*). (*Below*) Joe with Francis Cardinal George.

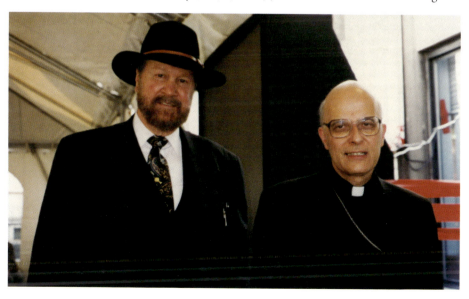

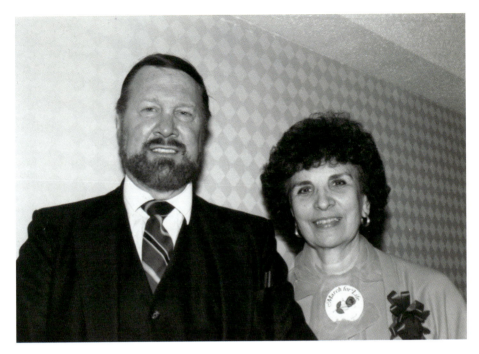

(*Above*) Joe with Nellie Gray, founder of the March for Life. (*Below left*) Joe with Dr. Bernard Nathanson, former abortionist who became a stalwart of the pro-life movement. (*Below right*) Joe with Dr. Mildred Jefferson and Dr. Jack Willke.

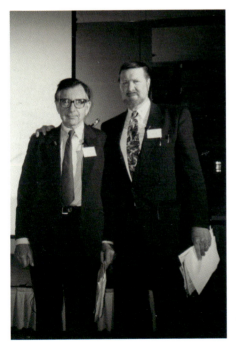

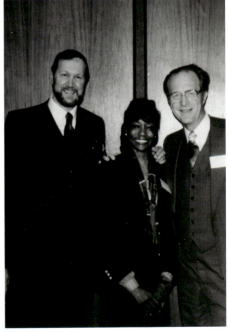

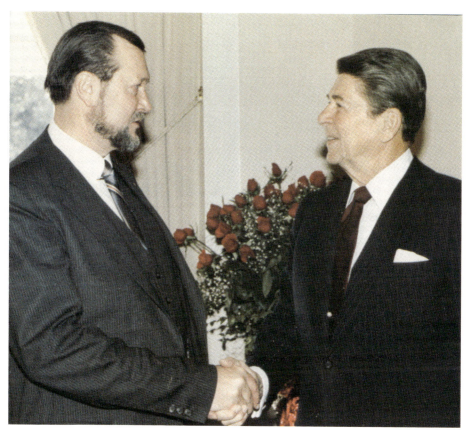

(*Above*) Joe with President Ronald Reagan at the White House, January 23, 1984. (*Below*) Joe appearing on the popular Phil Donahue show in 1984.

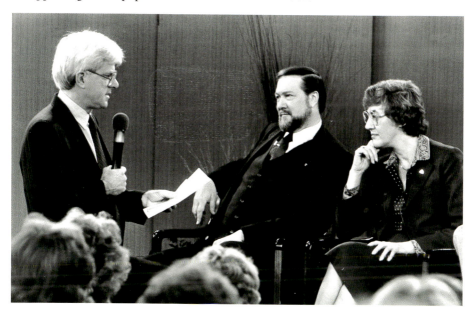

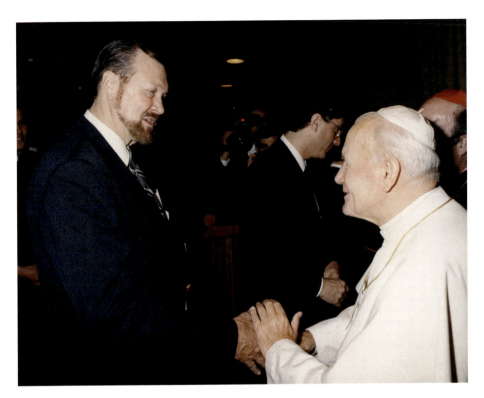

(*Above*) Joe meeting Pope John Paul II, 1991. (*Below*) Monica Miller and Joe in front of Planned Parenthood in Gary, IN.

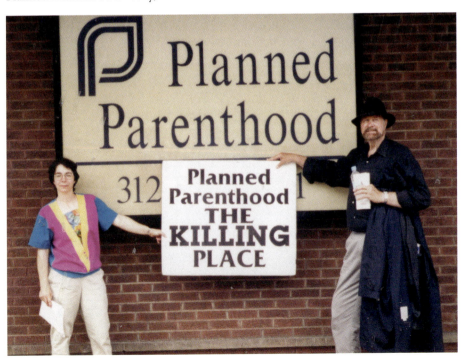

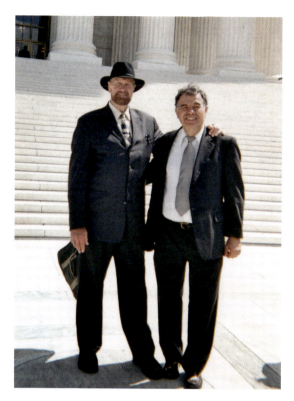

(*Above*) Joe with Jack Ames, director of Defend Life, at the US Supreme Court. (*Below*) Joe is interviewed after losing NOW v. Scheidler in federal court April 20, 1998; Tim Murphy is at his right.

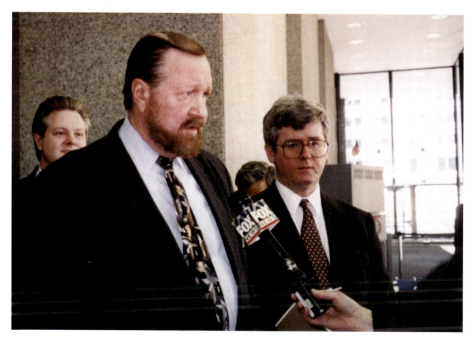

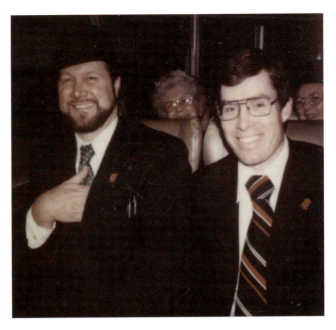

(*Above left*) Joe with Patrick Trueman. (*Below*) Joe meets Ramsay Clark in the Dirksen Federal Building in Chicago during the NOW v. Scheidler injunction hearing, July, 1998. (*Opposite*) In front of playhouse: Annie, Cathy, Sarah, Joe, holding Matthias, 1982.

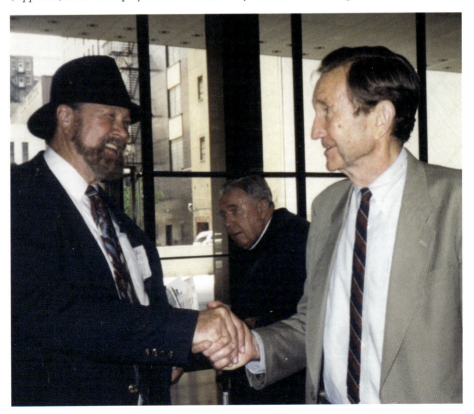

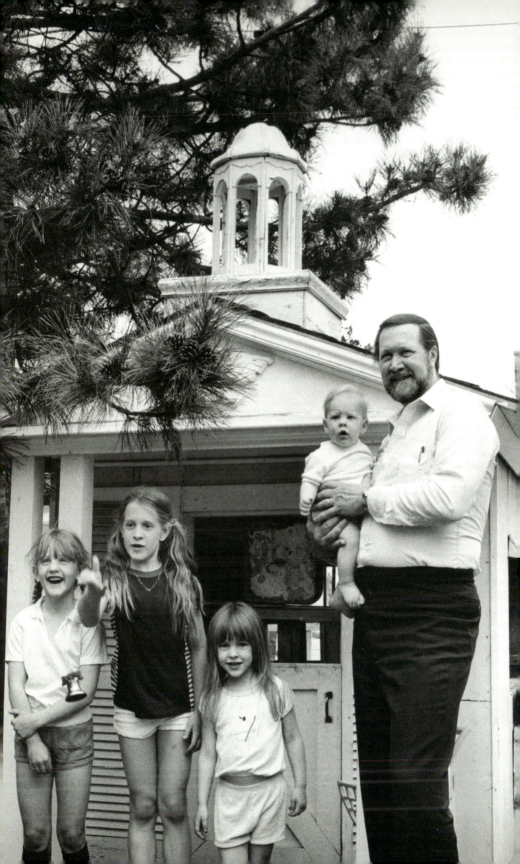

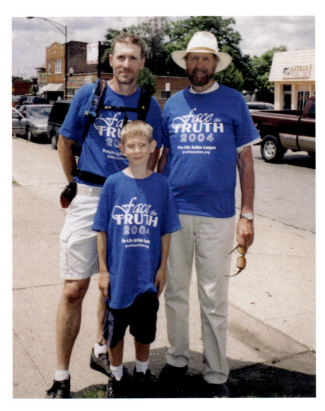

(*Above*) Son, Eric, and grandson, Nate, help Joe coordinate Face the Truth Tour in Maryland, 2003. (*Below*) Joe at a Christmas brunch with daughters, Cathy, Annie and Sarah.

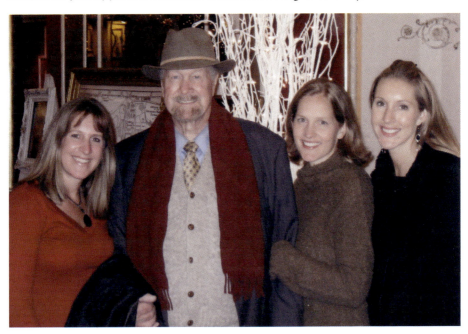

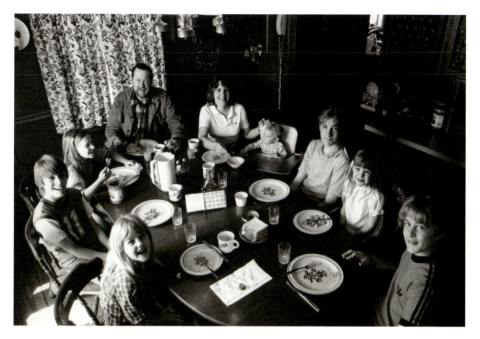

(*Above*) Scheidler family at breakfast: Joe, Ann, Matthias, Eric, Sarah, Joe Jr., Annie, Peter, Cathy. (*Below*) Entire Scheidler family at Joe and Ann's 50th wedding anniversary, Sept. 4, 2015, in front of their parish, Queen of All Saints Basilica.

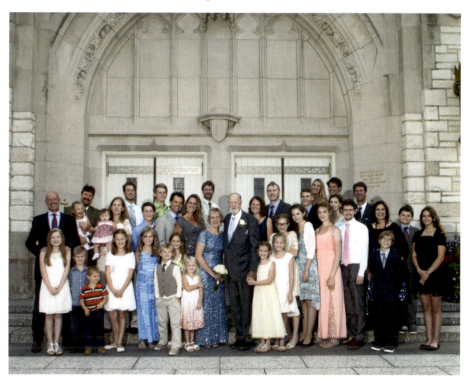

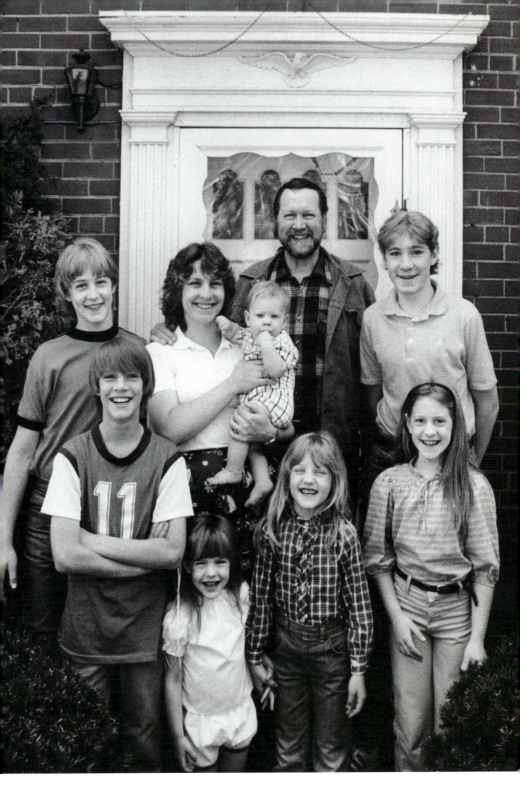

(*Above*) Scheidler family at home, 1982.

CHAPTER 25

# The Pro-Life Mafia

W hen *NOW v. Scheidler* was filed in 1986, three defendants were named: John Ryan, Joan Andrews, and me. Since we'd all openly professed that we intended to run abortionists out of business, the suit alleged that we violated federal antitrust laws. The Southern Poverty Law Center handled NOW's case, but after a couple years, they must have conceded that an antitrust case against protesters was never going to prevail, and they pulled out of the case.

NOW President and lawyer Patricia Ireland took over the case. She claims credit for coming up with the idea of racketeering charges, and she added the RICO claim, labeling us an organized crime syndicate. Years earlier, a reporter had dubbed me "the Godfather of the pro-life movement," and I was comfortable with the title. After our 1984 Fort Lauderdale activist convention, I wrote to John Cavanaugh O'Keefe about bringing new recruits into pro-life activism. In that letter, written a year before PLAN was named, I mentioned how beneficial it was that the nation's activists were forming themselves into a network. I joked that what we needed was a pro-life mafia.

Later that year when a group of activists met in Kansas City, six of us stopped by a photography studio and donned 1920s-era costumes. I sat in the middle with a Tommy gun, and the picture now hangs in my office. Another Mafioso-themed picture taken about that same time was reprinted in *Action News*. When I first met Randall Terry in Binghamton, New York, I noticed we were both wearing fedoras. We snapped a picture in front of Randy's home of the two of us standing side by side with Randy holding a bullhorn and me clutching his violin case.

When the lawsuit started, NOW subpoenaed all my files and correspondence. The AUL Legal Defense Fund represented us at that point, and having little experience with litigation, they handed over more information than the law required. The savvy thing to have done would be to challenge NOW's discovery requests, but the AUL handed over enough material for them to build a case that PLAN was a criminal enterprise. That material included a copy of my letter to John Cavanaugh O'Keefe, and the mafia remark may have given NOW the idea for the RICO charges.

When abortion became the law of the land in 1973, clinics opened their doors across the nation, and law enforcement officers nationwide were required to help them deal with any protests that might interfere with their business. As O'Keefe wrote in a pamphlet on pro-life civil disobedience, "Objectively, once we had acted to protect children, the cooperation of the police was a necessary and indispensable part of the process of killing them."

But there were some officers who could not comply. In Las Vegas, Officer Chet Gallagher received orders to haul rescuers away from a clinic. When he got to the demonstration, he looked at what the protesters were doing and—in full uniform—sat down with them. He was promptly fired. In Jackson, Mississippi, Officer Joe Daniels, a ten-year veteran of the child protective services division, was called to help arrest pro-lifers blockading the entrance at the Mississippi Women's Medical Center. As he transported the activists to the station in his squad car, they prayed aloud for him. In a letter he wrote to his commanding officer after the incident, Daniels said, "I have always taken pride in arresting the bad guys and bringing the scales of justice to balance. But in this case I have confused the good guys with the bad guys. I've failed God miserably. By carrying out my sworn duty as an officer, I realize I was helping abortionists ply their trade." The next day, he went in to deliver the letter and clean out his desk.

Still, it was rare that officers refused to arrest rescuers. As the rescue movement spread across the nation, pro-lifers started facing heavier charges and stiffer penalties. When Joe Wall was arrested with Joan Andrews at a rescue in Pittsburgh in late 1985, both were sentenced to two months in prison. During his trial, Joe was barred from even using the word "abortion."

After he was found guilty, Joe Wall chronicled America's tradition of civil disobedience in response to injustice. "The idea that you can separate a particular act in technical violation of a law from the reason for it makes no sense whatsoever," he wrote in his summary. "For anyone who thinks this way, a major part of American history is no more than a criminal conspiracy."

On Father's Day 1984, Father Ed Markley entered the Birmingham Women's Medical Center in Birmingham, Alabama, and smashed a suction machine with a hammer. He was convicted of burglary and handed a two-year sentence, but the sentence was suspended on the condition that he not go within five hundred yards of any abortion clinic in the fifty states for five years. Father Markley couldn't abide by the order. He felt called to save lives, and for him, staying away from the killing centers just wasn't possible. He went back. When clinic staff saw him praying outside their door, they reported him to the authorities. Father Markley's parole was revoked, and he was ordered to serve a five-year prison sentence.

In August 1986, I led a picket of the Alabama prison where Father Markley was incarcerated. The next day, I met with him at the prison. He told me he didn't regret anything he had done. Attacking the suction machine was illegal but morally correct, and returning to the clinic to counsel and pray was a moral imperative. In 1988, when he was again a free man, we honored Father Markley with the Pro-Life Action League's Protector Award at our annual banquet. I wrote in *Action News*, "We neither condone nor condemn his attack against an abortion machine. We honor him because of his strong convictions about the sanctity of life in the womb, and his willingness to sacrifice personal comfort for Jesus' sake. As a man of strong faith, Father Markley can serve as a model to all true right-to-life activists."

Two years after Father Markley attacked the suction machine in Birmingham with a hammer, Joan Andrews attacked one in Pensacola with her bare hands. The prosecutor asked for a one-year prison sentence, but Judge William Anderson sentenced Joan to five. The judge never expected her to actually serve it. John Burt, who had been arrested with Joan, received the same sentence, and both he and Joan could have had it suspended if they agreed to stay off the Ladies Center property.

John signed the form. He had a plan to purchase a strip of land adjacent to the clinic on which to counsel women. He bought the land, and when the Ladies Center put up a fence between their property and his, John built a platform so activists could still talk to women on their way into the clinic. He later added a statue dedicated to the unborn to the property.

Joan refused Judge Anderson's offer. She knew she couldn't stop participating in rescues, and she refused to cooperate in any way with those who supported the right to kill the unborn. Joan began serving her five-year sentence with a campaign of noncooperation. Complying with even the most trivial order while incarcerated, she said, amounted to compromising with abortion supporters. She went limp in prison. Guards carried her everywhere. Soon she was committed to permanent solitary confinement.

I wrote to Joan, asking her to cooperate and be released. "We need you out here," I wrote. "We need you to give seminars on activism, to be the speaker at pro-life gatherings, to testify with us on the loss of our civil rights, to help reactivate the movement." She wrote back that while she didn't expect anyone else to follow her example, she simply could not accept a release based on compromise. "The most important reason why I cannot compromise is that the very issue of compromise has become the basis and structure of the entire abortion holocaust," she wrote. But she made it clear that her prison stay was something she felt called to do, not something she expected of anyone else.

As a condition of having my own Florida burglary charge dropped, I agreed to stay out of Pensacola until John and Joan were sentenced, after which I was free to return. My son Joe and I flew down to Pensacola on Thanksgiving night 1986. The next morning, I joined a massive picket at the Ladies Center and led a picket at Judge Anderson's house. Then Joe and I left for New Orleans. That evening, Randall Terry called a meeting at a Western Sizzlin' restaurant to unveil a new protest strategy he wanted to discuss.

It seems I missed a rather spirited meeting. Randy circulated a document titled "Operation Rescue." The plan was to stage high-profile acts of civil disobedience in New York, Chicago, and Washington, DC. Activists would storm into a clinic, barricade the door, and unfurl a pro-life banner out the window. There was talk of trashing the clinics, dismantling the machines, hurling furniture out of windows, and perhaps disabling the elevators. But just about everybody there knew these tactics were far too drastic, and they convinced Randy that only a nonviolent movement could effectively manifest solidarity with the unborn victims. Randy took the advice. Operation Rescue would only blockade the exterior clinic doors.

Randy was fired up. He was willing to do something extreme for the cause. He wanted large crowds at his events, and the story of Joan Andrews's incarceration, combined with his connections with pastors and radio hosts across the country, helped him recruit new members into the rescue movement. Those of us who had been activists for a while understood that the most effective pro-life work is done one-on-one. Blocking access to a clinic would give sidewalk counselors more time to talk women out of abortion.

In the spring of 1987, PLAN held a convention in Atlanta. A rescue was planned. Some of the activists from St. Louis brought gold and silver star stickers for activists' nametags. The idea was to keep track of who was willing to be arrested and who would stand away from the entrance and pray. Those willing to go to jail got gold stars. As an organizing strategy, it made sense, but they probably should have chosen a different color code—the gold stars seemed to suggest that those willing to risk arrest were more dedicated to the cause than those with silver stars.

With resentment brewing, I was asked to speak at the convention on the importance of maintaining peace in the movement. Some considered that a strange topic for me, since for some pro-lifers I was too militant. I had joked that pro-lifers who disavowed activism were "Wimps for Life," and I'd had engagements canceled over concerns that my tactics were too aggressive. I'd even adopted the motto "No More Mister Nice Guy." But I'd always maintained my policy of not publicly criticizing anyone in the movement.

"The problem we have in this moment is that we are right!" I said in my talk. "We are absolutely right. And there is always the temptation to become righteous, to say, 'My way is right, and anyone who hasn't caught up to me is wrong.' We have to realize that God disposes. We propose, but God disposes. Tomorrow when we're out there, we will all be doing God's work."

I had no interest in getting a gold star. A year earlier, I had been charged with burglary for standing on a porch, and with the NOW lawsuit under way, my lawyers advised me to avoid getting arrested, especially out of state.

The next morning, I led a small group of protesters to Atlanta's Midtown Hospital, where late-term abortions were performed. The police followed us. By the time our protest was under way, 150 rescuers were blocking the doors to the clinic across town in Chamblee. By the time our picket ended, Chamblee police were hauling rescuers off to jail. Activists met at two other Atlanta-area clinics and saved at least three babies from death.

Randall Terry joined the Chamblee rescue. The next fall, he scheduled his first huge rescue in Philadelphia. He and Mike McMonagle recruited more than three hundred volunteers from twenty states to blockade the entrance to a clinic in Philadelphia. But the day of the event, they learned that all the clinics in town had police patrols that would make it impossible to blockade the doors. So they crossed the Delaware River and held their rescue in New Jersey. Three hundred protesters peacefully blocked the doors of the Cherry Hill Women's Center, shutting it down for the day. Two hundred were arrested.

After this successful test run, Randy was ready to launch the full Operation Rescue plan, which called for a series of clinic blockades over several days. In March 1988, he held a meeting at the Times Square Hotel in New York City, where participants planned to deploy an army of volunteers. Randy wanted lots of arrests—to pack the jails like the civil rights demonstrators had done in Birmingham in 1963 and to use the media to orchestrate a national campaign to end abortion.

Randy drew thousands into activism, but I worried that he wasn't being completely honest with them. During a break in our meeting at the Times Square Hotel, I met longtime friends Bill and Mary Tracey for lunch. I told them about the Operation Rescue meeting and the plan for mass arrests.

"They don't know what they're getting into," Mary said dismissively. "What are the police going to do with all those people? They're going to wind up on Rikers Island."

I thought about her comment. I spoke with Randy when I got back to the hotel.

"I'm hearing too much about arrests," I said. "That seems to be your whole plan."

"We're going to break the system," Randy said confidently. He was convinced that the size of the protesting crowds would overwhelm the police. "The system was here long before you were, Randy," I cautioned. "They can always get extra officers or have them work double shifts."

In my comments at the Atlanta PLAN meeting the previous year, I had mentioned John Ryan's hundreds of arrests. "Why does John have to go out and get arrested four hundred times?" I asked. "Why can't four hundred pro-lifers go out and each get arrested once?" I didn't mean all at once. Even though there were thousands of clinics across the country, there were hundreds of thousands of pro-lifers. If each one committed to counseling at a clinic once a year, thousands of lives could be saved.

Randy was recruiting hundreds of eager activists to the cause, but he seemed to have only one idea about how to deploy them. I worried that if these new recruits discovered that fighting abortion would mean arrest records and costly legal battles, many would find some other injustice to fight that carried less personal risk.

I've spent a large part of my career leading crowds, and crowds can be very useful. A crowd can raise awareness and keep abortion on the front page. Randy was assembling a huge mass of activists, but the crowds that answered his call were energized at the thought of risking arrest to protect the unborn. Randy had recruited them, and Operation Rescue was his plan—they weren't mine. Even though I thought that holding seminars to train the green activists in sidewalk counseling before sending them forth would be a more effective program, I supported Randy's overall effort.

I pitched an idea that I thought would be equally effective at temporarily closing clinics without mass arrests. As soon as police arrived, I suggested, protesters could start leaving—very slowly. With a crowd as large as Randy was confident he'd get, this could take nearly as long as hauling everyone away and save just as many lives. Randy wasn't interested.

On the final day of the New York conference, I left the meeting to attend an evening Mass at St. Patrick's Cathedral. St. Patrick's was only a few blocks away from the hotel, but it had started raining, so I hailed a cab. As I got in, Randy came running out of the hotel. He seemed agitated.

"Joe," he said, "I don't want you throwing a wet blanket on this. As of right now, I personally disinvite you from Operation Rescue."

"No," I replied, "I'll be there."

So I was there in May 1988 when Operation Rescue was officially launched. On Monday, May 2, six hundred rescuers arrived at the Times Square Hotel early in the morning. We split into several groups and headed for the subways, changing trains so our destination remained a mystery to the police and to counterdemonstrators. When we emerged near an Upper East Side clinic, it was clear that the ruse worked. By midmorning, hundreds of pro-lifers blocked access to the clinic entrance on east Eighty-Fifth Street. NOW protesters arrived and gathered across the street, shouting as we prayed. The police began pulling rescuers away. We had all agreed not to cooperate with the police, so they hauled us on stretchers to waiting busses.

I was among the 503 arrested that day. Given my lawyers' advice about avoiding arrest, that might seem like a risky move, but Randy's Cherry Hill rescue had shown that he would stay true to his plan of not trying to combine Operation Rescue events with clinic invasions. There was no chance of facing the kind of charges that I had faced in Wilmington and Pensacola. Frankly, there was also something to the idea of safety in numbers, at least for the time being.

All 503 of us were taken to the New York Police Academy auditorium and issued tickets. Then they let us go. Operation Rescue's lawyers handled all the paperwork, so there was no fine or court date for the protesters. Nobody wound up on Rikers.

The next day, I served as one of the Operation Rescue marshals, leading volunteers in a blockade of Queens Women's Medical Office, where 422 activists were arrested. All were charged with disorderly conduct, but those charges were soon dropped. The New York rescues were a resounding success. We had shut down clinics completely for four days in a row.

Two months later, Operation Rescue arrived in Philadelphia for two days of blockades. The second day resulted in just under six hundred arrests, taking police seven hours to haul away the protesters. Two weeks after that, Operation Rescue traveled to Atlanta, where the Democratic National Convention was meeting to nominate Michael Dukakis.

As with any demonstration where arrests are made, there was some concern that the peaceful pro-lifers would be made to look violent. To prevent this, rescuers were instructed to crawl, rather than walk, if they moved around during the blockade. They called it the "Atlanta crawl." Rescuers were also instructed to leave their IDs behind and, when arrested, to give their names as "Baby Doe." Both of these moves delayed the arrest process and highlighted the demonstrators' solidarity with the unborn victims.

Whereas Terry's rescues in New York and Philadelphia closed clinics for days, Atlanta police hauled away protesters in just a few hours, and the clinics were able to remain open. Meanwhile, hundreds of protesters who refused to give their real names stayed in jail up to forty days. Sergeant Carl Pyrdum was put in charge of arresting the pro-lifers. "This is never going to go the way you want it to go," he told Randall Terry at one rescue after quickly clearing the path to the clinic. "Every day you come out here, I am going to be here, and I'm going to put your people in jail as quickly as I did today."

Randy's plans had hit a snag, and Sgt. Pyrdum was showing other police departments how they could deal with Operation Rescue. But at the same time, the media coverage of the Atlanta rescues was huge. Pat Robertson praised the rescuers on *The 700 Club*, and Jerry Falwell came to Atlanta to present Randy and Operation Rescue with a ten-thousand-dollar check. "Nonviolent civil disobedience," he said, "is the only way to end the biological holocaust in this country."

NOW noticed that more and more people were donating money to Operation Rescue. They also knew that Joan Andrews and John Ryan had no assets, so when they changed their complaint from antitrust to RICO, they dropped John and Joan as defendants and added Operation Rescue and Randall Terry. The following spring, the Pro-life Action League gave Randall Terry the Protector Award.

While the League supported rescues, our style of activism usually didn't focus on getting large numbers of people arrested. One of our principal goals was, however, to get our message into newspapers and on TV.

Early one August morning in 1988, Tim Murphy, Toni Moriarty, and Don Treshman arrived at Park Medical Center in Chicago. Don was in town for a PLAN convention, and he had brought a cement block with a thick link from an anchor chain embedded in it. Don set the block in front of the door. Tim and Toni sat on the sidewalk, and Don locked both of them to the block with Kryptonite bike locks, Tim by his neck and Toni by her ankles.

Don left and took the keys with him. When the police came, they feared that trying to haul Tim away with the block attached to his neck would injure him, so they called the fire department to remove it. When the fire truck arrived, the fireman asked Tim and Toni if they wanted to be rescued. They declined, and the firemen left. Then the police called in a locksmith. When he couldn't pick the lock, he tried to drill it out, but he couldn't get through it.

We succeeded in keeping the clinic closed the entire day, but eventually Tim and Toni wanted out. The locksmith had damaged the lock, and Don's keys were useless. Tim and Toni were more stuck to the cement block than they intended to be. We got a hacksaw and cut through the steel ring, wondering all the while why the police hadn't tried that. Once the Kryptonite locks were cut from the block, Toni slipped her feet through. Tim was famished, so he strolled into a McDonald's with the bike lock still around his neck. After he had something to eat, we took him back to my garage. A mechanic friend came over with some high-powered tools and melted through the U-bar in a minute or two. Tim was a free man.

Then a Wichita, Kansas, rescue was organized by Reverend Keith Tucci. Wichita was a small town compared to the other cities where Operation Rescue had been, and instead of blocking multiple clinics throughout the city, there was only one where rescues could be staged: George Tiller's clinic. As the most notorious late-term abortionist in the nation, Tiller and his clinic drew activists from all over the country to join the events there. I went out three times. The original plan called for blockades over the course of a week, but the crowds kept coming, and the rescues went on for seven weeks. Pro-lifers began referring to it as "The Summer of Mercy."

During one rescue, police brought in U-Haul trucks to cart arrested protesters away. After they'd filled one van and latched the door, the officer who was supposed to drive it stepped away to talk with his commanding officer. Chet Kilgore, from Wisconsin, took advantage of the moment to open the van door. "Everybody out!" he announced. They all scattered. Chet was arrested and charged with helping prisoners escape.

In jail, rescuers were usually upbeat and spent a lot of time in song. Singing while under arrest became routine. Once when I was arrested at a rescue in Washington, DC, three of us in one cell were trying to form a barbershop quartet to sing some old tunes, but we were short a tenor. We asked one of the guards if he would join us, which he did—a perfect tenor. But in Wichita, the police were less appreciative of the singing, and many who were jailed during the Summer of Mercy discovered that their constant hymns aggravated the police into releasing them early.

In response to the rescue movement, pro-abortionists and their congressional allies pushed for a federal law to punish rescuers. Their initiative became the FACE Act. At first, FACE had very little support in Congress, since trespassing and resisting arrest are issues for state governments to handle, not the federal government.

But on a March morning in 1993, Pensacola abortionist David Gunn was shot and killed outside his clinic by Michael F. Griffin. Ten years earlier, Gunn had worked as a fertility specialist in Alabama. When the abortionist at Susan Hill's Columbus, Georgia, clinic fell ill, she searched for a replacement and found Gunn. He eventually gave up his Alabama practice and began traveling to several of Hill's clinics. Early in 1993, Gunn opened a clinic of his own in Pensacola. He had been raised in a family that belonged to the Church of Christ and opposed abortion. His family had no idea that he performed abortions until after he was shot.

Partially as a result of Gunn's killing, FACE sailed through Congress, and Bill Clinton signed it into law in 1994. Though the rescue movement was dedicated to nonviolence, and there was no connection between the clinic blockades and Gunn's murder, his killing was used to get the bill passed.

FACE effectively ended the rescue movement. The law threatens pro-lifers with jail terms of up to six months and fines of up to ten thousand dollars for a first offense. Second offenses carried three-year terms and fines up to twenty-five thousand dollars.

Sitting in jail for a few hours or even a few weeks can be a redemptive experience. It's gratifying to suffer for the unborn. But while we're in jail, children are still dying outside. Few of us can risk months or years of incarceration while we would be better out at the clinics and in the public square educating the public on the horror of abortion. The huge financial penalties that accompany a FACE violation would be better spent on other pro-life efforts.

Having been with civil rights marchers in the mid-'60s and with the pro-life rescuers of the '80s and '90s, I find both movements an answer to the call to defend human dignity. It's tragic that pro-lifers have to work around draconian laws designed to prevent our giving witness to the value of life and the horror of abortion.

But while the rescue movement drew a great deal of media attention, an increase in activist participation, and resulted in more than seventy thousand arrests from 1987 through 1994, the most effective ways to save lives are still those based on one-on-one interactions. That means everything from sidewalk counseling, working to convert providers, volunteering at a crisis pregnancy center, to simple conversations with friends to help them see the value of every human life. There is still a role for a mass movement and a powerful imperative to keep the issue in the public consciousness, but unless something changes, the era of mass blockades is over.

A new generation of pro-life activists is taking to the streets. Growing up in a society that not only tolerates but actually celebrates the killing of its posterity, the new recruits experience the evil of abortion in a deeply personal way. More than one-fourth of their classmates, their business acquaintances, and their social circle is missing. They were not allowed, as the earlier generation of pro-lifers was, to grow up in a country that values and protects unborn life.

Rescuers showed great ingenuity in the days before FACE, and these new pro-lifers are destined to come up with their own innovations. Some may pay a high price for their witness. But when their witness is ignored and their good intentions frustrated by an uncaring society, they can be assured they are in good company as they carry on the legacy of Father Paul Marx, John Cavanaugh O'Keefe,

Joan Andrews, John Ryan, Monica Migliorino Miller, Randall Terry, the late Father Norman Weslin, and the hundreds of others who formed the Old Guard.

For the new members of the "pro-life mafia," I share these inspiring words delivered at the 1981 Illinois Citizens for Life "Forget Me Not Ball." Though it was years before the full-fledged rescue movement took off, many activists already had endured jail time for staging sit-ins at clinics. Ann and I were sitting just a few feet from the podium when the keynote speaker, Congressman Henry Hyde, said:

> When the time comes, as it surely will, when we face that awesome moment, the final judgment, I've often thought, as Fulton Sheen wrote, that it is a moment of terrible loneliness.
>
> You have no advocates. You are there alone standing before God. And a terror will rip your soul like nothing you can imagine. But I really think that those in the pro-life movement will not be alone. I think there'll be a chorus of voices that have never been heard in this world but are heard beautifully and clearly in the next world—and they will plead for everyone who has been in this movement.
>
> They will say to God, "Spare him, because he loved us!"[1]

---

1    Henry Hyde, keynote speech at Illinois Citizens for Life at Indian Lakes Country Club, Bloomingdale, Il., November 12, 1977.

## Chapter 26

# The Seamless Garment

On October 22, 1962, President John F. Kennedy appeared on TV to tell the American people that there were Soviet missiles in Cuba. The United States had established a naval blockade around the island and was demanding their immediate removal. When a Russian convoy approached the American warships, many on both sides thought World War III was about to begin, but since a full-scale nuclear war would mean annihilation for both the United States and the USSR, it was in neither power's interest to fire the first shot. So while much of the nation was concerned over the naval maneuvers in the Caribbean, I was fairly confident we'd make it into 1963.

That same month, Pope John XXIII convened the Second Vatican Council. Because of the recent concern over the arms race, nuclear disarmament was a priority topic. One of the women in Rome to attend the Council and help draft some of its documents on world peace was a journalist and activist named Eileen Egan.

A generation earlier, when Germany invaded Poland and ignited World War Two, Egan was working in New York City with Dorothy Day's Catholic Worker Movement. Like Day, Egan was strongly committed to pacifism, and she criticized the just war doctrine as "an alien graft on the gospel of Jesus." The war produced unspeakable suffering, and Egan was eager to help its victims. She left New York to work with the US Bishops War Relief Services aiding refugees from Nazi aggression. In 1965, Egan joined civil rights activists on Dr. King's Selma to Montgomery March and faced the anger of Southern white supremacists.

In 1971, Egan met with British satirist Malcom Muggeridge, a one-time agnostic who had just published *Something Beautiful for God*, on the work Mother Teresa was doing in Calcutta. Egan also knew Mother Teresa, and in the course of their conversation, Muggeridge mentioned his strong opposition to the sexual revolution, particularly because it brought about legalized abortion, which the British Parliament enacted in 1967. While Egan held that Christians must oppose abortion, she also maintained that they could not condone war.

"Oh, no," Muggeridge objected, "you must defend your country."

"Well, you know," Eileen told Malcom, "the same goes for capital punishment. If you're against taking life, the life of the unborn or the life of the born, then it all goes together. The protection of life is a seamless garment. You can't protect some lives and not others."[1]

The "seamless garment" was a reference to Christ's tunic that the soldiers cast lots for at the foot of the cross. It was continuously woven, consistent throughout, and couldn't be divided without being torn. Egan was saying that to be against abortion but to favor killing in war or through the justice system was inconsistent. True consistency, she argued, requires a Christian to oppose all forms of killing.

In 1983, Joseph Cardinal Bernardin, the new chairman of the Pro-Life Committee of the US Council of Catholic Bishops, borrowed

---

1    A portion of this interview is reproduced in the "Consistent Life" video from the Consistent Life Network, http://www.consistentlifenetwork/org.

Egan's metaphor to articulate the US Bishops's position on a host of issues related to human life: abortion, euthanasia, poverty, immigration, and most prominently, the nuclear arms race.

The bishops met at the Palmer House in Chicago that May to approve the final draft on a pastoral letter on war and peace. Abortion had been the law of the land for ten years, with more than a million and a half babies aborted each year, but even though no one had been killed by a nuclear bomb in forty years, the bishops chose to announce that the nuclear arms race was the most serious issue facing the country.

When the bishops convened, a group of us went to the Palmer House and handed out copies of the *Human Life Review* edition that featured Ronald Reagan's "Abortion and the Conscience of a Nation." We also distributed copies of an appeal for the Center for the Documentation of the American Holocaust asking the bishops not to downplay the abortion issue. We talked with many bishops as they entered the Palmer House, urging them not to issue a statement implying that potential deaths were more alarming than actual deaths. Most of them took a copy of the *Human Life Review*, but very few took the American Holocaust handout.

Reagan's piece was all text, and given that many considered him responsible for the arms race, his article might not have carried too much weight at a meeting focused on the nuclear issue. The American Holocaust handout, however, contained photographs of some of the nearly seventeen thousand babies who had recently been found in a repossessed storage container in California. I knew the power of graphic photos firsthand, and so I was disappointed that so many of the bishops were unwilling to face the evidence that every month America was racking up a death toll equal to another Hiroshima.

The bishops met for three days. My cousin, Bishop Thomas Tschoepe of the Dallas Diocese, attended the meetings, and after the second day, he told me there had hardly been any discussion of the abortion issue. Since so few of the bishops had taken the American Holocaust handout, I wondered if they understood exactly what was at stake.

So on the third day, our pro-life group went back to the Palmer House and set up a large sign on a platform just outside their meeting room. It directly addressed the two bureaucracies who were meeting there: the National Conference of Catholic Bishops (NCCB) and the US Catholic Conference (USCC). Our sign featured a picture of a baby from the California body find whose legs had been nearly twisted off. His corpse had been laid on two crossed pieces of paper towel, and the photo resembled an image of a crucifixion. Above it, we put the words "NCCB-USCC: Why have you forsaken me?" This was one of the first times a photo of an abortion victim had been blown up to such a large size, and it's noteworthy that it was displayed, not to the general public, but to a group of bishops, who should have known better than the average person how serious an evil abortion is.

Bishop Tom congratulated us on our effort to keep the issue before the assembly, and Bishop Stanley Ott of Baton Rouge also said we were doing the right thing. But they were the only two bishops who stopped to commend our effort. Some of those walking past shot it a furtive glance, but they seemed embarrassed by our display.

However, in the final draft of their Pastoral Letter on War and Peace, they noted:

> Millions join us in our "no" to nuclear war, in the certainty that nuclear war would inevitably result in the killing of millions of innocent human beings, directly or indirectly. Yet many part ways with us in our efforts to reduce the horror of abortion and our "no" to war on innocent human life in the womb, killed not indirectly but directly.
>
> We must ask how long a nation willing to extend a constitutional guarantee to the "right" to kill defenseless human

beings by abortion is likely to refrain from adopting strategic warfare policies deliberately designed to kill millions of defenseless human beings, if adopting them should come to seem "expedient."[2]

It was good that the bishops acknowledged the link between the abortion mentality and a nuclear holocaust, but this statement appeared at the very end of a fifty-page document. Yet perhaps even this meager mention of abortion would never have appeared without our efforts to impress its importance on the bishops.

It was after this conference that Cardinal Bernardin started using the "seamless garment" metaphor in connection with his efforts to bridge the gap between "liberal" Catholics who favored disarmament but didn't view abortion as an important issue and the "conservatives" who opposed abortion but supported a strong nuclear arsenal. As he put it in a 1984 speech in St. Louis:

> Nuclear war *threatens* life on a previously unimaginable scale; abortion *takes* life daily on a horrendous scale. Public executions are fast becoming weekly events in the most advanced technological society in history, and euthanasia is now openly discussed and even advocated. Each of these assaults on life has its own meaning and morality; they cannot be collapsed into one problem, but they must be confronted as pieces of a larger pattern.
>
> The reason I have placed such stress on the idea of a consistent ethic of life from the beginning of my term as chairman of the Pro-Life Committee of the National Conference of Catholic

---

2    National Conference of Catholic Bishops, "The Challenge of Peace: God's Promise and Our Response, A Pastoral Letter on War and Peace by the National Conference of Catholic Bishops," May 3, 1983, http://www .usccb.org/upload/challenge-peace-gods-promise-our-response-1983.pdf.

Bishops is twofold: I am persuaded by the interrelatedness of these diverse problems, and I am convinced that the Catholic moral vision has the scope, the strength, and the subtlety to address this wide range of issues in an effective fashion. It is precisely the potential of our moral vision that is often not recognized even within the community of the Church. The case for a consistent ethic of life—one which stands for the protection of the right to life and the promotion of the rights which enhance life from womb to tomb—manifests the positive potential of the Catholic moral and social tradition.[3]

His idea that the Church, by taking the lead in the cause of disarmament, could help bring the antiwar crowd around to a pro-life position was an optimistic and, I thought, an unrealistic one. Political observers graded politicians on their "pro-life" positions by rating them on several issues in the "seamless garment" spectrum: capital punishment, welfare, abortion, immigration policy, the arms race, and euthanasia. They would assign a final grade on how "pro-life" each candidate was.

Conservatives tended to support just war logic, a strong military defense, and capital punishment, but they voted pro-life. Liberals on the other hand were usually against capital punishment and war, but they voted pro-abortion. A voter guide based on one of these seamless garment surveys gave Ted Kennedy and Charlie Schumer each a pro-life score of sixty-seven out of one hundred, while Henry Hyde only scored a thirty, and Jesse Helms got twenty-nine. Democrats used these results to sell pro-abortion candidates to Catholic

---

3    Joseph Cardinal Bernardin, "A Consistent Ethic of Life: Continuing the Dialogue," March 11, 1984, reproduced at Priests for Life, http://www .priestsforlife.org/magisterium/bernardinwade.html.

voters on the grounds that they were "pro-life" according to a range of Catholic social values.

Under Reagan, the country had finally had a pro-life president and Senate, but the House was still pro-abortion, and the seamless garment was hurting pro-life chances of changing that. Some of us started referring to the seamless garment as the crazy quilt. Bernardin seemed honestly surprised when it became clear that his metaphor actually worked *against* the pro-life cause.

At the time, Cardinal Bernardin had been the head of the Chicago Archdiocese for only a short while. His predecessor, John Cardinal Cody, who headed the Chicago Archdiocese when *Roe* was decided, disappointed pro-lifers on many occasions. One of the biggest issues was his support for the Crusade of Mercy, a United Way funding campaign. Catholic Charities was a fund recipient, and the Church promoted it at local parishes. Contributors signed up to have part of their paychecks go automatically into the fund.

Planned Parenthood also benefited from this fundraising drive, and when I started working with the IRLC, I tried to get Cardinal Cody to distance the archdiocese from any connection with Planned Parenthood. He didn't respond. In 1978, when Chicago Planned Parenthood sponsored a series of political cartoons mocking the Church's opposition to abortion, I renewed the effort.

It was in 1978 that Father Fiore, Tom Roeser, and I founded the FFL. When the Cardinal refused to sever ties with the Crusade of Mercy, or even threaten to do so unless Planned Parenthood was dropped from the fundraiser, we started working directly with local parishes to let parishioners know what the crusade supported. In 1980, Chicago's Crusade of Mercy was the only one in the nation that included both Planned Parenthood and the local Catholic diocese. Still Cardinal Cody refused to take a stand. It was during this battle that Pat Buchanan penned an editorial in which he dubbed me the "Green Beret" of the pro-life movement.

Cardinal Cody simply didn't give the abortion issue the attention it deserved. As Chairman of the Committee of Pro-Life Activities on the NCCB at a time when the Human Life Amendment was being considered, he urged pastors to seek support from their parishioners for the amendment. But when he failed to discipline a parish priest whose homily on Respect Life Sunday declared that a mother's rights always outweigh those of her unborn child and that abortion was permissible in a host of cases, we were discouraged. Then when the cardinal promoted that same priest to Dean of the School of Theology at St. Mary of the Lake in Mundelein, Illinois, we were incensed.

The Church's position on abortion is a major tenet of its moral theology. Abortion is also a human rights issue, but it differs from other human rights issues, most of which are social justice issues concerned with the *quality* of life. Abortion threatens life itself. Pro-lifers sometimes complain that they are more likely to be labeled single-issue people more than lobbyists or activists for any other issue. But that's how it should be. Our issue, the right to life, is the single most important issue there is.

Cardinal Cody couldn't see this, despite the fact that we had managed to garner the support of more than two hundred theologians, priests, bishops, doctors, and other experts in moral law and ethics who truly respected life and urged him to pull the diocese out of a campaign that supported pro-abortion groups.

After Cardinal Cody's death in 1982, Chicago pro-lifers were initially encouraged when Archbishop Joseph Bernardin was named to succeed him. Bernardin had made some strong pro-life statements, and I often quoted him on my hotline. When I heard of his appointment, I wrote him. "During the dark days of the mid-1970s," I said, "you were a shining light of the pro-life movement.

I have an enormous file of your powerful statements and a record of your zealous efforts on behalf of the unborn. *Bernardin*—a magic word to all of us. I hope the magic is still there and will be manifest in Chicago."

He took over in July 1982. The Crusade of Mercy drive was scheduled to begin on September 17. Archbishop Bernardin—who, we learned, would be elevated to cardinal by Pope John Paul II the following year—was to give the invocation at the Crusade's kickoff luncheon. I met with him a week before the event to discuss our concerns about the archdiocese continuing to join with Planned Parenthood in a fundraising effort. He told me he would consult his theologians and prepare a statement. This is what they came up with:

> There are within the Crusade groups which counsel for contra-ception and abortion. These groups I cannot support. There-fore I ask myself: "Am I cooperating in a moral evil by giving to the Crusade?" Traditional principles of moral theology in the Church tell us we cannot cooperate "formally" with moral evil, that is, intend and approve the evil. I hold with the Catholic Church that the dignity and life of an unborn baby are worth more than all the material goods in the world.

> But if my cooperation is "material," that is, not intending or approving the evil, then the Principle of Double Effect can be used. The Principle of Double Effect holds that one action can have two results: an overriding good result which I can choose, and a bad result which is not chosen or approved, but tolerated.

> I endorse the Crusade of Mercy according to the above principle. In no way can my endorsement be used to support groups who oppose Catholic teaching about the sacredness of human life and its transmission

Through proper Archdiocesan offices, I plan to stay in contact with the Crusade and with pro-life organizations to discuss questions which may arise as I familiarize myself further.

In alleviating suffering and promoting the common good, the Crusade deserves the support of all people of good will in Metropolitan Chicago.[4]

While the Archbishop delivered this message inside the Conrad Hilton on Michigan Avenue at the kickoff luncheon, I led a group of pro-lifers outside distributing flyers that pointed out that people of good will could *not* support the Crusade. I prepared a press release to convey our disappointment. It was titled "Bernardin Honeymoon Ends for Thousands of Pro-Life Catholics."

We told Archbishop Bernardin that he would be used by Planned Parenthood to promote their programs and their campaigning. We predicted that when a conscientious pro-lifer tries to withhold a part of his salary from the Crusade on the grounds that he can't cooperate in the funding of Planned Parenthood, the Archbishop's comments will be cited to him as evidence that such participation is not immoral. The pressure to contribute will be brutal.

We still think it is possible to get Planned Parenthood out, with or without the Archbishop's cooperation. But we would certainly welcome his help. We haven't closed any doors. We just wish the Archbishop would open a few.

I disagreed with Cardinal Bernardin's interpretation of the principle of double effect. That principle comes into play when a person is

---

4    Reproduced by the Pro-Life Action League, *Action News* 2, no. 5 (October 1982).

faced with the necessity of obtaining a good end even though an evil result will follow *and there is no alternative method* of effecting the good. The principle did not apply in regard to the Crusade of Mercy fund drive because another method of financing Catholic charities did exist: namely, an independent fund drive. I sent a letters explaining my position and urging a boycott of the Crusade to the *Wanderer* and the *Chicago Catholic*.

Eventually, Planned Parenthood did drop out of the Crusade of Mercy, but it wasn't through the Church's efforts. The year following Bernardin's talk at the kickoff luncheon, I walked into a Crusade board meeting and demanded a discussion on dropping Planned Parenthood. They escorted me out. Later, four of us went to the organizers' meeting room while they were out to lunch and stuffed their packets with literature explaining how deadly an organization Planned Parenthood is. The negative publicity the League helped generate led Planned Parenthood to voluntarily pull out of the Crusade of Mercy.

I wasn't thrilled with Cardinal Bernardin's first few years in office, but over the years, I couldn't help but note that any time I called or wrote to him, he always responded personally. We may not have been the best of friends, but the Cardinal and I sincerely respected one another. Throughout the fourteen years he served as leader of the Chicago Archdiocese, he proved himself on many occasions to be a good pro-lifer.

CHAPTER 27

# To Bury the Dead

Early in 1987, I got one of the most unusual phone calls I've ever received.

"Is this the Pro-Life Action League?" the caller asked. I told him it was.

"I'm John Smith. I do advertising for a clinic here on Michigan Avenue," he said. "I've got this huge budget." He told me the amount, and he wasn't kidding. The clinic that employed him did late-term abortions and advertised every day in papers all over the country.

John wasn't pro-life, but he was disturbed by the clinic's callous treatment of women. He knew that Aid for Women was right down the street from his clinic, and he called my friend Tom Bresler. In the course of their conversation, he also brought up another matter weighing on his conscience: the disposal of babies. Tom suggested he called me.

"I was wondering," John asked, "if you ever consider burying any of these babies we have here—the ones that are aborted?"

"We have, over the years," I said, "but they're hard to find."

"Well, every evening, after the abortions are done, each specimen" *victim*, I thought, but I let him go on—"is in a plastic bag with all the information: the woman, her age, how far along she was, which doctor did the abortion, that kind of thing, all on a little label. Then the bags get packed into a heavy cardboard box. They wrap the box in duct tape and put it out in the alley in a dumpster. A red dumpster. It's not locked. Anyway, I just don't think human beings should be used as landfill."

Tim Murphy and I met with John to assure ourselves that he was on the level. The following Saturday, Tim recruited Peter Krump, Jerry McCarthy, and Rudy Stefancik to go with him to the alley behind 30 South Michigan. They found the red dumpster just as John had described it, and they took the box of bodies and brought it to my garage. I was out of town that weekend and the next, but the four returned the following Sunday and retrieved more bodies. On the third occasion, March 14, I was able to join the crew. Monica Migliorino, Peter Krump, Andy Scholberg, Dick O'Connor, Jerry McCarthy, Edmund Miller, Rudy Stefancik, Tim Murphy, and I met at Blackie's Bar in the South Loop, less than a mile from the clinic. We ducked into the alley behind Michigan Avenue and located the red dumpster. Inside was another box wrapped in duct tape. We lifted it out and took it back to my garage, where we cut through the tape and opened the box. Inside we found two or three dozen small plastic bags, each holding the remains of an unborn baby and bearing a label with the infant's estimated gestational age and the name of the mother.

We continued visiting the alley behind 30 South Michigan for two months to collect bodies, eventually salvaging nearly six hundred. Rudy Stefancik was a pathologist at Rush Presbyterian St. Luke's Medical Center, and he examined the bodies and helped reassemble the pieces. We wanted to know whether the bags contained all the remains. If not, it would be safe to assume that the abortionist left fetal remains in the mother's uterus, which is extremely dangerous. But all the evidence suggested the abortions had been thorough. Some of the bags had four arms and four legs—twins.

We also wanted to see if the babies were in fact the same gestational age as the estimates on their labels. For the most part, they were: most were between six and fourteen weeks gestation. But one night, after removing the smaller bags from the box, we saw a much larger bag stuffed into the corner. This one had no label. Monica picked it up and looked through the fluid. Then she shifted the bag, and a severed arm appeared. It was a baby boy of at least six months gestation, cut to pieces by the abortionist. We took him and laid out his broken body on a paper towel. Andy Scholberg photographed the child. He laid a quarter and a ruler down on the paper towel to show the size of this perfectly formed child. It was so depressing that I had to leave the garage.

Andy and Monica photographed a number of the bodies. Some people think it macabre to take pictures of abortion victims. But we had to. For one thing, if this country ever comes to its senses and restores legal protection for the unborn, it will be essential that we have historical records so we'll never make the same mistake again. But that's far in the future. Though we live in a time of terrible slaughter, the victims are completely invisible. They are hidden in their mothers' wombs before the killing, then buried in landfills, incinerated, or ground up in garbage disposals and flushed away. The public needs to see what abortion is. As Father Frank Pavone says, "America will not reject abortion until it *sees* abortion."

We kept the bodies for a humane burial, but we had more to do than simply find a suitable resting place. As soon as we opened the first box, we knew we had to see to it that these beautiful children did not die in vain. On Wednesday, May 6, 1987, we held a press conference in front of the Michigan Avenue Medical Center. We set up a long table on the sidewalk. A hearse pulled up and we unloaded the bags containing the dead children and set them out in trays on the table. Behind them we set up large prints of the photographs we had taken.

The press couldn't just dismiss the pictures with the actual victims lying there in front of them. Many were respectful in their coverage. Some of the pro-abortion press, however, criticized us for exposing the brutality. "How dare those fanatic misnamed Right to Lifers show fetuses at a Michigan Avenue clinic?" wrote Ann Gerber of the *Lerner Newspapers*. "How sick and stupid. What kind of men or women would put on such a horrendous show as dragging out fetuses in plastic bags? They don't care about people. They are trying to alleviate their own guilts, inadequacies, and problems with their own sexuality, illuminate their drab, unhappy lives at the expense of women in trouble. They are dangerous clowns with hate in their hearts for the weak and sick. They should be put out on display in plastic bags marked '1987—Examples of Pathetic Nerds.'"[1]

Some of these photographs are still used in our demonstrations. We're often accused of having doctored them. Whenever that happens, I'm reminded of the summer of 1950, when I was traveling in Europe. I took a train from Heidelberg to Munich, arguing the whole time with a German about the Holocaust.

"It never happened," he insisted. "Those people died of influenza. The pictures with the big piles of bodies—faked. They stacked up department store mannequins and put some real bodies on top to make it look like a mass slaughter." He believed that. He had to.

After the press conference, the bodies were delivered to a South Side funeral home. Father Roger Coughlin arranged for them to be stored while their burial arrangements were being made. But the Chancery office contacted us and told us they would not be arranging for a burial, having received legal advice that one or more of

---

1    Ann Gerber, *Lerner Newspapers*, sec. 1, May 10, 1987, 7.

the mothers might sue the archdiocese for imposing religion on her dead baby if it got involved in handling these children's bodies.

We were shocked. Monica wrote Cardinal Bernardin, who then instructed Father Coughlin to go ahead and quietly arrange for the babies' burial. A few days after our press conference, I received a letter from Father Coughlin. "Dear Joe," it said, "I trust you will be happy to know that the bodies of the 500–600 victims of the 30 S. Michigan Avenue abortion mill have been laid to rest."

But we weren't happy. For one thing, those of us who had salvaged these bodies would have liked to attend the burial, but most pro-lifers were never invited. And while the archdiocese had buried them in consecrated ground—St. Mary's Cemetery in south suburban Evergreen Park—there had been no funeral, no ceremony. We thought this was an insult to these tiny victims. Finally, even though we could thank Cardinal Bernardin for having the archdiocese handle the burial, it had obviously been done in a semi-secret way to avoid any press coverage.

That was unacceptable. These children had suffered brutal deaths with the government's stamp of approval, and we'd been roundly criticized by the press for exposing that brutality. A public funeral could have granted these children reverence and respect, but without a final tribute, our decision to hold a press conference made it appear that we were exploiting these children, when in truth, we were hoping to spare others from the same gruesome fate.

The following winter, Conrad Wojnar, who operated a cluster of pregnancy centers in the Chicago area, received a call very similar to the one I'd gotten from John Smith. Conrad's caller worked at Vital Med Laboratories, a pathology lab in Northbrook, Illinois. The employee told him that several abortion clinics around the country were shipping their aborted babies to Vital Med. After conducting pathology on the victims, Vital Med put them in large barrels and left them on a loading dock to be collected by a disposal service. The employee was distraught that these tiny human beings were treated like garbage. Conrad notified Tim Murphy and me. Andy Scholberg called Monica, since she had helped with the retrieval of the babies from behind the Michigan Avenue Medical Center in 1987.

A few nights later, Tim Murphy and Bea Penovich went out to Vital Med and retrieved several boxes of aborted babies. That night, Tim came to my house with the boxes. I suppose it made sense for him to bring them to my place, since we'd brought the bodies from 30 South Michigan to my garage, but I wasn't prepared to store bodies at my home. I went out to the alley to take a look at what he and Bea had found at Vital Med.

"I'm not a mortician, Tim," I told him. "I don't have any space for this. You have to find some other place."

I thought that was the end of it, but on a Sunday afternoon in mid-March, Tim brought a barrel of aborted babies' remains and stashed it in my children's backyard playhouse. My daughter Annie's pet bunny had been missing for several days from his cage in the garage. When Tim put the barrel in the playhouse, he discovered the rabbit, frozen on the floor. He had apparently hopped in there and gotten trapped when a winter wind blew the door shut.

In their book on pro-life activism, *Wrath of Angels*, Jim Risen and Judy Thomas, intent on advancing the notion that all pro-lifers have psychological disorders, wrote, "When activists in his group covertly obtained a large number of aborted fetuses from a Chicago pathology laboratory used by a number of abortion clinics, Scheidler casually stored them in his children's playhouse in his backyard, waiting until he could use them for their shock value in protests."[2] But Risen and Thomas got it wrong. Our purpose in retrieving the abortion

---

2    Jim Risen and Judy Thomas, *Wrath of Angels* (New York: Basic Books, 1998), 103.

victims from the garbage dumpsters was to give them the dignity they deserve.

Monica photographed the Vital Med victims. Like the ones from Michigan Avenue, they were also sealed in individual specimen pouches with information about the patients and the babies. They also had information on where each abortion took place. In all, Tim, Monica, and others collected more than five thousand tiny victims. These victims came from clinics in Raleigh, Fargo, Fort Wayne, Fairfield, New Jersey, Tallahassee, Florida, Wilmington, Delaware, and Chicago.

All of the clinics named were members of Susan Hill's Women's Health Organization, and when NOW added their RICO charges to their lawsuit and added Monica and Tim as defendants, they also named Vital Med Laboratories as a codefendant. The allegation was that the lab had conspired with us in the theft of these bodies. NOW also claimed an additional RICO predicate act, interstate transport of stolen property of a value exceeding one hundred dollars, basing this charge on the fact that we sent the fetal remains to the states where they had been aborted for burial.

As we drew nearer to the trial, though, Vital Med was dropped as a defendant. A conspiracy charge may have been too hard to prove since our contact had been an employee, but I suspect the true reason was that the discussion of these thefts would force a definition of exactly what was stolen, and NOW's attorneys wanted to make certain that abortion victims were never presented to the jury.

We contacted pro-lifers in each of the cities listed on the bags and asked them to arrange funerals. The unborn victims were placed in several coffins handmade by Edmund Miller. These were shipped or driven to their point of origin, where they were laid to rest in dignified ceremonies.

We planned a funeral for the two thousand killed in the Chicago area. We wanted to avoid another secret burial. I met with Cardinal Bernardin in June 1988 in the Chancery Office. With me were prominent Chicago-area pro-life leaders: Eileen Dolehide, Dr. Eugene Diamond, Mary Ann Hacket, Nancy Czerwiec, Dr. John Kelly, Dick O'Connor, Jean Synovic, Pastor Denny Cadieux, Bonnie Quirke, and Ed Haberkorn. The Cardinal brought Father Francis Kane, Father Michael Place, and Jimmy Lago.

"Cardinal," I started, "we've uncovered another two thousand bodies of aborted babies. We want to hold a dignified funeral for them. We'd like you to help us do this."

"We did bury the six hundred you brought us last year," he said.

"Yes, and we appreciate that," I replied. "But what we need is a public ceremony that will show people that these are really human beings with dignity and value."

I followed up with a letter to Cardinal Bernardin, asking him to officiate at a burial service for the victims of abortion. The Cardinal not only allowed the archdiocese to hold a funeral ceremony, but he agreed to celebrate the Mass. On July 30, a thousand mourners gathered at the chapel at Queen of Heaven cemetery in Hillside, Illinois, for a memorial Mass to pay tribute to the two thousand infants in two white adult-sized coffins donated by a local funeral home.

"My brothers and sisters," the Cardinal prayed, "we have gathered this morning in witness to our belief that every human being is created in the image and likeness of God. This means every human life at every stage of development, from conception to natural death, and in all circumstances is sacred and beloved of God. As we mourn the aborted lives of the babies whose remains we bury with respect today, we also renew our firm commitment to protect and defend human life, especially those who are most vulnerable."

The burial at St. Mary's Cemetery received no media coverage, but the interment at Queen of Heaven was the lead story on the evening news, and it received substantial coverage in the local and national press. The ACLU criticized the service as a burial of "tissue" and criticized the Cardinal for being a pawn in a shameless publicity stunt. They insinuated that the bodies had been obtained illegally. When asked about these charges by a *Chicago Tribune* reporter, Cardinal Bernardin replied, "I didn't ask where the babies came from and I don't know what the legal consequences may be, but they pale in significance when compared to the taking of innocent human life. I knew what I was doing, and what I was doing was a corporal work of mercy done in a very beautiful religious ceremony."[3]

Five and a half years after the burial at Queen of Heaven, while I was preparing to appear before the Supreme Court, I received a phone call from Father Ken Velo, an aide to Cardinal Bernardin. Father Velo was an old friend who had been stationed at my parish, Queen of All Saints, and he was an extending an invitation from the Cardinal to join him at the Archbishop's Residence in Lincoln Park.

Oral arguments in *NOW v. Scheidler* were two days away. We were already deep in debt from legal bills. An unfavorable ruling from the court would only push those bills higher. In the press, NOW was making every effort to connect me with clinic bombings and arson. While I never lit any fuses or assaulted any clinic personnel myself, they argued, the bulk of the alleged violence in the abortion wars was directed by me—including the murders of abortionists.

Now the Cardinal was inviting me to come pray with him at the Residence and to bring any family members who wanted to come along. At the time, the Cardinal was himself the subject of a bogus lawsuit. A former seminarian, Stephen Cook, had filed charges of sexual abuse against a number of clergy, and he named Bernardin in the suit.

Ann and my son Matthias accompanied me to the Residence. It was a beautiful snowy evening, and the expansive lawn glistened as we walked up to the Victorian mansion. When we rang the bell, the Cardinal himself answered the door and took our coats, and he

---

3    Michael Hirsley, "Abortion Foes Hail Cardinal for Fetus Rite," *Chicago Tribune*, August 5, 1988.

showed us into a study where he had two prayer books opened to the same page. We sat and prayed together. Afterward, the Cardinal asked if we wanted to tour the downstairs and see his private chapel. We prayed there as well, each of us asking God that justice would be served and the charges against both of us would be proven false.

We talked more after our prayers about our respective lawsuits. "I know what it is to be accused of something you didn't do," the Cardinal said.

"I'd rather be accused of what I didn't do than what you didn't do," I told him.

"Me too," he replied.

The Supreme Court allowed the RICO case to proceed, and three and a half years later, I lost in federal court. I wouldn't be exonerated by the court until 2003. NOW's literature on the case says it was "overturned on a technicality." That technicality happens to be the First Amendment and the proper definition of extortion.

Cardinal Bernardin's vindication came much more quickly. Stephen Cook made the charge after undergoing hypnotic therapy, but three months later, Cook backpedaled, asserting he was "ninety-five percent sure he hadn't abused me." Others had—Cook didn't drop the case entirely—but he wanted to make sure the right defendants were named. Bernardin met with Cook in 1994. At that meeting, Cook was 100 percent certain the Cardinal was innocent. They prayed together, the Cardinal forgave Cook, and the two men reconciled.

The next year, in 1995, Cardinal Bernardin underwent surgery for pancreatic cancer. In 1996, he announced that his cancer had returned. It was in his liver, and it was inoperable. He wrote of his experiences accepting his impending death, and he closed it with the Prayer of St. Francis. It's a prayer that speaks in a special way to those working to save the unborn, to those ministering to mothers who may feel hopeless, trapped, or fearful. We work to begin a transformation from sadness into joy.

> Lord, make me an instrument of your peace.
> Where there is hatred, let me sow love.
> Where there is injury, pardon.
> Where there is doubt, faith.
> Where there is despair, hope.
> Where there is darkness, light.
> Where there is sadness, joy.
>
> O Divine Master, grant that I may not so much seek
> to be consoled, as to console;
> to be understood, as to understand;
> to be loved, as to love;
> for it is in giving that we receive,
> it is in pardoning that we are pardoned.
> It is in dying that we are born to eternal life.

On November 1, 1996, All Saints' Day, Joseph Cardinal Bernardin completed his book. Two weeks later, he passed into that eternal life.

## CHAPTER 28

# Vengeance Is Not Ours

In January 1993, David Gunn marked the twentieth anniversary of *Roe v. Wade* by setting up speakers in the windows of Susan Hill's Montgomery, Alabama, clinic to blast Tom Petty's "I Won't Back Down" at pro-life protesters.

At the same time in Pensacola, John Burt held a burial ceremony for two aborted babies on the strip of land he'd purchased adjacent to the Ladies Center where Gunn also did abortions. A newcomer to Pensacola turned up at Burt's ceremony. His name was Michael Griffin.

Six and a half weeks later, as John led a picket in front of the Pensacola Women's Medical Service Center, Griffin approached Gunn in the back of the clinic and fired four shots. He came around to the front of the clinic and went directly to the police, handing them his .38 revolver. "I've just shot a man behind the clinic," he said. "You need to call an ambulance." Gunn was rushed to the hospital and died later that day during surgery.

Gunn immediately became a martyr for the pro-abortion cause. Pro-life leaders across the country raced to denounce the killing and to distance themselves from Griffin—and, for a lot of them, from activism in general. John Burt, the outspoken activist who had protested the trial of clinic bombers and had been charged with burglary for invading the Ladies Center, was quickly vilified for brainwashing Griffin and encouraging the murder.

"Addressing oneself to the shooting of Dr. David Gunn," I wrote after the killing, "is a no-win situation. Unless one grieves uncontrollably for the death of this itinerant abortionist, who had at least thirty thousand abortion deaths to his credit and was about to perform another dozen, one is considered by the abortion crowd and the secular media to be unrepentant and supportive of the shooting. On the other hand, if we show too much regret, too much concern, and condemn the killing, we run the risk of minimizing the reality of what this man did for a living. Six days a week for the past five years, he murdered unborn babies."

I suspected Griffin would try to argue a defense of necessity. "One problem with this argument," I wrote, "is that the abortionist is not the immediate aggressor against the unborn. He is an auxiliary hired by the primary aborter: the mother herself, or the boyfriend, husband, or family members forcing her to have an abortion. Dr. Gunn would not have been doing those abortions if he had not been hired by those who wanted the babies killed. The abortionist is the hit man. Even when he is stopped, the goal of saving the child's life is not likely to be achieved. The woman can always hire another abortionist to destroy her child."

But not everyone in the movement saw it that way. A Presbyterian minister in Pensacola, Paul Hill, argued that Griffin had committed a justifiable homicide. I had met Hill in October 1986 when I was the keynote speaker at the Mississippi Right to Life convention, where he was honored with a Pro-Life Friend of the Year award. But that was the only time I had heard of him until the Gunn killing.

After the shooting, Hill began carrying a large sign outside the Ladies Center with modified text of God's covenant to Noah from Genesis:

"Whoever sheds (unborn) man's blood, by man will his blood be shed." He had added the word to make it clear he considered abortionists guilty of murder—and subject to capital punishment. Hill began recruiting other pro-lifers to sign a statement that Griffin's actions were justified. He composed a document titled "Defensive Action."

> We the undersigned declare the justice of taking all godly action necessary to defend innocent human life, including the use of force. We proclaim that whatever force is legitimate to defend the life of a born child is legitimate to defend the life of an unborn child. We assert that if Michael Griffin did in fact kill David Gunn, his use of lethal force was justifiable provided it was carried out for the purpose of defending the lives of unborn children. Therefore, he ought to be acquitted of the charges against him.[1]

Hill only got a few people to sign his petition, but he got himself a great deal of media attention. Talk show hosts, eager to dazzle audiences, gave Hill and his theory far more attention than they deserved.

Six months after Gunn was killed, Shelley Shannon shot George Tiller outside his Wichita clinic. She thought she was taking a more nuanced approach than Griffin had, since she shot him in the arms so he couldn't perform abortions, but Tiller recovered and went right back to his practice. I had met Shelley several times at various pro-life events, and I was shocked when I heard she had shot Tiller.

Shelley managed to get away from Tiller's clinic after the shooting and was a fugitive for several weeks, but eventually another pro-lifer convinced her to turn herself in. Despite the claim that she had sought only to injure Tiller, she was tried for attempted murder. During her trial, her connection to other incidents came

---

1    Paul Hill, "Defensive Action Statement," http://www.armyofgod.com/defense.html.

out. Shelly had set some fires and committed several "acid attacks," which evokes images of a terrorist flinging acid in someone's face, but in this case involved squirting butyric acid into mail slots. The acid has a rancid vomit smell, but it's completely harmless. She got a ten-year sentence for the shooting, with another eleven tacked on for the stink bomb and arson incidents.

Paul Hill, meanwhile, added support for Shelley to his Defensive Action document. He eventually got twenty-four others to sign his list. Some signatories had already been convicted for attacks on real estate, but Paul was asking them to condone attacks on *people*. As I told the *Los Angeles Times* in September 1993, "I'm not a wimp, but I'm not with the arson and bomb squad, either. Guys I've worked with for years who've shared my views are saying, 'wait a minute, maybe it's time to get a little more forceful.' I used to be able to sit around a table and say, without any prevarication, that these were nonviolent people. I can't say that anymore."[2]

One doctor was killed and another wounded. People I knew either had done the shooting or were accused of encouraging it. Now with some pro-lifers endorsing the shooters' actions, something had definitely changed, and the ripples from that change would impact activism all over the country. The Pro-Life Action League and other pro-life leaders decided it was time to host a closed-door meeting of activists to discuss how we should respond to these shootings and to impress on new recruits to the pro-life movement that declaring oneself judge, jury, and executioner was not only immoral but disastrous to our cause as well as our image.

Held at the Purple Hotel in Chicago, it was a tense meeting. Federal laws were being enacted against activists. The Supreme Court had ruled to allow my RICO case to proceed, and FACE, which transformed local

---

2      John Balzar, "Abortion Foes Test the Limits," *Los Angeles Times*, September 30, 1993.

trespass misdemeanors into federal felonies, had sailed through both houses of Congress and was awaiting Clinton's signature. But none of these difficulties was as serious as the emerging image of pro-life activists as gun-wielding maniacs. We discussed why violence could never become an acceptable part of the pro-life movement. The majority was adamantly against any use of violence—bombing, arson, threats, anything aiming to hurt or kill abortion providers.

But Paul Hill showed up at the meeting. He brought his Defensive Action document with him, looking for signatures. I didn't have any contact with Hill at that meeting, but shortly afterward he called my office to try to convince me to sign his statement. I asked Ann and two volunteers, Penny and Eileen, to come into my office to listen to the conversation. I turned on the speaker. Hill maintained his theory as just that: a theory, one based on biblical principles. I asked him directly, "Would you ever pull the trigger?"

"No," he replied. "It's just a theory."

"That's good," I said. "But it's not a theory I can support." I declined to add my name to the document.

But it wasn't just a theory. The Ladies Center hired abortionist John Britton to replace David Gunn, and the following July, Paul Hill pulled a shotgun on Britton and his bodyguard, James Barrett, killing both of them. He was convicted and sentenced to death by lethal injection, a sentence that was carried out in 2003. In addition to being tried for murder in the Florida court system, Paul Hill became the first person in America prosecuted under FACE. It's ironic that the first use of a law designed to outlaw peaceful protests—a law passed because an abortionist was murdered—was used in the case of another murdered abortionist.

Hill was sentenced to death early in December 1994. At the end of that month, two more killings occurred. Twenty-two-year-old John Salvi entered a Planned Parenthood clinic in Brookline, Massachusetts, a suburb of Boston, and fatally shot the receptionist. He then went across town to another Planned Parenthood clinic and killed the receptionist there. Five others were wounded in Salvi's shooting spree. He was convicted and sentenced to prison without parole. He committed suicide in his cell in 1996.

Immediately after these shootings, Boston's Bernard Cardinal Law called for a moratorium on all pro-life activities at abortion clinics, including sidewalk counseling. I thought this was a bad idea—why stop trying to save babies' lives because of the actions of one fanatic? I called pro-lifers in Boston to see whether they were going to heed the Cardinal's suggestion. They were. None were willing to go to the clinics.

At that time, my niece, Elsa Scheidler, was in graduate school at Boston College, a Jesuit university. She had been spending her Saturday mornings at local clinics praying and counseling. I called her to ask if she would be willing to go to a clinic where she usually counseled.

"But the Cardinal told us not to go out," she said.

"It's not an order," I said. "It's only a suggestion. The fact is, we've done nothing wrong. Pro-lifers don't kill people. We're not responsible for those deaths. Staying away from clinics is conceding guilt. Women will still go to those clinics and babies will still die if nobody is there."

"You don't think anyone else will be out there?" she asked.

"I've called everyone I know in Boston. None of them will go. It looks like the Cardinal has scared them off. But if your conscience tells you to be out there trying to counsel women, don't let him stop you. And the press is definitely going to be out there. If there are no pro-lifers there, the only ones who they'll be interviewing are the pro-aborts. Someone needs to be there to speak for our side to let them know we don't condone these shootings."

Elsa agreed to go and was enthusiastic about it. The next morning, she and her friend Michael Patrick went to a Boston clinic—the only pro-lifers in the city willing to ignore Cardinal Law's suggestion.

The press was also there. "Didn't your bishop order you not to be here?" asked one reporter.

"I don't owe the Cardinal political allegiance," Elsa answered. "I owe him spiritual obedience. Nothing I'm doing here violates my spiritual obedience to the Church. I'm following my conscience as a Catholic by being here trying to save lives."

Nine months later, abortionist Barnett Slepian was warming a pot of soup in his suburban Buffalo, New York, kitchen when a bullet tore through the window, striking him in the back. He died two hours later. Investigators identified pro-lifer James Charles Kopp as the main suspect. Kopp disappeared. The FBI put him on their Ten Most Wanted list.

I had met Kopp in New York City in 1985. He was dating a dental assistant at the time, and they were talking about getting married, but they decided to dedicate themselves to pro-life work for a few years first. A year later, I ran into Kopp again at an activist convention in San Francisco.

I met Jim a third time in 1989. By now the dental assistant had married a doctor, and Jim had begun using the one-man rescue technique known as the "Lock and Block." His first blockade was on a clinic staircase, where he'd cuffed his ankles together around the steps and kept the clinic closed all day. Kopp and I spent hours driving around to various junkyards in Oakland and Berkeley looking for materials he could use in other "Lock and Blocks." We spent the evening discussing how closing clinics didn't require the large number of protesters that Randall Terry and other Rescue leaders thought were essential. A one-man "Lock and Block" could do the job.

When I heard Kopp was suspected in the Slepian killing, I was certain the FBI had the wrong man. Kopp eluded capture for two years, fleeing to Mexico and then Ireland before he was arrested in France in 2001. He declared his innocence, and I believed him.

But in the end, Kopp confessed, claiming he'd only tried to wound Slepian. What made the killing especially tragic was that pro-lifers had gained some ground in their attempts to convert Slepian. In the last speech he ever gave, Slepian told a group of Medical Students for Choice that abortion is undeniably the taking of potential life. "It is not pretty. It is not easy. And in a perfect world, it would not be necessary."[3]

Pro-lifers have converted a number of abortion providers, and if not for Kopp's actions, Barnett Slepian could have joined the ranks of former abortionists who now advocate for life.

In 2009, George Tiller was shot again, this time at his church by Scott Philip Roeder. The shooter was not aiming to wound. Tiller is now the most famous of the slain abortion providers. Pro-abortion demonstrators sometimes sing a little rhyme in his memory: "Pro-life, you're a killer; we remember Dr. Tiller." We remember him too, and we pray for his soul.

The struggle to restore protection to the unborn is not just about stopping abortion providers. It's about creating a culture that welcomes and respects human life. The pro-life movement has powerful tools at its disposal: prayer, compassion, crisis pregnancy centers, sidewalk and postabortion counseling, street activists, legislators and lobbyists, and the energy of a young generation.

We don't need violence. We have the truth.

---

3    John Wells, *Sniper: The True Story of Anti-Abortion Killer James A. Kopp* (New York: Wiley, 2008), 108.

## CHAPTER 29

# The Road to Damascus

D r. Bernard Nathanson entered the abortion business long before *Roe v. Wade*. He was one of the main speakers at the inaugural NARAL meeting at Chicago's Drake Hotel in February 1969. He had no qualms with abortion and even aborted his own child when his girlfriend got pregnant. When New York passed its permissive abortion law a year later, Nathanson knew women would flock to the state from all across the country. He opened a clinic in Manhattan that he bragged was the largest in the world. Dr. Nathanson provided the data introduced in the *Roe* case that claimed there were nearly a million back-alley abortions in America each year, with ten thousand maternal deaths annually.

But in 1974, Bernard Nathanson quit doing abortions. That same year, he published an article in the *New England Journal of Medicine* about his career in which he confessed his "increased certainty that I had in fact presided over 60,000 deaths." In his 1979 book, *Aborting America*, he admitted that the pre-*Roe* data he and NARAL had publicized were fictions: The true figures, he said, were about one-tenth as many illegal abortions as he had reported and fewer than 300 abortion-related deaths per year. He knew these smaller numbers wouldn't convince people that America needed "safe, legal" abortion, and so he falsified the data.

After his conversion, Dr. Nathanson became a big name in pro-life circles. When he spoke at various events, he received standing ovations. I never stood. *Wait a minute*, I thought. *This is a* doctor. *He knew what he was doing.*

One evening, when Dr. Nathanson and I were staying in the same hotel during a pro-life conference in Indianapolis, he approached me in the lobby and asked if I'd have a drink with him. As we sat at the bar, I told him that I didn't trust him when he said he hadn't known it was a baby.

"Sure, that ten-thousand figure was phony," he said, "but some women *were* dying from back-alley abortions, and I thought the safest thing to do was to get abortion legalized."

He was trying to avoid talking about the babies.

"But you killed sixty thousand people," I said. "And think about the children *they* would have had. You wiped out a whole city!"

He looked down at his drink. "You're right, Joe," he said. "It's so awful I can't dwell on it. Suicide runs in my family, you know. I can't let myself believe I actually knew what I was doing."

I began to understand Nathanson a little better. He seemed to revel in the applause at pro-life events, but under it all, he was anguishing over what he had done. After our conversation, I started to feel compassion for him. We eventually became good friends.

When I shared the cab ride with George Tiller on my way to my first NAF convention and he told me about using ultrasounds to do abortions, I suspected that such a film would be a powerful tool for pro-life work. I hadn't seen his footage, but after the convention, I called some former abortionists I knew to see if anyone could get a copy of the film. I had no luck. However, just a few months later, Dr. Nathanson talked to one of his abortionist colleagues. "Do me a favor," he said. "Next time you're doing an abortion, put an ultrasound device on the mother and tape it for me."

Nathanson and the doctor watched the film together. It was the last time that doctor ever performed an abortion. Nathanson narrated a film that used the ultrasound abortion footage, *The Silent Scream*. It shows a baby at twelve weeks gestation trying to get away from the suction cannula and then struggling and opening its mouth in agony as the abortionist rips its limbs off. The film had a tremendous impact worldwide. President Reagan himself praised it as a valuable educational tool for teaching the truth about abortion.

Nathanson used to describe himself as a "Jewish atheist," but in December 1996, he called to tell me he was converting to Catholicism. He was baptized on the Feast of the Immaculate Conception by John Cardinal O'Connor in New York. Joan Andrews was his godmother. He invited me to come, but I had a speaking engagement that day and I couldn't break it.

A reporter once asked Nathanson why he had converted. "No religion matches the special role for forgiveness that is afforded by the Catholic Church," he said.[1] He was able to confess the evil he had done, and he had found the path to forgiveness.

When I was arrested in Denver in 1986 on the Florida burglary warrant, I missed Carol Everett's talk at the National Right to Life Convention. She had operated five abortion clinics in Texas, earning close to a million dollars a year. But now she had joined the pro-life cause, and I wanted to hear her story.

I bought the tape from the conference and listened to it on the plane ride home. She recounted how a financial advisor she worked with helped her get out of the industry. As I listened to her story, I thought of other abortionists I'd known who had quit, and it

---

1    Nathanson quoted by Joseph Pearce, *C. S. Lewis and the Catholic Church* (Charlotte, NC: St. Benedict Press, 2013).

occurred to me that we could set up a whole conference of reformed abortionists. Such a conference could give other pro-lifers ideas for how to appeal to abortionists and urge them to quit. One of the chapters I'd written for *CLOSED* is entitled "Adopt an Abortionist," and it offers suggestions for getting physicians to give up their grisly trade, but a conference of this sort would be much more effective, since the testimony would be coming firsthand.

I started looking for ex-abortionists who might be willing to testify at such a conference. Carol was happy to be on the panel, and Adele Nathanson, Bernard's wife, supplied us with other names, including that of Dr. Anthony Levatino of New York. In addition to Carol Everett and Tony Levatino, we invited Debby Henry, a clinic worker from Detroit, and Dr. Joseph Randall from Atlanta. We held the conference in November 1987 at the Hyatt Regency O'Hare and called it "Meet the Abortion Providers."

When I started promoting the conference, I caught some objections from dedicated pro-life friends. "Why should I listen to anything a baby killer has to say?" they asked. I explained that we had to know more about why these doctors and nurses went into the abortion business, what it was like working in the industry, and why they quit. If we got some inside information, we could better reach out to current providers.

I drew up a graphic for the event that borrowed from the 1978 "Meet the Abortion Profiteers" series in the *Chicago Sun-Times*. Theirs featured a doctor with a surgical mask and thick eyebrows and a sinister gaze. We didn't want our image to be quite as eerie. I removed the mask, groomed the eyebrows, gave him glasses, and added a nurse. After we started publicizing the conference, I got a letter from the *Sun-Times* accusing me of stealing their picture. I reminded them that the whole "Profiteers" exposé had been my idea in the first place and that they'd sent a spy to my office. They let the matter drop.

Tony Levatino gave a particularly memorable talk. He spoke about his daughter who had died after being hit by a car at age five. The loss of his own child made him reconsider the work he did every day, eliminating other people's children. It was the first time he had publicly told the story of why he'd left the abortion business, and he had to stop for a while to compose himself. His talk, and indeed the whole conference, was very powerful. My friends who had been skeptical all agreed it was a very worthwhile effort.

We held a second "Meet the Abortion Providers" conference in February 1989 at the Marriott O'Hare. The evening before it began, I met with the speakers to discuss their talks. As before, they planned to describe what it was like to work in a killing center and why they had to quit. At the end of our meeting, I told them, "People are going to be hanging on your every word, so don't hold back. Though abortion is technically classified as homicide, since it's legal, it would be very effective if you called it murder."

Our first speaker was Dr. MacArthur Hill. He stepped to the podium and began his talk, saying, "I am here to tell you that I am a murderer. I have taken the lives of innocent babies."

He recounted a recurring nightmare he started having when he was working as an abortionist. He'd be delivering a healthy baby, then would present it to a jury of faceless people to see whether the baby was to live or die. Every night, the jurors would give the baby a thumbs down, and he'd wake up in a panic.

Dr. Hill spoke of how he'd gotten into the business. "I wasn't an avid abortion proponent," he said, "but a reluctant puppet in a world gone mad." His clinic had never been picketed, but he told the story of a colleague whose clinic *was* picketed and who wanted his name off the picket signs. "'Simple,'" Hill told his colleague. "'Stop doing abortions.'" Hill encouraged the assembly to keep up their pressure on abortionists. He said he wished someone had put that kind of pressure on him. It would have gotten him out of the business sooner—"and," he said, "it can help them save their souls."[2]

When we held the first of these conferences, I hadn't thought to film the presentations, but one of the attendees, Roger McZura, a videographer from Hell, Michigan, asked if he could set up his cameras.

"Sure," I said, "just don't get in the way."

Roger filmed the second conference as well, and Ann and I met with him in Detroit to produce an hour-long video of the highlights from these two conferences. We'd rented the studio for only one day, and we had to work long into the night to get it done.

We did a fundraiser to help us send copies of our *Meet the Abortion Providers* video to crisis pregnancy centers all across the country. Several pregnant women opted to choose life after seeing and hearing testimony from former abortionists about exactly what goes on in clinics and the consequences of abortion. They'd never hear this from abortion clinic counselors.

We held two more conferences featuring former clinic workers: nurses, administrators, guards, and doctors. Dr. Beverly McMillan, who had opened Mississippi's first abortion clinic in 1975, spoke at our 1989 conference about why she was now pro-life. She'd even sat in with rescuers at clinics where she once performed abortions. In November 1997, we held a conference in New York City. The day of the event, I stepped outside and saw none other than Dr. Bernard Nathanson coming down the sidewalk. I explained what we were doing in town, and he asked if he could come up and address the crowd. The 1997 conference featured some of the speakers who had first told their stories at the earlier conferences. In these

---

2    "Former Abortionist MacArthur Hill," *Pro-Life Action League*, http://prolifeaction.org/providers/hill.php.

presentations, they spoke more about the attitudes pro-lifers can adopt that can better encourage the conversion of an abortionist.

Roger produced a second video, *Abortion: the Inside Story*, from these later events.

In 1994, the abortion war saw one of the most dramatic conversions of any movement in history when Norma McCorvey—*Jane Roe* of the infamous 1973 *Roe v. Wade* ruling—became pro-life. Sandra Cano, the plaintiff from *Doe v. Bolton*, had long been a critic of the forces who used her to dismantle American abortion laws. Both Norma and Sandra testified at our fifth Meet the Abortion Providers conference. Both had agonized for years over the part they had played in legalizing abortion. They had been cruelly used by the instigators of the move to legalize abortion. They found solace in the pro-life movement.

In 2012, the Pro-Life Action League held another conference of former abortion providers, "Converted: From Abortion Provider to Pro-Life Activist." Many who once campaigned for the right to choose now support the pro-life cause. But I've yet to hear of any pro-life leader who has gone over to the other side. When the doctor who campaigned ardently to legalize abortion on demand can stand on a stage and be introduced as "the Saint Paul of the pro-life movement," there is hope that one day we will be able to call all abortion providers "former."

## CHAPTER 30

# Ora et Labora

In the fall of 1973, just after I founded the Chicago Office for Pro-Life Publicity, Ann and I contacted our pastor at Queen of All Saints to ask if we could speak to the parishioners on Respect Life Sunday. Ann addressed the congregation while she held our four-month-old daughter Catherine. She explained that just a few months earlier, while Catherine was still in the womb, it would have been legal to have her killed. It's fitting that our first pro-life talks were in a church. Pro-life activism has to be prayerful work. At the root of the right-to-life movement is a profound respect for the Author of life and a desire to see His will carried out.

At the Benedictine monastery I attended in the '50s, we lived by St. Benedict's motto: *ora et labora*—pray and work. Prayer first, then work. It's a perfect formula for pro-life activism. When I started out in my pro-life mission, I was motivated by the horror of abortion, its cruelty and its inhumanity. But as I delved more into the anti-life mentality and began spending more time at clinics and talking with abortionists, I began to recognize the evil that drives the abortion machine. I suspect that few who advocate for abortion realize just how evil it really is. After all, it's difficult to choose evil without first dressing it up in something that looks good, such as "reproductive freedom."

But there are times when the evil is palpable, and in those times, we have no recourse but prayer. This battle is fundamentally a spiritual one. Our work must be based in prayer if we are going to accomplish anything.

At a rescue rally in South Bend, Indiana, a young man came up and asked if he could have his picture taken with me. I said sure, and we took the photo. Then I asked him why he was interested in being photographed with me.

"Because until a few days ago, you were the person I hated most in the world," he said. "I have a picture of you on my dartboard back home."

"Where's that?" I asked.

"Ohio. I worked as a clinic escort back there."

"What happened?"

"I was hitchhiking out here to protest you guys," he told me. "A couple of ministers picked me up. They talked about abortion the whole way here. They converted me."

He went on to describe his experience at the clinic he worked for, and he told me that at that particular one, some of the staff were Satanists. They considered their work pleasing to Satan. The abortion was an "offering" to Satan.

In Chicago, in the mid-'90s, the virulently pro-abortion group Refuse and Resist specialized in harassing pro-lifers. From time to time, one of their leaders, a woman named Sunny, came out to counterprotest with the word *witch* written across her forehead. She held a voodoo doll that she claimed was me, and she stabbed it repeatedly with a large needle. I don't know enough about it to critique her technique, but I never felt a thing.

In March 2004, while on a Face the Truth Tour at local colleges, Refuse and Resist came out in force to harass us. One of their members sneaked up behind me with a can of black ink. When I turned, she whipped it at me with a paintbrush. It splattered all over me, and some of it got in my eye. I had to go to the hospital to have the ink cleaned off the inside of my eyelid.

When Kansas native Allison Jurczyk came to Chicago in 1996 to study law, she contacted the League office looking to join in some activist work with us. I suggested she go undercover and infiltrate Refuse and Resist to keep us informed when they planned to counter our demonstrations. She liked the idea and stayed with them for about a year.

Allison was with them during the months we endured their most hostile opposition, which we encountered when we came out to the American Women's Medical Center on Western Avenue in Chicago. A man named Jonathan was one of their regulars, and he was without a doubt one of the most unpleasant people I'd ever met. He was there just about every time we were to insult us, berate us, and try to frustrate our efforts to save lives. Some days he would dress up as a priest and pretend to consecrate his coffee and mock our prayers.

Jonathon was so hateful that we were concerned he would cross the line. We started videotaping his antics. One day, as I stood by the clinic fence praying, he walked up and began shouting in my face. I could feel his spittle on my cheeks. Suddenly, without even thinking, I punched him—something I'd pledged never to do. He was more shocked than hurt, but he ran over to a squad car parked near the clinic. I quickly left the scene.

When I got home, I called the police precinct near the clinic to file a complaint. I hoped I could get my version of the story reported first, but they told me that if I wanted to file a report I had to do it in person. When I got to the station, I noticed that the last entry in the book was Jonathon, reporting that I struck him.

A few weeks later, I received a summons to appear in Cook County Criminal Court to stand trial for battery. When I arrived, neither the judge nor my accuser was in the courtroom. Then the door to the judge's chambers opened, and I heard laughter. The judge came out chuckling, and right behind him walked the man who had incited me to punch him. I realized I had no chance of getting a fair trial from that judge, so I demanded a change of venue.

The morning of the rescheduled trial, Allison Jurczyk called the office. She was still spying on Refuse and Resist for us, and she'd just learned that the man's attorney ordered a subpoena of the video footage shot the day of the incident. When I called my office to check in, I learned they were demanding the tape. I hadn't seen the film yet, but I wanted to make sure that what was shown in court would also include his aggressive and offensive behavior. We asked for a jury trial to buy some extra time. In the hours it took to assemble the jury, the activist who shot the video, Brian Martens, compiled a greatest-hits version of the man's harassment of pro-lifers over the past year. At the end was my blow to his jaw.

Once the video was ready, we told the judge that we no longer wanted a jury trial. He permitted a bench trial, but he made a point of letting us know he was pro-choice. While I was on the stand, I listed a number of the accuser's antics: mocking us as we prayed, dressing as a priest, shouting down pro-lifers. He took the stand and denied doing any of those things. Then they demanded the video be shown. On the first showing, it was clear he had lied on the stand. His attorney was visibly upset.

The judge came down from his bench and asked to view the video again. After doing so for a second time, he asked to see the video a third time. Then he went back up to the bench and told Jonathon that he deserved whatever he got for the kind of insults and harassment he'd hurled at us.

"Don't you dare use my courtroom to fight your political battles," he said. He dismissed the charges against me and sent my accuser away, telling him that if he ever saw him in his courtroom again, he would find him in contempt. We went out and celebrated.

Not long after his case against me was dismissed, Jonathon got very ill. A large boil on his neck burst and he got blood poisoning. Two young women from my staff went to his hospital room with a get-well card, but he refused to see them and called hospital security to throw them out. His condition worsened, and he died not long after that. I think of him every time I pray at the American Women's Medical Center.

Pro-life activists are used to being in the minority in front of clinics. Often a lone pro-life counselor will be on the sidewalk while several escorts usher women into the clinic before they can say a word. But there's one event where pro-lifers can always be certain of being in the majority. The March for Life in Washington, DC, continues to draw hundreds of thousands of pro-lifers from all over the country every year. I've marched in nearly all of them.

Each year, the march opens with many Masses celebrated across DC, but the most notable is the one held at the Basilica of the National Shrine of the Immaculate Conception the night before the march. Several hundred clergy process down the aisle into the sanctuary. They are joined by hundreds of seminarians, deacons, priests, Eastern Rite patriarchs, and Roman Catholic bishops and cardinals. It takes nearly an hour for the procession to enter the sanctuary. Thousands of pilgrims begin their *Roe v. Wade* memorial and protest at this powerful prayer vigil.

The following morning, after Masses, breakfasts, and talks, thousands file out onto Constitution Avenue, where members of pro-life clubs from high schools and colleges are gathered with their banners and flags, joining with Right to Life organizations from all fifty states and many national groups. Together they form one of the largest marches seen each year in the nation's capital. In recent years, estimates have marked attendance at more than half a million.

Marches are held in other parts of the country as well, such as San Francisco's Walk for Life West Coast and March for Life Chicago.

Impressive as the March for Life is, dedication to the pro-life cause cannot be fulfilled one day each year. In 2007, the Pro-Life Action League produced a handout that we circulated near the Supreme Court building. "Congratulations," it said. "Today you marched for life. How about tomorrow?" On the back of the card, we listed a dozen possible activities to keep supporting the cause throughout the year, from sidewalk counseling to supporting a crisis pregnancy center to organizing a prayer vigil. It was a miniature outline of the ideas in *CLOSED*. With some help from friends, we handed out twenty-five thousand cards. We were giving the marchers some ideas for *labora* to put their pro-life enthusiasm into action throughout the year.

My father did well in his many businesses and had given his children a moderate amount of stock. When I quit my public relations job and got involved in pro-life work, I had to sell off those assets to make ends meet. Pro-life activism is not a lucrative field. When I consider all the prayers we've offered to keep the office going, to make payroll for our small staff, and see how consistently those prayers have been answered—so often at the last minute—I can't help but believe that God wants this work done.

Creativity, combined with prayer and hard work, is the key to success in pro-life activism. Ann and I start every day with Mass. Our staff says morning prayers in our office chapel every morning. Then we get down to the nitty-gritty work that must be done, whether that is a Truth Day out on the streets with our victim photos, sidewalk counseling and praying in front of a clinic, or meeting with a pro-abortion writer. We take a break at 3 PM for the Divine Mercy Chaplet, and then it's back to *labora*.

Being arrested in Denver brought me to the daily rosary and a closer relationship with our Blessed Mother. I never let a day pass without saying the rosary. I've also made it a habit to pray for abortionists every day. Whenever I'm meditating on the Joyful, Luminous, Sorrowful, or Glorious Mysteries, the third is where I include a prayer for the abortionists.

After a series of attacks on our storefront office on LeMai Avenue, just a block from my home, our landlord refused to renew our lease, so we moved the Pro-Life Action League into a six-story building on Cicero Avenue, about a mile east of our first office.

In our new office, we had a room that we used for morning prayers. I decided to convert it into a proper chapel. My friend Penny Kleiner knew that the Trappist Monks at New Mallory Abbey near Dubuque replaced their choir stalls and stored the old ones in a barn. We drove up to Dubuque to see if we could buy some of them. Brother Felix went up into the loft and found about a hundred choir stalls covered in dust. The abbot allowed us to take the ones we wanted. We selected eleven, took them back to Chicago, and had them stripped and refinished.

A carpenter friend, Noel Naughton, paneled the room and put in risers for the altar and choir stalls. I spent evenings making wooden detail pieces for the windows. A small closet became a sacristy.

We found a set of Stations of the Cross at a secondhand store. One station was missing so we got a good price. The missing station was the twelfth: Jesus dies on the cross. A few days later, Tim Murphy called me to tell me he had found the twelfth station. It was from a different set but was an exact match with ours.

A friend donated a tabernacle. The chancellor of the Chicago Archdiocese sent a representative of the archbishop to see the space. He was impressed and suggested we could keep the Blessed Sacrament in the chapel if we could bolt down the tabernacle, add a sanctuary lamp, and have Mass celebrated there at least once a month.

We gather in the "St. Joseph Chapel" each day to pray—for the children threatened by abortion; for the women considering it or suffering from their decisions; for any intentions people ask us to remember in prayer; for our donors, counselors, and volunteers; and for the conversion of abortion providers.

In 1991, I was invited to a conference on family life at the Vatican. I flew to Rome and stayed in a little pension run by an order of nuns. Speakers came in from all over the world. It was a three-day conference, and for several of the events, I was grouped with delegates from Canada, Australia, and other English-speaking countries. Near the end of the conference, Pope John Paul II entered the auditorium. After his talk, we lined up to meet him. When the Pope made his first visit to Chicago in 1979, Ann and I were fortunate enough to have been selected for the choir that sang at his Mass in Grant Park. But I had yet to meet him personally. I'd brought along a copy of our *Meet the Abortion Providers* video to give him.

I shook hands with Pope John Paul II in my turn. He asked where I was from. When I replied that I was from Chicago, he said, "Oh, yes, Chicago is a very pro-life city."

It was an awesome experience, being in the presence of the Pope. Even though the room was crowded, when I was talking with him, I had a sense of immediate contact, an instant friendliness, as if we'd known each other all our lives. I've often wondered how it must have felt two millennia ago for those who met Christ face to face. That day, I got a sense of what it must have been like.

Frequently when I'm giving a talk, I'll tell the audience, "We're going to have a little Latin lesson. We are going to learn the three most important words that sum up our philosophy of the pro-life movement. Repeat after me: *ora et labora*."

## CHAPTER 31

# Tidings of Great Joy

When executives at NBC first saw *A Charlie Brown Christmas* in 1965, they thought it would be a flop. Throughout the cartoon, Charlie Brown complains about all the commercialization surrounding the holiday. The NBC execs didn't think viewers would relate to a kid who couldn't get into the Christmas spirit. They planned to run it once and cut their losses. They were way off. Of all the Christmas specials the networks have produced, none has been as successful as *A Charlie Brown Christmas*.

Near the end of the show, after being ridiculed for buying a puny tree for the Christmas pageant the kids put on, Charlie Brown yells, "Isn't there anyone who knows what Christmas is all about?" Linus says he can tell him. He walks to the middle of the stage and says, "Lights, please," before pausing in the glow of a spotlight as the auditorium dims. He then recites the story from the Gospel of Luke about the angels appearing to the shepherds.

Of the many Christmas specials that run each year, this is one of the scant few that make even a passing reference to the birth of Jesus. When he finishes the story, Linus walks off the stage and says, "That's what Christmas is all about, Charlie Brown." Charlie takes his puny tree and walks out into the snow with a smile on his face. As the stars twinkle overhead, we hear Linus repeating the gospel story.

Vince Guaraldi's jazz score for the show is now a staple of the season, but the final song, which runs through the closing credits, isn't jazz. It's the classic "Hark the Herald Angels Sing," a song about the very story Linus has just told.[1]

It is interesting that Charles Schultz had Linus tell that part of the nativity story. He could have recited the part about not finding room at the inn or the angel telling Mary about the child she would bear. But he chose to focus the story about how the coming of the messiah was revealed to the world. The Christmas story isn't just about Jesus. And—what was so troubling to Charlie Brown—Christmas isn't just about us, either. It's about both: about God incarnate choosing to be like us, so that we might be able to be like Him.

When the angel appears to the shepherds, it's the third time an angel announces the arrival of the Prince of Peace. The first time, the angel Gabriel visits Mary in Nazareth and tells her of the plan. Mary, aware of the hardship in store, trusts God. Her assent, "be it done unto me according to thy word," is an example for us all. God has a plan for each of us, and we can only achieve true happiness if we strive to live in harmony with His plan.

The second time, an angel visits Joseph in a dream, telling him to not be afraid to take Mary and the child into his care. The news of this pregnancy was not something either of them had expected. To some degree, this story is relevant to any couple surprised by an unplanned pregnancy.

When Mary goes to visit her cousin Elizabeth, who is pregnant with John the Baptist, Elizabeth hears Mary's greeting, and the baby in her womb leaps for joy. The Church Feast of the Visitation

---

1    *A Charlie Brown Christmas*, directed by Bill Melendez and written by Charles M. Schulz (Hollywood, CA: Paramount Pictures, 2000), DVD.

celebrates this event, and it reminds us that the Incarnation occurred not when Jesus was born but when he was conceived. In fact, when the Anno Domini calendar era was first devised, the start of the new year was not placed close to Jesus' birth but nine months earlier, on March 25, the Feast of the Annunciation. The word was not made flesh on Christmas, but when Jesus was conceived in Mary's womb.

In 2012, Ann and I made a pilgrimage to the Holy Land. The last night of the trip, Father Simon Braganza asked each of us what holy site touched us the most. For some, it was seeing where Jesus was baptized in the Jordan. For others, Jesus' path through Jerusalem to His crucifixion was most moving. For me, the most intense moment of the pilgrimage was being in Nazareth at the site of the Annunciation, the very spot where God became man. Inscribed on the altar at the Church of the Annunciation in Nazareth is the phrase "Verbum caro hic factum est"—"the word was made flesh here."

After the nativity, when it came time to announce to those outside the Holy Family that the Savior had been born, the angel appeared to shepherds: common people. Later, royalty from outside the Jewish community recognized the infant Jesus as a king. The tradition of gift-giving that we've taken to such extremes was originally done to commemorate the gifts of the three kings.

After the Magi leave, the Angel of the Lord comes again to Joseph in a second dream, warning him to leave Judea, since King Herod is out to kill the child. On the Feast of the Holy Innocents, just days after Christmas, we remember the babies killed by Herod. This was one of the Bible stories that really disturbed me as a child, and I still find it intriguing that even as the great news of a savior is revealed, those invested in denying Christ begin by slaughtering innocent children.

Chicago used to be full of nativity sets. City Hall had a beautiful set donated by the Plasterer's Union. It stood in the center of the building where the two hallways intersect. Then suddenly, it was gone one year. There used to be a gorgeous crèche near the historic Water Tower surrounded with trees. When atheists launched their campaign against it, the city posted a sign that the city of Chicago did not sponsor the display. I crawled under the fence and removed the sign. The next year, the set was gone.

The ACLU was one of the forces behind this concerted effort to twist the meaning of the First Amendment into a freedom *from* religion. They are also a heavily pro-abortion group, and so several of us made a point of visiting the ACLU offices in Chicago to sing Christmas carols. Of course, we couldn't go on Christmas Day, because oddly enough, the ACLU closes on Christmas, but we brought along a nativity set so that, at least for a while, there was a nativity display at the ACLU offices. We balanced the baby Jesus on the US Postal Service mail drop box, so for a moment, there was even a nativity set on federal property.

The first time we caroled at the ACLU offices, they called the cops. When the officer told us they wanted us to leave, we asked if he wanted to sing with us. He just smiled and held the door. We came again the next year, and this time, the ACLU had cookies for us. So it is possible to warm people's hearts—even if it's only at Christmas. Our caroling expanded, and we began visiting the Chicago offices of Planned Parenthood and NOW. Neither welcomed us with cookies.

After the display in City Hall vanished, a local businessman named Bill Grutzmacher and Reverend Hiram Crawford got a permit to erect one across the street at Daley Plaza. When the American Jewish Congress complained, the city revoked the permit. A few days before Christmas in 1987, I got a call that it was being torn down. Upon reflection, it might seem strange to see a crèche being dismantled and thinking, "Hey, I gotta call that pro-life guy to do something about this." But I wouldn't want it any other way.

As soon as I got the call, I gathered a group and raced down to the Daley Center. City workers were already tossing the statues into a dumpster. About half the statues were in the trash. Joseph and the shepherds were already gone. Each of us grabbed what we could and held on tight.

Television crews arrived, and the struggle made the national news that evening. The workers left, thinking we'd leave, but we didn't. I held the angel with the "Gloria in Excelsis Deo" banner. Passersby joined in, and we called in others to help relieve our crew. We held the statues all through the night. The next day, schoolchildren stopped by, and we let them hold the baby Jesus statue. Meanwhile, pro-life attorney Jennifer Neubauer went to court and got a temporary restraining order from federal judge James Parsons, halting the city's efforts to tear down the set.

By the next year, Neubauer had secured a federal injunction barring discrimination against religious symbols in the public square. So the scene could stay, not just that year, but in future years as well: not just in Chicago, but wherever citizens are inspired to celebrate the birth of Christ—or Hanukkah, or any other religious observance. The atheists have even begun displaying a large *A* in Daley Plaza near the nativity scene. Every year on the Saturday after Thanksgiving, a crew we call the "God Squad" arrives at Daly Plaza to erect the nativity scene.

Just over a year after our Daley Plaza adventure, the Berlin Wall fell. Energized by his project of keeping the Holy Family visible in public, Bill Grutzmacher decided he was going to put up the first nativity set in Red Square after the Iron Curtain came down, and he asked me to come along.

We set up meetings with pro-life leaders in Russia. Transitioning from a totalitarian state to a more democratic society allowed citizens there more freedom to demonstrate, but abortion had been legal in the USSR since 1920, and there was almost no opportunity to protest it. It was difficult finding Russians who considered abortion wrong after having lived with it for so long. It had become routine.

This told me how critical our work in America is. All but the most hardened pro-abortionists in the United States see their way to an argument that abortion destroys life. But some societies have lost even that. Once it goes, it's hard to get back. Nevertheless, some people are called to protect the most helpless members of the human family, and the pro-lifers I met in Russia were dedicated to restoring a culture of life there.

Bill and I put up our nativity set in Red Square. For Russians, we were introducing something new. Eastern Christian churches emphasize icons, not statues, so it's unlikely that nativity sets had been prominent in Russian Orthodox churches, and they certainly hadn't been found in the public square. Ours wasn't just the first nativity set in Red Square since the fall of communism: It might have been the first one ever. Passersby seemed to like it a great deal.

Our weeklong visit to Russia was an eye-opener for me. The reemergence of religion there fascinated me. The communists had converted a number of church buildings into warehouses and factories, and we saw many of these being restored while we were there. The first thing they'd do was erect the cross atop the church, then begin restoring the dome before working their way downward. There'd been a top-down implementation of atheism in the eastern bloc, so it was interesting to watch as the restoration of the churches followed literally the same pattern.

In the United States, we have to work from the bottom up to keep religion in the public square. The idea that your faith is something private, something you need to hide away, is the antithesis of the American way. Working to keep nativity scenes visible at Christmas is one way to do something for the cause of life and truth.

Another program with a pro-life message that airs at Christmas every year is *It's a Wonderful Life*. That film is such a favorite with my family that one year I wrote a trivia quiz for them based on the film. I picked some minute details—the number on George Bailey's football jersey that he wore after the dance (3), what's framed in the Bailey dining room (butterflies), the headline on the paper Burt is reading when George gets his suitcase (Smith Wins Nomination). It was impossible to stump the kids. They got them all right.

When George is visited by his guardian angel, Clarence, George wishes he'd never been born, and he gets his wish. The world he sees shocks him: his hometown overrun by vice, the townsfolk poisoned by anger and mistrust. Near the end of the film, George discovers the grave of his younger brother Harry. Without George, Harry would have died, and hundreds of other lives would also have been lost without Harry. George goes to see his mother, who doesn't recognize him. Clarence is nearby, leaning on a mailbox. "Strange, isn't it?" he said. "Each man's life touches so many other lives. When he isn't around he leaves an awful hole, doesn't he?"[2]

Multiply that hole by sixty million.

One Christmas, I bought the house for an evening's showing of the Goodman Theater's production of Charles Dickens's *A Christmas Carol*. We sold tickets as a fundraiser for the Pro-Life Action League. Before the play began, I told the audience to watch for the scene where the Ghost of Christmas Present opens his robe to reveal two shivering children. In Dickens's story, Scrooge asks the ghost who they are. "They are Man's," is the reply. "This boy is Ignorance. This girl is Want. Beware them both, and all of their degree, but most of all beware this boy, for on his brow I see that written which is Doom, unless the writing be erased."

2 *It's a Wonderful Life*, Frank Capra, Frances Goodrich, James Stewart et al. (Los Angeles: Republic Entertainment, 1998), DVD.

After the ghosts leave, Scrooge awakens ready to start a new life of generosity. Like Scrooge, we have work to do to stamp out the ignorance that threatens society. Every Christmas, we take that calling into the streets. We tour the local abortion clinics with an empty manger, singing our medley of Christmas carols. Dan Gura made a large banner that reads, "All I want for Christmas . . . is an end to abortion." The pro-abortion line is that pro-lifers are angry and aggressive at clinics, especially as a group. Our Empty Manger Caroling suggests otherwise.

One year while we were caroling at the American Women's Medical Center, a couple got out of their car and asked Father Steve Lesniewski if he remembered them from months before. They asked if he would baptize their baby whom he'd saved from abortion. Father Steve said yes, of course, and the little baby was baptized that Christmas Day. At another clinic, a woman in the waiting room heard us caroling. She came out to tell us that our carols got her wondering: "What if Mary had aborted baby Jesus?" She chose life for her baby.

Empty Manger Caroling is catching on nationwide, and it's even spread internationally. In New Zealand, Mary O'Neill dresses up as Santa and visits hospital abortion wards, handing out treats along with fetal models.

Jesus' coming into the world as a baby reminds us that human life is sacred, and that it is indeed, as the angel said and as Linus reminds us every year, a tiding of great joy.

## CHAPTER 32

# The Pro-Life Family

The pro-life activist family isn't exactly your typical American family. On the one hand, we looked like *Leave It to Beaver*, with a stay-at-home mom who regularly baked cookies and managed the home, though with a few more kids than the Cleavers. Maybe we were more of a *Brady Bunch* crew. But often enough, the entire family climbed into the station wagon to go to a pro-life picket. Many Saturdays, Ann headed to an abortion clinic to sidewalk counsel.

I was often out of town giving talks and leading protests and marches. As word spread about my mission, my children were often questioned about what their dad did for a living. For the older ones, it wasn't an easy question, and it generally resulted in a debate or an argument. It may have been an opportunity to evangelize, but it also put my kids in a difficult position. I recall Sarah recounting a day in the second grade when the teacher asked the students to tell what their parents did for a living. They went around the class, each student rattling off his or her parents' professions. Sarah said she wished her father was a dentist.

There were difficult times. A pro-life family can become isolated in a neighborhood. As a movement leader, my situation was different from someone who has a separate profession that provides an income and who does pro-life work on the side. People not directly involved in pro-life tended to think of me as an extremist. Of course, having protesters show up at my house routinely didn't do much to dispel that impression. Little by little, I discovered that my only real friends were other pro-lifers. Nice, well-meaning people at my parish—including the priests—would ask, "How's your cause going?" Sometimes I'd say that it wasn't *my* cause—it should be everyone's cause—but usually I'd just reply that it was keeping me busy.

By the time I founded the Pro-Life Action League, my two older boys were young teens. I found a storefront office just around the corner from our house, and the boys helped me set it up for my new office. Joey, thirteen, had a real knack for organization. His bedroom desk looked like it belonged to a CEO, with little compartments for pens and paperclips. He took on the task of preparing our fundraising mailings. I had a pretty good list of supporters, about a thousand, on three-by-five cards. Together we created a set of mailing labels and duplicated the letters.

Joey recruited his brothers and some friends. They set up an assembly line to fold, stuff, seal, and stamp the letters. One of the incentives to get his friends to help was that we had a VCR in the office, a Betamax. Hardly anyone had those in their homes yet, so it was a treat to be able to come over and watch a movie on the Betamax when the work was done.

The kids also helped us with yard sales. The office was located just off a major Chicago street and had a nice lawn next to it. We borrowed tables from everyone we knew, and people donated all sorts of items. Ann and the kids and I, along with board member Rosie Stokes, manned the tables. The sales were always a success, and the proceeds kept the League going for another couple of months.

Among donations to the League was a 1976 Buick LeSabre. It wasn't in very good shape, and the seats were a mess, but a set of seat covers fixed that. The body had dents and rust, but the car ran—most of the time. I called it the "Brown Dream." My daughter Cathy was mortified to be seen in that Buick, and she'd usually crouch down in the back so nobody would see her when we were driving through the neighborhood.

I decided to buy the car from the League and let Eric use it when he got his license, but eventually the car could only make about forty miles per hour, and it arrived at its destination in a cloud of smoke. Finally, when the car was on its last legs, a pro-life mechanic who was also a Chicago fireman told me to bring it to his house to see if he could breathe some life into it. He lived on the South Side, about twenty miles from our neighborhood. I drove the Brown Dream, and Ann followed me. By the time we got to the mechanic's house, you couldn't even see the car. The mechanic wasn't home, so we just left it on the street in front of his house. He couldn't bring it back to life, so it went to the junkyard.

In the mid-'80s, Linda Witt, a *Chicago Tribune* reporter, did a story on the Scheidler family, complete with photos of all of us. We were delighted to cooperate. I have good-looking kids, and they thought being featured in Chicago's major newspaper was exciting. Linda came to our house to interview Ann and me and each of the kids, asking them what it was like to belong to an anti-abortion family.

A photographer took group pictures in our living room and at the breakfast table. In the backyard, we took a picture in front of the same playhouse I'd built for the kids where just a few years later Tim Murphy would stash a barrel of aborted babies. We took one more on the front steps of the house. The next Sunday, the camera crew joined us at Queen of All Saints. Ann and I were in the choir, and they snapped pictures of us in the loft.

The story was fair, although it started with a comment from one of our fellow choir members that "he thinks he's doing a good thing."[1] The woman had lost a daughter to cancer at nineteen, and she was bitter about it. She couldn't understand caring about anyone else's child. But otherwise, the story was basically about an average middle-class American family that had taken on a large fight, a fight that could last for many, many years. Ms. Witt caught the family ethos that abortion was wrong and that we had to fight it.

I've always felt it an honor that people look to the Scheidlers as a pro-life family, a family with a very definite cause: to change our society and bring back appreciation for life. And my kids seemed to take on the pro-life cause as a natural part of life. Of course, the younger ones never knew anything else. At first, they probably thought that everyone went out to picket clinics. They held signs and small caskets, chanted slogans, and fielded insults. Eric was sidewalk counseling as a teenager. He was good at it.

Over the years, though, we've been the target of some vicious attacks. It became fairly common to receive death threats by phone. One of my children would answer the phone only to be told I would be shot. Once Ann answered and was told to come down to the morgue to identify my body. As she'd just hung up from talking with me a moment before, she knew I was perfectly fine.

Refuse and Resist picketed my home several times. They leafleted the neighborhood with flyers claiming I hate "womyn." Once when they came early in the morning and woke the kids, I went out and invited them in for doughnuts. They refused, saying I'd probably poison them. They decided instead to lie down on the sidewalk in front of the house. But Annie, my middle daughter, irritated that they'd awakened her, noticed that our sprinkler was out on the front lawn. She went out the back way and turned on the water, dousing the group.

Another time, abortion advocates visited my home during the night to put plastic hangers in the trees and bushes and tape posters

---

1    Linda Witt, "Man with a Mission," *Chicago Tribune*, August 11, 1985.

to my front door and columns. These were easy enough to clean up, but another time, they vandalized my home while we were all out of town. They'd alerted the media that they planned to spray paint our house and garage. The results appeared on WGN evening news, complete with my home address plastered across the TV screen. The program was even seen by some friends in Frankfurt, Germany. One night, in their zeal to brand me a "womyn" hater, someone was sent to spray anti-Joe slogans all over my garage—but it was my neighbor's garage, not mine. That was embarrassing. I quickly sent Tim Murphy over to scrub and repaint their garage. My neighbors actually took it pretty well.

When my son Peter was attending graduate school at Virginia Tech, a friend came out to visit him. They visited a local bookstore together, and Peter picked up a copy of *Spy Magazine* that ran a story about pro-lifers stockpiling aborted babies. The story, called "Fetus Frenzy," mentioned our backyard playhouse and had a picture of Ann and me. Peter showed the story to his friend. About an hour later, out of the blue, the friend asked Peter, "Are you okay, man?"

"Yeah," he answered, puzzled. "Why?"

"My dad's an electrician. I couldn't imagine opening a magazine and finding a story slamming my parents. You sure you're all right?"

Peter was fine. That kind of story was old news to him.

In 1993, while Annie was at Southern Illinois University (SIU), we all went down to Carbondale for a family weekend. Comedian Richard Jeni was entertaining there as a part of the weekend activities. Annie was excited about our visit and bought tickets for the whole family. We had seats in row three.

Jeni started off with a couple of snide remarks about religion, and I hoped that would be it. It wasn't. He became increasingly crude, and after a string of anti-Catholic jokes, I whispered to Ann that I was leaving. I rose and started walking down the long aisle to the back of the auditorium. "Where are you going?" Jeni called out.

I decided not to duck the issue. "Your jokes are foul, and I don't have to stay and listen to you." He launched into a barrage of vulgarity, mocking me for walking out. At that point, the rest of my family got up to leave as well, along with several other members of the audience. Jeni continued to deride everyone leaving.

Annie demanded a refund on the tickets. She was mortified that the event turned into such a fiasco. She wrote a letter to the school newspaper, *The Egyptian*, which then ran articles and letters for a week about the controversy. I received a letter from the SIU chancellor, as well as one from a professor emeritus, apologizing for the entertainment being so inappropriate for a family audience.

One year, my son Matthias accompanied Ann and me to the March for Life in Washington, DC. Matt was a quiet kid. I hadn't heard him say much about abortion. As I got to the march's terminus at the steps of the Supreme Court building, I overheard a discussion between a young pro-lifer and a knot of feminists. I stood to the side and eavesdropped. For every argument that abortion is vital for women or that the unborn aren't human, the boy had a solid retort. I remember thinking he was winning the debate. I turned to get a look and discovered that it was none other than Matt.

Even my grandchildren have joined the fight for life. My daughter Cathy had taken a picture of her eighteen-month-old son Aaron picking up a stone to throw in a puddle in the alley behind our house. It was such a captivating picture that we selected it for a billboard campaign that ran in several states around the nation. The billboard featured Aaron's photo, the words "see the world through your child's eyes," and the message "Choose Life," along with phone number of a pregnancy help line—800-848-LOVE. The local crisis pregnancy centers reported significant increases in calls for assistance wherever the billboards appeared.

Aaron and his brothers Aiden and Noah have traveled to Washington, DC, with the Crusaders for Life for the March for Life, and have joined me on my radio program to discuss the role of young people in the pro-life movement.

Eric's sons Nate and Sam became integral parts of the Face the Truth team, with Sam serving as the League's official photographer. Liza and Clare have also joined the crew, as has Aaron. And all my grandchildren have held signs and witnessed to the beauty of life.

One December night in 2010, Ann and I were awakened by a loud crash downstairs, followed by a second crash. We thought a shelf had collapsed, and we went downstairs to look around. Nothing seemed amiss, so we went back to bed. When we came down in the morning to go to Mass, we noticed the house felt awfully cold. In the morning light, we discovered what had caused the noise: Someone had thrown two huge chunks of asphalt through our front windows. One of the missiles was wrapped in paper with a message from "angry feminists" stating that we'd never take their rights away.

We called the police and put out a press release about the vandalism. The Illinois Choice Action Team had held a training meeting nearby the same night, so we suspected them, but the police seemed disinterested in following that lead.

Two days later, I got a call from Gilkey Windows. The owner, Mike Gilkey, read online about what happened to our house and wanted to replace our windows free of charge. Gilkey knew me—I'd stayed at his father's house in Cincinnati once when I was speaking there. Gilkey didn't just replace the smashed windows. He also replaced our old windows in that part of the house for free. Our home is much more comfortable now—and our heating bills are lower.

After completing his master's degree at Yale, my son Joe worked in the business world for several years. Once when he went in for a job interview, the interviewer told him, "You won't believe this, but I Googled your name, and what came up was this crazy anti-abortion guy."

"Yes, that's my father," answered Joe. He didn't apologize for the fact that his dad was a crazy anti-abortion guy. He got the job.

My daughter Annie took on the activist mantle during her college days at Loyola University and went on to become a youth minister. She applied for a position at a parish in Winnetka, an upscale Chicago suburb. The parish board saw the Scheidler name and got spooked, fearing that all a Scheidler would do was talk about abortion. But the religious education director was in Annie's camp, so they invited her for an interview. They loved her. They even hired her sister Sarah to teach fourth grade at the parish school.

As hard as it was for my children to belong to a pro-life activist family, I do believe it taught them an important lesson. When something is very wrong in society, we have a Christian obligation to do something about it. It's not good enough to wait for someone else to do it. We have to step up and do it ourselves.

## Chapter 33

# Decisions, Decisions

In the spring of 1997, just a few months before Tom Brejcha had to leave Abramson & Fox to found the Thomas More Society, Ann and I accompanied him and his wife, Debbie, to the Institute on Religious Life banquet in Mundelein, Illinois.

The keynote speaker that night was Supreme Court Justice Antonin Scalia. I wanted to talk to Scalia about the court's unanimous decision to uphold an injunction against right-to-lifers in New York State that established buffer zones around abortion clinics. I got my chance after dinner, and I made my case that bubble zone rules violated our freedom of speech.

"But the injunction doesn't prevent protests from taking place," he explained. "It only requires that they take place away from the clinic. Freedom of speech can be exercised just as effectively from across the street."

"Freedom of shouting, maybe," I said. "But speech also includes trying to start a civil conversation with someone, doesn't it? That's what our sidewalk counselors try to do in front of these clinics. Your bubble zone rule makes it illegal for us to do that."

Scalia seemed genuinely surprised to learn that sidewalk conversations outside of clinics can persuade women to choose life, but the bubble zones continued to gag pro-lifers. Three years after my conversation with Scalia, the court again ruled against pro-lifers in *Hill v. Colorado*. Sidewalk counselor Jeanie Hill had sought an injunction against Colorado's bubble zone law on the grounds that it violated freedom of speech, but the court upheld the law. This time, however, three Justices dissented, citing First Amendment concerns. Scalia authored one of the minority opinions.

In 2008, George W. Bush invited nearly a hundred pro-life leaders to a breakfast at the White House before the March for Life. It was the first time in over twenty years I'd been invited to the White House, and Ann and my son Eric joined me. When we arrived in the morning at the White House gate, the guards checked their list and guided us through a metal detector. It was easier to get into the White House than onto an airplane.

Once inside, we were free to roam the first floor: the Green Room, the Red Room, and the State Dining Room, the rooms famously redecorated by Jackie Kennedy. The views from the windows, even in the dead of winter, were beautiful. A marine in full dress uniform played the grand piano. A beautiful buffet breakfast was served in the dining room.

We were invited into the East Room, where President Bush came in and thanked us for our commitment to life. He specifically thanked Nellie Gray for organizing the March for Life for so many years. Then we were led through the lower level of the White House to the library, where we were welcome to take pictures and peruse the books. And so we did. We felt very much at home.

That was the last March for Life of Bush's presidency. Little did we know that the next fall Americans would elect the most proabortion president in history. Barack Obama served in the Illinois Senate in 1997 when the Illinois partial birth abortion ban was passed with overwhelming support. The future president voted "present" to keep his support for near-infanticide off the record and preserve his 100 percent pro-abortion rating from groups like NARAL, NOW, and Planned Parenthood. He also opposed the Illinois Born-Alive Infants Protection Act in 2001 and 2002. There was no doubt he was firmly pro-abortion.

When Obama launched his presidential campaign, the Pro-Life Action League was the first group to publicly oppose him. He announced his candidacy from the steps of the old capitol building in Springfield, the same spot where Abraham Lincoln announced his candidacy in 1860. It was a bitterly cold day. More than a hundred pro-lifers turned out to chant, "Life, yes! Obama, no!" at the rally. The new candidate had worked hard to earn that 100 percent rating, and we wanted to make sure he knew he would be vigorously opposed on this critical issue.

Just days after taking the oath of office, Obama began building on his pro-abortion record by rescinding the Mexico City Policy that had been put in place by Ronald Reagan, and which prohibited funding for international family planning programs that included abortion. He then embarked on an array of appointments and executive orders that advanced a pro-abortion agenda.

Obama's book, *The Audacity of Hope*, includes a chapter titled "Faith." In it, he cites the story of Abraham and Isaac. "If any of us saw a twenty-first century Abraham raising the knife on the roof of his apartment building," he writes, "we would call the police; we would wrestle him down; even if we saw him lower the knife at the last minute, we would expect the Department of Children and Family Services to take Isaac away and charge Abraham with child abuse." But, Obama explains, Abraham was acting on faith, and the intervening angel speaks only to Abraham. Faith is such a personal matter, he says, that public rules need to be based on something more general. "The best we can possibly do," he concludes, "is act in accordance with those things that are possible for all of us to know."[1]

Obama's words suggest that any belief about when human life begins—and what that should mean legally, politically, and culturally—can only be based on faith. But even before the court established abortion as a constitutional right and before Blackmun wrote that the question of when life begins was difficult and "an unknown," medical science was quietly concluding that human life began long before the law said it did. Obama's use of the sacrifice story to argue that faith-based beliefs are a poor basis for public policy is ironically contradictory: After all, the heart of his proof is a belief that the law *should* protect a child's right to life, even against a parent's wishes.

One of Obama's signature achievements was the 2010 passage of the Affordable Care Act, nicknamed "Obamacare." The bill was intended to increase the quality and affordability of health insurance, but a number of specific measures seem designed to target the Catholic Church. The Health and Human Services (HHS) Department mandated that birth control, abortifacient drugs and devices, and certain kinds of sterilization must be covered under *all* health plans, including those offered by Catholic institutions. The HHS Department would only consider churches eligible for exemption, but not other religious institutions like schools or hospitals. Numerous legal challenges were brought against the HHS Department by Christian businesses and Catholic institutions, forcing the nation's courts to address the issue of religious liberty. Monica Miller and my son Eric took the lead in organizing "Stand Up for Religious Freedom" rallies across the nation to protest the policy and focus media attention on the controversy.

The night of the 2012 election, my daughter Catherine and her family came over to watch the returns. The next morning, I joked

---

1      Barack Obama, *The Audacity of Hope* (New York: Crown, 2006), 220.

with my granddaughters, "I just had the worst nightmare. Obama was reelected."

"That wasn't a nightmare, Grandpa," my granddaughter Hope said. "It really happened."

But for pro-lifers, it was a nightmare. First Justice Stevens retired and was replaced by Elena Kagan, and then Justice Souter left and Sonia Sotomayor filled his seat. Those were abortion votes replaced with abortion votes, but the 2016 death of Antonin Scalia opened up a new vacancy. As of this writing, the Senate has declined to hold hearings to even consider President Obama's nominee to fill Scalia's spot on the Court.

Two years before his death, during arguments in the Massachusetts bubble zone case of *McCullen v. Coakley*, Justice Scalia interrupted the lawyer who was defending the bubble zone. "This is not a protest case," he said. "These people don't want to protest abortion. They want to talk to the women who are about to get abortions and try to talk them out of it. I think it is a distortion to say that what they want to do is protest abortion." However his vacancy is filled, Scalia's death dealt a severe blow to the pro-life remnants on the court.

Justice Samuel Alito began serving on the court in January 2006, and so he was not involved when the court ruled in *Hill v. Colorado*. But in oral arguments for *McCullen*, Alito posed this scenario to the attorney representing Massachusetts:

> A woman is approaching the door of a clinic, and she enters
> the zone. Two other women approach her. One is an employee
> of the facility, the other is not. The first, who is an employee of
> the facility, says, "Good morning—this is a safe facility." The
> other one, who's not an employee, says, "Good morning—
> this is not a safe facility." Now, under this statute, the first one
> has not committed a crime. The second one *has* committed a

crime, and the only difference between the two is that they've expressed a different viewpoint. One says it's safe; one says it's not safe. Now, how can a statute like that be considered viewpoint-neutral?

Alito was describing our Chicago Method of sidewalk counseling, the very same thing I'd described to Scalia in 1997. In June 2014, the court ruled that the Massachusetts buffer zone violated pro-lifers' First Amendment rights. The finding was unanimous. So while the court didn't reevaluate the mistakes of *Roe*, at least it expressed respect for one of the other founding rights and allowed those of us who believe the unborn have a right to live to continue working to save them. Perhaps this recognition that the pro-life perspective is protected under the First Amendment is a step toward not just permitting it but promoting it.

*Roe* is still settled law—for now. The 7–2 court that voted in abortion on demand dropped to a 5–4 court, and with Scalia's passing, the numbers are dead even. But even if *Roe* was overturned, legalized abortion in the United States would not suddenly be overturned. The legal battle would then shift theater to the states. And the battle for minds and hearts would continue as it always has.

These political and judicial battles are an important part of our pro-life work, but they aren't the most critical. A government has an obligation to uphold the right to life, and we will oppose them whenever they shirk or contravene that responsibility, but true pro-life work is not merely to make abortion unlawful. The real work is to strive for a world where all life can be accepted, loved, and supported.

The right to life will continue to be an issue in every presidential election, in every new appointment to the high court, and before every legislative assembly in the nation. And if these issues aren't raised loudly enough, pro-lifers will be there to turn up the volume. With a bullhorn, if necessary.

CHAPTER 34

# Conspiracy Theory

Twelve years after I was first served notice of the NOW lawsuit, I finally stood trial in federal court.

Jury selection in *NOW v. Scheidler* began on March 2, 1998. There was a large media turnout, and I spent much of my time giving interviews in the lobby. Ann worked as Tom Brejcha's paralegal and stayed in the courtroom as eighty potential jurors were brought in and questioned over two days.

The case was a class action suit brought by two groups: clinics and their patients. NOW's lawyer, Fay Clayton, represented the class of women who had ever visited or would visit a "reproductive health center." Her husband, Lowell Sachnoff, represented the clinics. NOW sought a nationwide injunction against pro-life protests. Since FACE had passed four years prior, rescues were no longer taking place the way they had in the early '90s. We worried that an injunction would be used to ban picketing or even sidewalk counseling.

The suit also named Randall Terry as a defendant. Just weeks before we went to trial, Randy accepted a deal from NOW that was essentially identical to the nationwide injunction they sought. He

explained to me that he had to take the deal because he was planning to mount a political campaign and couldn't spare the time and
publicity of a trial. But even though Randy and Operation Rescue
were listed as "settling defendants," Judge David Coar ruled that
Operation Rescue would be kept as a defendant.

This was a serious blow. Having a group without its leader listed
as a defendant would make it appear to the jury that Operation
Rescue was simply a front for *our* activities. The fact that I—not
Randy—coined the phrase "National Day of Rescue" and that I
attended the planning meetings and the first rescues in New York
would surely come out in the trial. Randy promised me that he'd
come to Chicago to testify that Operation Rescue was his own
group and that I hadn't coordinated his events, but a few weeks
later, when we needed his testimony, his lawyers advised him not to
take the stand.

Attorney Larry Crain represented Operation Rescue. The remaining defendants were from the Pro-Life Action League: me; my assistant director, Tim Murphy; and my former assistant director, Andy
Scholberg. We were all represented by Tom Brejcha.

Our lawyers and theirs had spent days hammering out a questionnaire to vet potential jurors, but Judge Coar refused to strike
questions about what schools they'd attended and what clubs they
belonged to, which provided a loophole through the ban on questions about religion. NOW's lawyers would use their peremptory
challenges to automatically reject candidates who were members of
Catholic organizations or who had attended Catholic schools.

The questionnaire included inquiries into candidates' positions on
abortion, as well as others about objectivity. As Judge Coar scanned
the questionnaires completed by the jury candidates, he called Tom
Brejcha to the bench. "Your own people aren't doing you any favors,
Mr. Brejcha," Judge Coar said. "They're too honest." He was telling
Tom that while abortion supporters professed impartiality, pro-life

candidates said they thought we were innocent, already stacking the pool of "objective" jurors against us.[1]

Criminal trials have twelve jurors, but ours was a civil trial, which required only six. Judge Coar was certain the case would be over within a month, but Tom was sure it would take twice that long. Worried that exhausted jurors would take out their frustration on the side that presented its case last—us—Tom wanted to make sure they knew they were in for a long trial.

The judge allowed four alternate jurors. All ten would hear the whole case, but only the six officially on the jury would decide the verdict. On the final day of jury selection, Judge Coar advised the pool they would receive phone calls that evening if they were selected and to prepare to serve for several weeks. Opening statements were set for the next day.

During the night, Chicago was hit by a blizzard. The next day, half the jurors were late. Finally, when all but two had shown up, the judge sent federal marshals to track them down. The marshals were only able to find one, and the first alternate was seated in the missing juror's place.

Susan Hill, president of the principal plaintiff WHO, arrived at the Dirksen Federal Building that morning with a brawny six-foot-four bodyguard. I sat at the defendants' table with Tim, Andy, Ann, Tom, and Tom's cocounsel, Debbie Fischer. My son Eric and daughters Cathy and Annie joined us. Judge Coar was clearly annoyed by Susan Hill's burly media ploy and ordered the bodyguard to take a seat in the gallery. We never saw him again.

Clayton began her opening statement by introducing NOW President Patricia Ireland to the jury, calling her "The NOW Representative

---

1    Quotations here and in subsequent chapters are taken from the trial transcripts compiled by court reporter Tracey McCullough. Transcripts are on file at and available from the Pro-Life Action League (www.plal.org) and the Thomas More Society (www.thomasmoresociety.org).

of the Day." The ceremony was repeated every morning and afternoon, with a new person presented each time, so that the jury could
see the broad array of women represented in the class action suit. The
daily NOW rep had a seat at the plaintiffs' table.

"NOW brought this lawsuit," Clayton explained, "but didn't
bring it for itself." She described how NOW wasn't seeking monetary damages but an "order of protection" for women who would
visit abortion clinics in the future: a nationwide injunction to keep
pro-lifers away from clinics. Clayton set up her "PLAN Leadership
Council" flowchart and started telling the jury about my efforts to
build a network of radical groups to fight abortion.

"The thing that differentiated all these groups that came together
to form PLAN from groups like the National Right to Life Committee," she told the jury, "is that these groups were committed to using
all means necessary—to breaking the law, every method available—to
prevent women from obtaining abortions."

She then launched into descriptions of arsons, bombings, and
kidnappings. In pretrial discussions, Judge Coar ruled that because
there was no evidence linking us to these events, the plaintiffs could
not reference them in their opening statements. Both Larry Crain
and Tom Brejcha objected. Judge Coar let her continue.

While Clayton spoke, I erected a small cardboard grotto to the
Blessed Mother. Hidden behind the volumes of binders stacked on
the defendants' table, my shrine housed a statue of Our Lady. Tim,
Andy, and I placed our rosaries in front of it.

As Clayton continued, she again brought up arsons and bombs,
and again our attorneys objected. This time Judge Coar reminded
her about his ruling. At the fifth reference, he finally called a sidebar.
"There is to be no reference to arson or bombing during the opening
statements, period," he told Clayton.

"Your Honor, I—"

"Period. Period."

When Clayton finished her statement, Lowell Sachnoff began his.

"Ladies and gentlemen of the jury," he began, "I'd like to introduce Susan Hill. Miss Hill is the representative of the national class of women's health clinics, over a thousand such clinics which provide a wide range of health services, including abortion."

"The defendants' campaign of fear, force, and violence to shut down every clinic in America that provides abortion services," Sachnoff continued, "involves acts specifically made illegal under RICO. These are threats of bodily harm, threats of arson and murder, and actual violence and extortion of the clinics' legally-protected right to provide a wide variety of health services for—"

"Your Honor," interjected Tom, "I'm going to object."

"Overrule the objection. Go ahead, Mr. Sachnoff."

I was stunned. Judge Coar had just told Clayton she couldn't make any references to arson or bombing, but now he was letting Sachnoff do just that—and to add murder into the mix.

Sachnoff described the services provided by the clinics—mammograms, pap smears, annual physicals, prenatal care, and most importantly, counseling. The familiar hardship cases, Sachnoff said—maternal health, severe birth defects, poverty, rape, incest—explained why these clinics occasionally performed abortions.

"Now, the RICO statute that you have heard so much about for the last couple of days is designed to prevent an enterprise like PLAN from organizing as a vehicle to commit illegal acts," Sachnoff continued. "That's the basis of RICO. And these acts include not only murder, arson, bombings, and extortion, but they also include threats of committing those illegal acts."

"Your Honor," Tom interrupted, "if I may object. Again a reference to overt acts of violence."

"There's no prohibition against that," Judge Coar answered. "Go ahead, Mr. Sachnoff."

Because of the weather delay, we couldn't present our opening statements until the following day. That's not the way it's supposed to work—the defendant's case should be the last thing the jury hears. But that day, jurors went home with claims of murder and terrorism ringing in their ears.

That evening, Tom Brejcha prepared a formal motion for a mistrial based on the deferred opening statement and Judge Coar's flip-flop on what language was and wasn't permitted. The next morning, Judge Coar denied the motion. Tom knew the judge didn't like him, so he had his cocounsel, Debbie Fischer, make our opening remarks, thinking the judge might not be as quick to sustain NOW's objections if Debbie were presenting our case.

It was Debbie's first trial, and she was nervous about being the first one to address the jury. Her opening statement largely focused on the extortion allegation. She explained that, by definition, extortion is the use of fear and intimidation to obtain another's property and that our witnesses who had left the business—and NOW's own witnesses still in it—would testify that, though they may have despised us, they never feared us.

Following Debbie's opening, Tom Brejcha addressed the jury:

> As you hear the evidence unravel, please keep in mind why it is that the National Organization for Women, a massive 250,000-member organization, and the entire abortion industry, represented here by Miss Hill, have picked out these defendants.
>
> Why we are in here in Chicago trying to have these people adjudicated as racketeers—extortionists—isn't because they deal in violence or threats of violence. It's because these people are very, very effective in getting out a message that the abortion industry cannot stand. It's a very simple, straightforward message.

In opening, Mr. Sachnoff said that we all believe every child should be a wanted child. The defendants here believe the *unwanted* child has a right to life, that the poor child, the child who has some medical flaws, that the homeless, anonymous, outcast, alien—that all these people have a right to live.

But that is not what this case is about. What this case is about is the right to speak out, the right to get your message across and to leave it to your audience to decide whether they agree with you or whether they don't.

The plaintiffs are fearful. We concede it. Our clients are proud of it. Because they're fearful of the message that the Pro-Life Action League and others with whom it works gets out. The message is one directed to women, a message that has a lot to do with the experience of other women who have had legal abortions in the generation that's passed since *Roe v. Wade*.

Many of those women are active in support of the Pro-Life Action League or any of the other hundreds or thousands of groups around the country. You may call them converts, you may call them victims. You will hear from some of them, many of them.

In addition to those named as defendants, NOW had labeled dozens of other pro-life activists coconspirators. Tom Brejcha explained that PLAN didn't constitute the enterprise necessary for a RICO violation, and he asked why those who'd actually carried out violent acts weren't being sued. He explained that NOW's case employed a new interpretation of RICO and that a fear of being labeled a coconspirator infringed on freedom of association.

Next came Operation Rescue attorney Larry Crain, whose opening statement described the case as "an attempt by one side of this debate, those who profit from abortion, to silence the opposition."

With opening statements concluded, Lowell Sachnoff called the
first witness: Susan Hill. She had run a dozen clinics throughout
the country, and in 1998, she had eight, two of which were named
in *NOW v. Scheidler* as representing the whole class of clinics nationwide. These two were Summit in Milwaukee and Delaware Women's
Health in Wilmington.

Hill's testimony began with a story of how she entered the abortion business as a counselor at a Florida clinic that opened the week
*Roe* was announced. She explained that back then she worked closely
with the CCS. Judge Coar called a sidebar to find out if Hill's background information had any bearing on the case. Apparently, it
did. Sachnoff and Hill then went on to discuss the WHO's extensive counseling program, which prompted another sidebar about
relevance.

We broke for lunch. When we got back to the courtroom, Susan
Hill resumed her testimony. She seemed to have rehearsed her
routine over the break, and when we finally got around to some
allegations—taking fetal remains from Vital Med labs, she said:
"There were announcements that there were patients' names that
the defendants had in this case, and threats to our patients that those
names were going to be disclosed."

This was pure invention. The names had been on the bags, so
we had them, but we had made no such threat, and both Hill
and Sachnoff knew it. Those bodies were taken so they could be
buried properly—an act of mercy, not harassment. Tom Brejcha
objected, and Judge Coar sustained his objection.

Hill described a sit-in that took place at her Wilmington clinic
in 1985. She mentioned Joan Andrews by name. She also discussed
my 1986 visit to her clinic with Jerry, Norm, and a local pastor. She
admitted she hadn't been present for either event, and explained her
company's policy of calling her right after calling the police whenever an incident occurred.

"Miss Hill," asked Sachnoff, "did any of the defendants in this case or people associated with PLAN ever personally threaten you?"

"Yes. I have received personal threats from several of the people associated with PLAN."

"Would you describe for the jury the first such threat that you can recall?"

"Well," she said, "the day after Mr. Scheidler entered the building in Delaware—stormed into the building," she corrected herself, "I was present at the protest he had organized and was speaking at, and he threatened me that he would make sure the clinic was closed down, and that he was there to make Delaware an abortion-free state."

Next, she described being the guest on a radio call-in show when Randall Terry called.

"Could you in your own words describe what happened in connection with a threat made to you by Mr. Terry?" Sachnoff asked.

"When I was on the phone, we were discussing some of the violence that had occurred right around that time, and it was during the conversation that Mr. Scheidler—that Mr. Terry, I'm sorry, I apologize—threatened me and said: 'That's right, Ms. Hill. We know where you are, where you live, and we're coming to get you.'"

Randy had settled his part of the case. Why was he still on trial—and why had my name been swapped with his? I doubted that it was an innocent mistake. My fears of a setup, of taking a fall for others, surged back.

"Now, Ms. Hill," Sachnoff continued, "Did you take those words to be a threat to you?"

"Yes, I had to take them as a serious threat. There had been violence occurring very close to me at that point, and people that I had been associated with had been gravely injured. I had to take every threat that was made by Mr. Terry or anyone else as a serious threat at that point."

"Who was the person who was closely associated with you who had been gravely injured?"

"Dr. David Gunn."

Sachnoff started to ask another question, but Tom rose to object. "Withdrawn," Sachnoff said, cutting of the objection.

"Shortly before you received that threat from Mr. Terry," Sachnoff went on, "what, if anything, was involved with Dr. Gunn?"

"Dr. Gunn was shot in Pensacola and was murdered," Hill said.

Hill testified that during a 1995 rescue, Roy McMillan from Rescue America, a part of PLAN, threatened her, telling her she wouldn't live if she entered the clinic.

"Why did you view that statement as a threat to you?" Sachnoff asked.

"I knew that Mr. McMillan was a signer of a petition called Defensive Action that endorsed justifiable homicide."

That was Paul Hill's petition, which he wrote after Michael Griffin shot David Gunn. Though the court had spent hours in pretrial proceedings on the Defensive Action statement, we still weren't certain whether Judge Coar would allow it to be introduced into evidence. The plaintiffs had been sternly warned not to introduce the Britton killing. Crain and Brejcha both objected when Hill raised the subject, and the sidebar was so long that the judge invited everyone in the courtroom to stand up and stretch.

In the end, Sachnoff pledged he wouldn't mention that Paul Hill had killed an abortionist, nor lead Susan Hill to do so, and the judge allowed the Defensive Action statement to be admitted. When the questioning resumed, the prosecution displayed Paul Hill's petition on the overhead projector, and Susan Hill read aloud that Griffin's "use of lethal force was justifiable."

Now that he'd managed to introduce the topic of murder, Sachnoff led Susan Hill back to events that directly involved me—demonstrations and rescues. "Did Mr. Scheidler have any role in terms of leading the protest or blockade?" he asked.

"Well, he was the star when he was there," she said. "He was the person that all the other people appeared to look up to, and they were thrilled—and were thrilled for weeks before—that Mr. Scheidler was coming to town, and continued to tell us that he was coming to town."

"Your Honor," Tom interjected, "move to strike. Too general, vague, no foundation as to how everybody was thrilled."

"Well, all right," said Judge Coar. "I sustain that objection. How this witness knows whether people were thrilled or not is not evidence."

Sachnoff had Hill read excerpts from my testimony at the House Subcommittee Hearings on Clinic Violence and passages from my newsletters and hotlines. She said she called my hotline "hundreds of times" to keep up with our plans. They selected snippets suggesting I supported arson and bombing.

Larry Crain and Tom Brejcha's cross-examinations of Hill were tedious. Tom kept trying to get her to admit she'd never seen me do anything violent. She had to allow that I'd been acquitted of the harassment charge at her Delaware clinic and that the demonstrations where I was the "star" were all peaceful.

In the middle of Hill's cross-examination, NOW's attorneys asked that she be excused from the stand temporarily. They had a witness who was scheduled to leave town and had to take the stand before the end of the day. She was the first of four anonymous witnesses NOW planned to call—women who claimed they couldn't reveal their identity for fear of retaliation from pro-lifers.

Permitting a witness to remain anonymous is almost unheard-of, but we had agreed to it because we wanted to present women who chose life after talking to sidewalk counselors to testify that most pro-life activism, and sidewalk counseling specifically, isn't harassment. Naturally, these women didn't want their children to learn they had been minutes from being aborted, so we thought allowing anonymous witnesses could benefit us.

NOW's first anonymous witness said she'd been pregnant with a baby whose heart was malformed, and she went for a late-term abortion at George Tiller's Wichita clinic. NOW called her "Witness A." Privately, we referred to her as "Ms. Wichita." She testified that she arrived at the clinic during an Operation Rescue demonstration in July 1991—the Summer of Mercy. She told the jury that the clinic sent a car to her hotel, which picked up two other passengers, both rape victims. As they pulled into the clinic, she said, protesters crowded around the car, and Randall Terry screamed at them through a bullhorn.

Randy had spent most of that time in a Wichita jail for tearing up Judge Kelly's injunction in front of TV cameras. Since Terry wasn't in the courtroom, we couldn't know whether he'd been out of jail and in the demonstration in time to greet Ms. Wichita's arrival.

The car couldn't get through the crowd, so it returned to the hotel. They tried again for the next two days. On the third day, Ms. Wichita said, she saw me at Tiller's clinic.

"Did you have any personal contact with Mr. Scheidler on that occasion when you saw him at the clinic in Wichita?" Fay Clayton asked.

"Yes, ma'am."

"Would you please describe that for the ladies and gentlemen of the jury?"

"Just basically the same thing, speaking to us through the window, saying things, you know, screaming at us 'don't do this' and that sort of thing."

As soon as they got into the clinic, Ms. Wichita testified, they had to leave again. "All of us had to get up, and we all had—some people had to get dressed—and we all had to get out into what's kind of like a courtyard. Where the entrance was, there was this fenced-in area. So we all had to walk out there while the policemen went in to check for bombs."

When Debbie Fischer cross-examined Ms. Wichita, she asked if she could recall my exact words.

"He was screaming, 'Don't kill your babies, we want them, you're murderers.'"

"Did he threaten you?" Debbie asked.

"He didn't threaten us verbally," Ms. Wichita answered. "It was more the physical presence of all the people, plus him on top of us in this car that scared me."

Debbie asked what she meant by "on top of us."

"Well, we were in a subcompact kind of car," she explained. "And all these hundreds of people were surrounding our car. He's a very tall man, so he's kind of leaning over us. Everybody is screaming, and the mean faces, you know, and banging on the windows is what caused me to be terrified."

I was at Tiller's clinic three times during the Summer of Mercy in '91. The first time I got there, I was immediately handed an injunction, and I obeyed it. Had I gone anywhere near the blockaders that summer, I'd have been arrested. There was no chance I had gone anywhere near Ms. Wichita's car.

Because Ms. Wichita testified anonymously, her name hadn't appeared on the witness list, so our side hadn't been able to interview her before she testified. We naively assumed she would testify to the facts of the case, so we didn't have a copy of the injunction handy to refute her testimony. Her bomb scare story sounded odd, since no bomb squad would pen evacuees in a courtyard. We checked police reports after the fact and found no record of a bomb scare at Tiller's clinic that summer.

On Fridays during the trial, lawyers would meet with the judge to go over motions and evidence. Jurors and litigants were excused. That first weekend, I traveled to St. Louis to give a talk and join protests—or, as NOW would have it, engage in racketeering. On Monday, I was back in the courtroom, where Fay Clayton called NOW employee Maureen Burke to the stand.

"When you became an employee at NOW," she asked, "what was your title?"

"Special Projects Coordinator."

"Will you please tell us what that entailed?"

"Among other things, I headed up a program called Project Stand Up for Women," Burke explained. "That was a program that NOW developed to monitor the activities of the defendants and other people around the country."

Burke brought with her a thick notebook of documents, and she was the one who had provided all the evidence of every PLAN meeting, every rescue with arrests, and every detail intended to convince the jury I'd led a national conspiracy to illegally deny clinics the right to provide abortions and the right of women to visit them.

The lawyers had haggled for weeks over which portions of which documents would be admitted. Among the items in Burke's notebook were the answers I had sent to Carol Kleiman of *Ms. Magazine* when our interview was cut short by her son's car accident—not the article, but the notes I'd sent to Kleiman's *Chicago Tribune* office. NOW wanted to introduce half a sentence from my response to a question about the necessity defense.

Judge Coar was inclined to admit the phrase NOW wanted Burke to read, but he didn't want to allow any discussion of the necessity defense. "You hear that every day in philosophy classes not just at Loyola and Notre Dame and St. John's and Georgetown," Tom explained in the judge's chambers. "You hear it at the University of Chicago, you hear it at Harvard."

"I never heard it at the University of Chicago," said Sachnoff's colleague Kerry Miller.

"Well, go back and take a philosophy course," Tom retorted. Tom insisted that enough of my statement be read to the jury to make it sound reasonable. Judge Coar eventually permitted a few other lines from my notes to Kleiman to be admitted.

In the courtroom, Clayton led Burke through a recollection of how "concerned" Burke had been when she tracked our coordinated activism, beginning with the first National Day of Rescue in 1980.

They continued in chronological order, but after covering references to the rash of bombings and arsons in 1984 and 1985, Clayton directed Burke to the phrase from the *Ms. Magazine* notes from 1983.

Burke read: "Violence is permissible as a last resort."

Larry Crain objected. He asked that the entire statement be quoted. Burke read:

> Violence is permissible as a last resort, when it must be used to prevent or stop a greater violence. If I saw a mother chain whipping her three-year-old to death, I would feel compelled to try to stop her, even if I had to break her arm to accomplish that. Self-defense might involve violence, but it would be justified to forestall an unjust aggressor.
>
> While I would not use violence against an abortion clinic, I can understand the arguments of those who might feel differently. But I have always argued against a use of violence regarding abortion because of the peculiar nature of the abortion situation.
>
> The doctor is the major and immediate aggressor, but he is operating on both a willing subject, the mother, and an unwilling victim, the unborn child. The child is being aborted, but the mother is consenting to the abortion. You can't just grab the child away. The child is dependent on the one who wants it killed.

That's where Maureen Burke stopped reading. Judge Coar had excluded the very next line: "I have actually talked people out of using physical violence on one or two occasions when it was suggested."

Clayton and Burke continued to present a series of out-of-context statements from me spanning a twenty-year period. Hours were spent on objections and sidebars as attorneys wrangled over what was allowable testimony and what wasn't.

They spent a lot of time on a quote from me in the 1978 *Chicago Sun-Times* "Profiteers" series: "You can try for fifty years to do it the nice, polite way, or you can do it next week the nasty way." The "nasty way" meant taking to the streets—fighting abortion where it took place rather than writing to politicians. But I wasn't advocating violence. That statement was made at a time when my pro-life work was almost exclusively local, and a time when clinic arson and vandalism was almost unheard-of—and years before the 1982 Zevallos kidnapping that prompted Kleiman's questions about pro-life radicalism. By jumping from the '80s back to the '70s, Clayton presented her own narrative of history to the jury.

Clayton and Burke then focused on a press release from the April 1985 Appleton pro-life convention that declared the next twelve months a "year of pain and fear for the abortion industry." I was out doing radio programs in Appleton when that release was issued, and when I saw the wording I knew it would invite allegations of violence. In the next issue of *Action News*, which previewed the upcoming year's coordinated events, I wrote, "The twelve month period was designated as 'a year of pain and fear for America's abortion providers.' The pain refers to their loss of revenue due to pro-life efforts to convert women away from their facilities, and the fear refers to their concern over pro-life's growing membership and sophistication."

Burke never read that passage aloud. I had explained what those words meant several times on my hotline and in speeches and interviews, but Clayton repeatedly insinuated "pain and fear" were tacit instructions to my terrorist network. I would eventually get a chance to defend myself, but for now, the jury was fed a steady stream of false accusations against me.

The rest of Burke's testimony used issues of *Action News* and my daily hotlines to prove we held PLAN conventions every year from 1985 to 1997, quoting my reports on demonstrations that resulted in arrests, alleging that the purpose of our conventions was to conspire to break laws. These exhibits summed up NOW's evidence that I was the kingpin of a criminal enterprise, guilty of extortion against abortionists.

"Is it your testimony," Tom Brejcha asked Burke on cross-examination, "that you reviewed these documents about the time they were produced?"

"They were requested by our attorneys," Burke answered.

"Were you trying to give the jury a complete picture of Mr. Scheidler or only a partial picture?"

"Enough of a picture for purposes of—of—of the lawsuit."

Tom then asked Burke to read some other portion of the notes I had sent Carol Kleiman, including my response to the question, "What is the moral responsibility of individuals under the present circumstances?"

> The moral responsibility is to resist the decision legalizing abortion, point out its error, encourage a greater respect for all human life, educate, support, march, picket, sit in, and generally do all in one's power to negate the effect of that decision with the exception of violence. Violence would do the cause no good and would only give pro-life a bad name. Besides, it is not productive, and it would hand a public relations tool to the enemy and be used against all pro-life groups. I would never condone violence.

To the question of whether I envisioned small activist groups "uniting," as Kleiman phrased it, "into a larger and more activist anti-choice organization," Burke read:

I hope not. Rather, I would like to see the larger, cumbersome, and often poorly managed larger groups break up into lots of smaller activist organizations. It is important to keep the activist groups relatively small and local, although in touch with one another to coordinate activities.

My policy is to organize Pro-Life Action Leagues all over the country. And in every community where I visit I try to get the already existing organization to adopt my policies, subscribe to my *Action News*, call my Hotline, et cetera. In the same spirit I try to learn from other groups more active and effective than mine.

But organizing into a large cumbersome organization with a long distance director—I don't buy that.

We hoped these pieces of evidence might cripple NOW's claims that I was the shadow director of the national pro-life movement and that I encouraged attacks on clinics. PLAN was never anything more than a locus for sharing ideas and keeping the abortion issue on the front page. Attacking it with the RICO statute seemed absurd. And yet here we were.

Up next was NOW's Anonymous Witness B. After the experience with Ms. Wichita's questionable testimony about the bomb scare and being verbally assaulted by me, Tom Brejcha and Larry Crain appealed to Judge Coar to require the plaintiffs to provide more information on what the anonymous witnesses would present and to be permitted a twenty-minute interview with each before their testimony.

"These are very vulnerable women who have been through hell and back," Clayton argued. "They have been brutalized by the defendants themselves and their co-conspirators, and to force them to go through a twenty-minute interview on the eve of their testimony could be unbearable, and make it impossible for them to go through with it."

Judge Coar ordered NOW attorneys to supply a detailed statement as to what each witness would say and that our attorneys be allowed fifteen minutes with each of the remaining anonymous witnesses prior to their taking the stand.

Anonymous Witness B testified that she went for an abortion in 1993 at Aware Woman in Melbourne, Florida. Operation Rescue protesters blocked her way, she said, delaying her by about fifteen minutes. But the clinic escorts were helpful, she said, and the clinic personnel were kind and sensitive.

NOW's last witness on that day was Cathy Conner, administrator of the Delaware Women's Health Clinic. She provided essentially the same detail Susan Hill had but added that she was very scared.

"I felt very threatened," she explained. "I was by myself. These four men walked in. As I said, I had heard about Mr. Scheidler. He's quite a large man, very tall man, very threatening, intimidating. I was frightened."

Up to this point, all of NOW's witnesses had been women. Every morning and afternoon, Clayton's "NOW Representative of the Day" would take a seat at the plaintiff's table. I was often joined by family members at the defendants' table, including my three daughters. The day after Cathy Conner testified, my son Joe and his wife, Amy, joined me. Evidently, the abortionists thought it hurt their case to have their racketeer accompanied by attractive young women. NOW's attorneys complained to the marshals about the number of people at the defendants' table. Judge Coar ruled that those not directly involved as defendants had to sit in the gallery. Joan Andrews and Monica Miller had been dropped as defendants, and it occurred to us that they'd been dropped so the case could appear as a matter of big, scary men intimidating vulnerable women and explained why they wanted to keep my daughters and daughter-in-law from sitting with me.

Later that day, Dido Hasper of the Feminist Women's Health Centers took the stand. She was questioned by Sara Love, an associate of Fay Clayton. Gesturing to an exhibit displayed by the projector, Love asked, "Do you recognize this?"

It was my business card.

"Yes," Hasper said. "He'd written on the back, 'Sorry I missed you, I'll be back.'"

"What was your reaction to seeing this card?" Love asked.

"We were scared."

"And why were you scared?"

"We'd already had some vandalism and some threats," Hasper said, "and we were worried that a national leader was coming to our clinic and what might follow."

The questions turned to a protest I'd attended nearly a year later, at Hasper's clinic in Chico.

"Did you have any contact with Mr. Scheidler that morning?" Love asked.

"When I saw him, I recognized him, and I was very scared and shocked because I didn't want him in front of my clinic," Hasper explained. "I immediately went over and served him with an injunction."

"What did Mr. Scheidler do when you handed him that court order?"

"He dropped it on the ground."

"And was Mr. Scheidler arrested for his activities that day?" Love asked.

"Yes, he was," Hasper answered.

It was true. I was standing on the sidewalk doing an interview with Gary Wills of *Time* magazine some distance from the demonstrators when a police officer came over and told us to move. Wills and I moved off the sidewalk into the street. Another officer told me I couldn't stand in the street, so Wills and I stepped back on the sidewalk. I was then arrested, apparently for failure to hover.

After I had been booked, I was given a court date. I didn't want to have to come back to California for trial, so I pled no contest and paid a small fine. In the meanwhile, Gary Wills—who escaped arrest, despite sharing the same patch of sidewalk—went off to interview some Operation Rescue activists. When the article came out, I wasn't even mentioned. So much for Hasper's theory that I had been in charge.

Linda Taggart took the stand to be questioned by Sachnoff's associate Judi Lamble. First they brought up the 1984 bombings. Crain objected.

"We'll move on," Lamble said—but they didn't. Tom asked for a sidebar, but Judge Coar declined, choosing instead to instruct the jury to disregard the bombing comments.

After establishing that the Ladies Center had been bombed, Lamble asked Taggart if I'd ever been to her clinic. I had left my business card there in 1985 when I was in town to attend the bombers' trial. At Lamble's prompting, Taggart read my handwriting on the back of my business card displayed on the projector: "Linda, choose life—Joe Scheidler, Chicago."

## Chapter 35

# Perjury

O n cross-examination, Tom asked Linda Taggart how she reacted
when she saw my business card.

"I didn't know how to interpret it," she said.

"Could you have reasonably interpreted it to be that you should
stop being involved in the abortion industry and do something else?"

"No, sir."

Tom questioned Taggart about the consequences of the March
1986 clinic invasion in Pensacola and the result of the burglary and
assault charges that followed. Taggart said that John Burt and Karisa
Epperly both received probation and that Joan Andrews refused probation and spent two years in a Florida prison.

"Was a portion of her sentence served in solitary confinement?"
Tom asked.

"I don't know, sir."

"You don't know? You didn't look into that?"

Lamble objected.

"Sustained."

"The jury found that there was an assault committed against your
person?" Tom asked.

"I'll tell you what," Taggart said. "I wasn't quite sure what the jury found after the instructions from the judge. I was very confused."

"One of the charges was thrown out, correct?"

"I believe so."

"And the charge that was thrown out was that you were assaulted?" Tom asked.

"They threw out the entire assault and battery charge, all right?" Taggart shot back. "But that doesn't mean it didn't occur!"

Judge Coar called a sidebar.

"I will limit each witness to an answer," he told Tom, "but if you keep testifying and commenting on the answers, then I'm going to let the witness have at you. Fair is fair, and if we're going to play rough, then the gloves are going to come off and it's going to be a free-for-all."

I wasn't sure how Judge Coar was under the impression that the gloves were still *on*.

The next testimony came from John Burt's deposition. Lamble read from a script with one of the plaintiffs' lawyers on the stand reading John Burt's part. Lamble asked "Burt" if he'd ever heard the phrase "Lilypads for Life."

"Yes."

"Who came up with that phrase?"

"Joe."

"Did you ever discuss the comment with Joe?" Lamble asked.

"I'm sure we laughed about it," the lawyer deadpanned. He was a poor substitute for John. "Lilypads for Life are pro-lifers who just float around in the pond and do nothing but look pretty."

"Did Joe Scheidler consider people who picketed but didn't block-ade clinics to be Lilypads for Life?" Lamble asked.

"Of course not."

"Did you and Joe Scheidler agree that trying to prevent abortion through the legislative process would be ineffective?"

"*Was* ineffective, yes."

"Did you and Mr. Scheidler agree that other tactics were required to prevent abortions?" Lamble asked.

"Yes."

"What other tactics did you agree were necessary to prevent abortions?"

"Rescue. Sidewalk counsel."

Faux Burt was asked about PLAN conventions he'd attended and whether Rescues took place in those cities at those times. They had, of course. Then Lamble asked, "Did you have a sign at an event in Jackson, Mississippi that said, 'Which is worse, one doctor or 4,500 babies a day?'"

"Yes."

"You've agreed with Mr. Scheidler, haven't—excuse me. We'll have no further deposition designations at this time."

Naming me at the end was a dirty trick—and there were more to come.

When the third anonymous witness was sworn in, she recounted her visit to a Los Angeles clinic on Pico Boulevard for follow-up care to check the incisions made during a surgery to remove ovarian cysts. She was too weak to drive, so her pastor "Pops" drove her. She testified that her seat was reclined, so she didn't see the crowd at the clinic, and when they arrived, Pops got out and came around to her side of the car. He helped her out, and as she leaned against the car, Pops went to open the clinic door.

"What happened as you were leaning against the car there in the parking lot by the clinic?" Fay Clayton asked.

All of a sudden, a crowd of people came running from both sides of the building towards the parking lot, towards us. I didn't know who they were or what they wanted. They just rushed up on us so fast. I noticed that some of the people were carrying posters, at least I thought they were posters, and they were carrying signs and were shouting things at us.

They were shouting "murderer, baby murderer." I remember a gentleman walked up to me and Pops and asked was I going into the clinic, and I was shaking my head yes, and Pops was telling him that I was sick. Then another gentleman that was three or four people behind the first gentleman yelled, "Nobody's going to get in this clinic, not today."

Then right about that time, somebody grabbed me by the back of my hair, and I fell against the car. Then I just saw all of these people, and they were grabbing their arms and grabbing at me. I didn't know what was happening, and I was yelling for Pops to help me. Then Pops was pushing the people away, and they were fighting Pops.

I remember trying to move, but I was in between the open door. Then I remember rolling down the side of the car, and the people were hitting me. Then I remember looking up to call out to ask God to help me. As I looked up and yelled "Oh, God, help me," a man hit me in the head with a big old sign. It was at this point that I grabbed Pops' arm and Pops grabbed me, and I put my arm around Pops' waist. Then Pops was pushing the people away, and they were still grabbing and pulling at me.

Then I felt myself going down, and I got real scared, real scared. It was just so many people, and they were fighting and grabbing at me, and they were yelling things like "murderer." I wondered, who did I kill? Who did I hurt?

As I remember going down, Pops grabbed me by the waist, and the last thing I remember I just saw feet. Then I passed out.

"You mentioned the man with the sign who hit you with the sign," Fay said. "Do you have any recollection of what was depicted on that sign?"

"I remember the sign was colored. It was a colored picture of body parts. I remember seeing feets and arms, and that's all I can remember, just feets and arms, and the poster was red, like blood."

Clayton asked if she remembered regaining consciousness.

"When I opened my eyes, I was up in the air. They had lifted me up above the people."

"Now, who was it that had lifted you up above the people?"

"Pops had the upper part of my body. There were people in orange vests. They had these orange vests, and they had my legs and my lower hips. There was a woman in all white, so I knew she was a nurse, and they had lifted my body up above the crowd. The people were still grabbing, trying to grab at me, and they were moving me up over the heads of the crowd."

Clayton showed her a vest. "Can you tell me if this was similar to the vests that those people were wearing that day?"

"Yes, it's similar to those vests."

"Did the vests that you saw on the people who were helping lift you say 'escort' or some word like that?"

"It had—"

"Objection," interrupted Crain. "Leading."

"Don't lead, please," said Judge Coar.

"Okay," Clayton said. "Did it have any words on it?"

"It had big block letters across the chest area of it," the witness said.

"Do you recall what the words were?"

"It was 'E' something. . . ."

"Okay," Clayton said. "Was it—"

"Escorts!"

"Did you ever find out what had been going on at the clinic that day?" Clayton asked.

"On the news, I saw myself being attacked by a mob of people who were clawing and pawing at me, and they were carrying big old signs and posters, and the news told me who the people were."

Clayton asked if she saw any signs on the TV coverage and to describe them if she could.

"I saw a big round sign that was blue with white writing that said 'Operation Rescue.'"

That design should sound familiar to anyone who follows abortion protests. Round blue signs with white letters are still prominent at demonstrations, but the text is "Keep Abortion Legal," and they are made by the NOW.

With all this creative narrative, we began calling this witness "Miss Hollywood."

On cross, Debbie Fischer asked Miss Hollywood if she was a NOW member. She was not.

"How were you contacted to testify in this suit?" Debbie asked.

"I was contacted via phone call."

"How did NOW become aware of your story of this incident?"

Judge Coar sustained an objection from Clayton.

"Is it your testimony that someone contacted you, and that you did not contact them?" Debbie asked.

"Someone contacted me."

"Thank you. No further questions."

The witness had been tearing up throughout her testimony, and more spilled as she stepped down from the witness stand. A woman from NOW's side of the gallery rushed forward to embrace her in front of the jury box. Judge Coar didn't say a word.

In chambers, Tom Brejcha asked Judge Coar to sign a subpoena for news coverage of the fracas the witness described.

"What authority would I have to order a television station in Los Angeles to produce records?" he asked. Tom reminded him of the nationwide subpoena power under RICO, and the judge reminded Tom that this power applied to cases brought by the US government. Tom told Judge Coar that although a federal judge had dismissed this case in 1991, it had been reopened by the US Supreme Court in

1994, so Judge Coar had federal subpoena power. Judge Coar asked why the defense was seeking this footage now and not before the trial.

"This evidence came through an anonymous witness!" Brejcha replied. He told the judge that the plaintiffs hadn't provided us with any chance to depose the witness before trial.

"Well, you know," Judge Coar said, "nobody raised that with me until now, and we're not going to make it up as we go along. If you wish to go out to California and obtain the information, go right ahead."

"All right, but we can't do it without a subpoena, your honor."

"Well, go out and ask a California court to issue it," the judge replied. "Anything else?"

Tom contacted Life Legal Defense attorney Andy Zepeda in California to seek the order, but without Judge Coar's signature, we couldn't get one, and so we couldn't refute Miss Hollywood's testimony in court. But after the trial, Tim Murphy made three trips to California and spent days at the UCLA Film and Television Archive combing through coverage of Operation Rescue events in the Los Angeles area and interviewing activists involved in the events. Nothing he uncovered looked like what the third anonymous witness described. In fact, reporters commented on how peaceful the demonstrations were. Tim also found coverage of the Summer of Mercy that clearly showed Ms. Wichita screaming at demonstrators outside Tiller's clinic and walking in unimpeded.

Meanwhile, attorney Katie Short found old court papers from an earlier California lawsuit against Operation Rescue, *National Abortion Federation v. Operation Rescue*. The case, filed right after the Pico Boulevard rescue, resulted in a statewide injunction against any further rescues in California, and the plaintiff in that case recounted a story—which she had sworn to in an affidavit—that was both strikingly similar and yet tellingly contrary to the story told in our case over a decade later by the third anonymous witness, Miss Hollywood. While she swore in the earlier case that the rescue prevented her from getting into the clinic, she said nothing about any violence, let alone getting beaten bloodily and losing consciousness.

After further digging, in February 2000, we discovered that Miss Hollywood *was* the same plaintiff from the California case and that she made a habit of filing lawsuits. She'd bragged to a neighbor about making "a bunch of money" from a federal case in Chicago, and during an interview by Lynn Vincent of *World Magazine*, she showed Vincent a photo of herself with Fay Clayton and Patricia Ireland. They were attending a victory celebration after the *NOW v. Scheidler* verdict at Kent College of Law in Chicago, Clayton's alma mater.

Miss Hollywood was a tough act to follow. NOW's final anonymous witness testified that she'd been delayed a few minutes by a demonstration when she went to a clinic to get birth control pills. After Miss Hollywood's dramatic tale, it was anticlimactic.

With only three exceptions, the remainder of the plaintiffs' witnesses were women who worked in clinics. Each provided testimony about scary pro-life activists and compassionate abortion providers. Several mentioned that they knew protesters were associated with Operation Rescue because of their Operation Rescue T-shirts, and they made sure to list all the services the clinics offered, occasionally neglecting to mention abortions. Nearly all made allegations of verbal assault, misconstruing or misrepresenting our concern for the emotional, physical, and spiritual wellbeing of the providers and their patients. Allegations of physical assaults were made with no evidence—no police reports, no medical records—to substantiate the claims.

The three exceptions were the male witnesses. The first was Lt. Carl Pyrdum of the Atlanta Police Department, who jailed thousands of rescuers during the 1988 Democratic convention.

The other two were my codefendants, Andy Scholberg and Tim Murphy. Since this was a civil trial, they could be summoned to testify by the plaintiffs. I wasn't called, so I had to wait to present my side. Tim and Andy were questioned about whether they'd received paychecks from the Pro-Life Action League and whether PLAN conventions included "field training."

Our trial was suspended for a few days near the end of the plaintiff's case. Judge Coar took a trip to the Caribbean. When he came back, he was very excited about an analogy stemming from his trip, where he had apparently seen divers hunting sunken treasure.

"Let me give you the example I've come up with," he told the lawyers before the jury entered. "It's not perfect. I'm still working on it."

Suppose there was a group that opposed some of these treasure hunters in the Caribbean on the grounds that they use techniques that disrupt the ocean floor and create ecological damage, and one of the ways that the opposition combatted this activity was to chum the waters around where they were working to attract sharks. They weren't always sure if it would attract sharks, but the fact was that it could cause fear among those who were engaged in the activity. Suppose the chummers said: "We don't want anybody to get hurt, and nobody will get hurt if they just get out of the water."

But they also said: "If the sharks come along and if they don't get out of the water, it's their own fault. If the sharks eat somebody, then I'm not going to be too sad about that either. That's not my purpose. My purpose is simply to stop the activity."

In fairness, Coar *did* admit his analogy wasn't perfect. Taking innocent life isn't recovering buried treasure, and sharks aren't quite the moral agents human beings are.

"Let me just add that I've been skimming Mr. Scheidler's book," he added, "and some of the things he says in the book are consistent with, I think, this analogy. He talks about using inflammatory rhetoric, for example. Rhetoric like, 'year of fear and pain,' and 'we know where you live,' and 'the goal is to close abortion clinics by any means necessary,' and the unwanted posters. It seems very much like chumming."

"Skimming" was right—that chapter on rhetoric is less than two pages, and it's about using terms like "baby" and "mother" instead of "fetus" and "patient." And I hadn't produced any of the "chum" he referenced. I wondered—had he been paying attention to *anything*?

The plaintiffs called Susan Hill back to the stand to detail how pro-life activism had increased her business costs. She spent a great deal of time describing the decision to use an armored car to deliver weekly cash deposits to the bank. Despite all the rhetoric about routine medical visits, for years many clinics only accepted cash payments, and many clients still don't want it to show up on a credit card statement.

Much of NOW's case hinged on my Wilmington and Pensacola arrests, and the plaintiffs devoted substantial attention to Joan Andrews's arrests at the same clinics. As their case unfolded, Tom decided it would be useful to bring Joan to Chicago to testify that she'd acted on her own and never blocked or entered a clinic or refused to cooperate with the law on my orders or advice. But at that time, Joan was in prison in Pennsylvania for failing to register for parole—the same parole she had finally received after two years in prison over the whole Pensacola mess.

Tom prepared a writ of habeas corpus that would permit Joan to interrupt her sentence to come to Chicago. When Clayton heard that, she pulled a paper from her file that I was shocked to see. It was a statement I had prepared for my attorneys in 1986 after the Ladies Center invasion. That document was supposed to be protected under attorney-client privilege—Clayton should never have seen it—but our AUL lawyers complied far too willingly with NOW's discovery requests.

The statement indicated I'd heard John Burt and Joan Andrews planning their blitz and said I didn't want to be involved. Clayton convinced Judge Coar that my statement proved the invasion had been planned and that if Joan Andrews testified to acting on her own, she'd commit perjury. He refused to sign the writ.

On March 25, the Feast of the Annunciation, the plaintiffs rested their case. Larry Crain asked the court to dismiss charges against Operation Rescue on various technicalities and argued that NOW hadn't proven any RICO violation by Operation Rescue. Tom Brejcha argued that the case should be summarily dismissed on First Amendment grounds. Judge Coar denied all motions to dismiss. The racketeering trial would go on for four more weeks.

Now it was our turn.

## CHAPTER 36

# Defense

Operation Rescue presented its case first. Their witnesses were mostly evangelical Christians. Their frequent references to God, prayer, and the need for "spiritual strength" drew a barrage of "Objection"—"Sustained," "Objection"—"Sustained." The hours of dull testimony were at least peppered with a few comical moments, such as when Judge Coar reminded Pastor Johnny Hunter seven or eight times not to mention that he was moved by the Lord.

Since the first set of witnesses testified about Operation Rescue, Larry Crain conducted their direct examination. Debbie Fischer and Tom Brejcha each asked on cross-examination whether they'd seen Tim, Andy, or me break any laws or encourage anyone else to do so. None had.

Fay Clayton's cross-examination of Operation Rescue witnesses focused on violence, conspiracy, and lawbreaking. "Are you aware," she asked Pastor Hunter, "that Mr. Scheidler has repeatedly refused to condemn the arson and bombing of clinics?"

"I understand he refuses to condemn anyone," Hunter answered. "Even former abortionists are his friends."

She asked if he'd ever heard me say, "Sometimes you have to singe these people," meaning clinic workers.

"No," he replied. "I have not heard him use those exact words."

On redirect, Tom Brejcha asked Pastor Hunter to read part of a taped interview, listed as plaintiff's exhibit 435A: "I always try diplomacy first, and if it doesn't work, then I try something a little more fun. I sometimes hope it won't work, because I think sometimes you have to singe these people a little bit. So I went up into the bleachers and when Birch Bayh started his speech, I took my liturgical bag and pulled out my bullhorn and I gave my speech. And my speech was better than Birch's." Tom asked, "This doesn't refer to singeing people in an abortion clinic, does it?"

"Objection."

"Sustained."

During Keith Tucci's cross-examination, Lowell Sachnoff centered on the fact that the Operation Rescue member once sold used cars, as had Randall Terry. The idea was to associate pro-lifers with swindlers. Crain asked Tucci about the details of his Summer of Mercy arrest.

"I was convicted of conspiracy to commit loitering," he said. The audience chuckled, but the crack annoyed Judge Coar.

"Ladies and gentlemen," he scolded the gallery, "it is distracting and inappropriate to laugh, snicker, or comment during testimony."

Sachnoff kept Tucci on the stand for two full days. He accused Tucci of trying to evade questions, and in a sidebar, Judge Coar declared that Tucci could "stay on the stand until hell freezes over, but he's going to answer the questions."

At one point, the judge told the lawyers that listening to Tucci's testimony was like watching paint dry. Tom mentioned his words to a reporter, and when Judge Coar read his quip in the next morning's paper, he was furious. He told Tom if he wanted to make statements to the press, he'd do it himself.

NOW's lawyers knew that Norma McCorvey, the "Roe" of *Roe v. Wade*, had flown to Chicago to testify on our behalf. We'd been told the jury could hear her real name but not her pseudonym. Concerned that jurors might recognize her, NOW wanted to prolong the proceedings so she'd miss the chance to testify. They succeeded in the short term, but Norma returned to testify later in the trial.

After a series of witnesses defending Operation Rescue, we brought our first witness to the stand on April 1. Lucy O'Keefe Hancock answered Tom's questions about her education and employment. She was a Harvard graduate with degrees in astronomy and astrophysics and worked as a consultant with the World Bank.

"Can you tell us why we are having so much trouble with El Niño?" Judge Coar asked her jokingly.

"Yes," she replied.

"In that vein," Tom piped up, "may I ask: have you ever sold used cars?"

"No," Lucy said. She testified to joining sit-ins in 1977 with the PNAP three years before the Pro-Life Action League was established and a decade before Operation Rescue arrived on the scene. Our attorneys wanted to refute the charge that all clinic protests were the brainchild of the League, PLAN, or Operation Rescue. When Tom asked her about her protests, she objected to the word: "When you think of a protest, you think of someone who's looking to tomorrow, looking to the TV cameras. And we weren't. We were trying to make an appeal specifically that day for those people, there and then. And so I don't see it as a protest. It wasn't a symbol. It wasn't a demonstration. It was an appeal to save those lives there that day. I see it as different." Lucy testified to being arrested fourteen times for blocking clinic entrances. On cross-examination, Fay Clayton asked Lucy, "Is it fair to assume that when you were doing those rescues or sit-ins back in the '70s, your purpose in sitting outside the door was to prevent any women from getting in?"

"That's not exactly right," Lucy answered. "I knew that they could if they walked over me."

"But they would have to walk over you, right?"

"Which they did."

"My question is," Clayton clarified, "was that your purpose—to prevent them from getting in without having to walk over you?"

"My purpose was to make an appeal by sitting there. You asked my purpose, and that is what it was. Perhaps it was formless or stupid, but that is what it was."

"Ms. Hancock, yes or no, was your purpose to prevent women getting into that procedure room without having to step over you?"

"No."

Clayton then asked whether anyone in her group ever used Kryptonite locks.

"I don't know what you mean by 'my group.' Do you mean PNAP?"

"No, no," Clayton said. "The group you—the loose association— that worked in the 1970s, either before or after it developed a name."

"The loose group with whom I worked?" Lucy asked. "That's, like, all the pro-lifers in the country."

Clayton might have thought she couldn't wrest any answers from Lucy O'Keefe Hancock, but it was pretty clear to the defense table that the rules of Clayton's worldview prevented her from grasping Lucy's meaning. She explained perfectly what rescuers were trying to accomplish for the unborn.

Our next witness was Dr. Jack Willke, former president of the NRLC. Clayton had mentioned the NRLC in her opening statement and even claimed to admire the group.

"Have you heard Mr. Scheidler either in an address or otherwise advocate any form of violence or violent tactics to oppose abortion?" Tom asked.

"Quite the contrary," Dr. Willke answered. "He's totally opposed to it. He feels it's counterproductive and shouldn't be done, and it's wrong. I share that view."

On cross-examination, Clayton asked, "Are you aware that Mr. Scheidler spoke out against you on several occasions in the mid-1980s?"

"Over twenty-five years I think we probably both criticized each other one time or another," Dr. Willke answered.

Clayton showed Willke the picture of the Appleton activists beside their "Have a Blast" marquee. "Now, you weren't invited and you didn't attend this convention in Appleton, Wisconsin, in 1985, did you?" she asked.

"I didn't know there was one."

"And you don't approve of that kind of language in the context of opposing abortion, do you, sir?"

"I don't know what it means," he answered. "Did they have a dance or something?"

"As President of the National Right to Life," she asked, "wasn't it important for you to pay attention to such a powerful new organization that was opposing abortion?"

"Objection, your honor," said Tom. "She is testifying that it was a powerful organization. That is what this case is about, and I object to her testifying."

"Overruled."

"If it had been more powerful," he answered, "I certainly would have paid more attention to it."

Clayton stuck with Dr. Willke's role as head of the NRLC and asked about the committee's refusal to allow vendors to sell *CLOSED* at the 1985 NRLC convention.

"Do you have any recollection that one of the reasons for turning down his request was that the book proposed the commission of illegal activity?"

"Certainly I have no memory of that," he answered. "And I personally would have disputed that if it had been brought to me. I would not have seen that as a reason to exclude him."

Throughout our defense, Clayton used her cross-examinations as a vehicle to make more insinuations that I condoned violence and lawlessness. She asked Dr. Willke whether it would surprise him that during an appearance on Ted Koppel's program, in response to a question about whether I would go along with the law of the land, I replied, "No, never."

"I'd like to hear the whole program before making a judgment, ma'am," Dr. Willke replied.

"Wait a minute," Judge Coar interjected. "The question was, 'would it surprise you?' The question was not what was your judgment. The question was, 'would it surprise you?'"

"I don't think I can answer in that context, ma'am," Willke told Clayton. After that, we heard "Would it surprise you?" dozens of times. It became a favorite gimmick of Fay's during cross-examinations.

On redirect, Tom Brejcha handed Dr. Willke a transcript of the Koppel interview and asked him to read it. He obliged.

"No, never," he read. "We will *change* the law eventually by constitutional amendment, but until then we've got to save human lives. And I feel that when I've talked a woman out of an abortion and she has her baby, so far as that baby is concerned, there never was a 1973 Supreme Court decision."

John Cavanaugh O'Keefe followed Dr. Willke on the stand. A veteran of clinic arrests, he mentioned that he'd saved several children, one at the first sit-in he ever did. When asked how he knew there had been a save, he explained that part of how he won exonerations on the necessity defense was that the mother who chose life testified at his trials that violating trespass laws saved lives.

When Clayton cross-examined O'Keefe, she asked if he'd ever seen anyone take property at a rescue.

"No."

"You are aware, aren't you," she asked, "that 'property' includes the right to go to your doctor? You are aware of that?"

"Sure, all right."

Clayton went on, "You are also aware that 'property' under the law includes the right of clinics to provide medical services aren't you?"

O'Keefe answered, "To provide medical services, yes."

Clayton pressed, "And you saw those interfered with, didn't you sir?"

O'Keefe was straightforward with his answer: "We did certainly interfere with abortions."

NOW's entire case rested on this question. Despite all their emphasis on violence, NOW merely had to convince the jury that the right to perform and receive abortions was an actual thing that could be taken away, even if only for a few minutes. Establishing this new definition of extortion was the key to their victory.

Clayton pressed O'Keefe about PLAN's structure. He answered that it didn't really have one. On redirect, Tom asked him to clarify.

"You say PLAN is not an organization. What does that mean?"

"Well, quite seriously," O'Keefe answered, "one could say this trial is the most recent meeting of PLAN. I mean, there are pro-life activists from around the country meeting here, talking about what has happened and what to do in the future."

O'Keefe's testimony focused on the rescue movement's philosophy and its nonviolent emphasis. Our next witness, Christie Ann Collins Dickson, also testified to peaceful protests, but she described the details of her own arrests to assert that pro-lifers were the ones being harassed. She'd been arrested fifty-two times. Debbie Fischer asked her to list the charges brought against her. Dickson listed trespass and noise ordinances as well as one count of "violating airspace," for reaching over a fence at a Falls Church, Virginia, clinic to hand a patient a pamphlet. She'd been arrested three times on that charge.

Dickson continued: "I've been arrested for interstate transportation of—"

"That's ruled out of this case," Debbie cautioned. Dickson was talking about the aborted babies whose bodies were collected in one state but were sent back to the states in which they were killed to be laid to rest.

Dickson returned to the airspace violations, explaining how she'd received a sixty-day jail sentence for the first one but was acquitted on that charge the other two times. As Debbie was asking about other arrests, Clayton objected. Judge Coar called a sidebar. Clayton wanted to ensure that the next arrest included a conviction, not an acquittal, to emphasize that rescuers were scofflaws.

Judge Coar indicated that his jury instructions at the end of the trial would make it clear that an arrest without a conviction does not prove anything.

"Well, your honor," Clayton said, "I request that you tell the jury that the mere fact of a dismissal doesn't establish anything either." But Clayton knew it wasn't a principle any lawyer or judge could support. The judge joked that it hardly mattered anymore whether he applied the law competently. "Mr. Cavanaugh O'Keefe has just ruined my chances of being on the Supreme Court," he said. "I can just see the hearing now where they say that Coar hosted a PLAN conference."

After the sidebar, Debbie asked Christie Dickson about her interactions with the administrator of the Falls Church clinic, Joan Appleton.

"Well, after about a year of inviting her out to lunch, one time she agreed to join me," she said.

"Was it a pleasant occasion?" Debbie asked.

"I wouldn't describe it as pleasant. It was—it was a real difficult conversation. It was confrontational, but it was cordial. We were there to discuss each other's opinions and ideas and philosophies."

"Did you use forceful language with Joan Appleton at that event?" Debbie asked.

"I did."

"Would you give me an example of what you mean by 'forceful'?"

"Objection."

"Sustained."

Joan Appleton herself testified next. Because of Christie Dickson's concern and the prayers and support of other pro-lifers, Appleton left the industry. On the stand, she recounted how, during rescues, she called patients and helped them schedule their abortions at other clinics. Then she'd call other abortion supporters and have them come to her clinic pretending to be patients to put on a show for the media.

Joan once snapped a picture of me smiling and waving while we protested from a platform on the other side of her fence in 1987. When she left the industry, she gave me a copy of the picture, which I included in the 1992 edition of *CLOSED*. Joan identified the picture on the stand.

Jerry Horn was our next witness. He'd worked for the League in the late 1980s, and by the time the trial took place, he had become a Catholic and worked for Priests for Life. Jerry is an organizational master. We borrowed him to help us coordinate the arrival of witnesses and arrange their hotels. He also managed our media relations during the trial.

On the stand, Jerry described the circumstances behind the "Have a Blast" marquee. Clayton questioned him about it on cross-examination, asking him to name the people in the picture. Jerry had already testified that his duties at the hotel kept him from spending much time at the conference, and so he only knew a few of the names.

But Clayton knew them, and named them for Jerry. "Is that Monica Migliorino Miller? And is this John Ryan?"

"Excuse me, your honor," Jerry said. "May I ask a question?"

"Yes, sir."

"She's asking me to identify the people and then she's telling me who they are. Doesn't that seem a little bit unfair?"

"No, it does not," Judge Coar answered. "She's entitled to lead you on cross-examination. Please answer the question."

"I believe this is John Ryan, this one I can't remember. But this is Harry Hand, and this is Jesse Helm's—"

"Earl Appleby," Clayton interjected. After a while, she brought up the issue of the marquee's message.

"You testified on direct a moment ago that someone from the conference actually came to you and criticized the sign," she said. "Is that right?"

"Okay, first of all," Jerry began, "I didn't say someone from the conference, I said someone from the hotel. Mrs. Stone asked me, and I said if they wanted to change it, fine, but I thought it was stupid then, and I think it's stupid now, for someone to draw that kind of conclusion from a colloquial term, and if this case is built on that, then I think it's ridiculous as well."

"Mr. Horn," warned Judge Coar.

"I'm sorry, your honor," Jerry said. "I apologize."

Earlier, in answer to Tom's questions, Jerry had described our visit with Cathy Conner at the DWHO in 1986 as pleasant. He testified that Ms. Conner didn't seem at all scared and that she hadn't called the police and that she wasn't alone—someone else was in the waiting room.

"You have a vivid recollection of that?" Clayton asked during her cross.

"Absolute recollection of it."

"In any event," Clayton continued, "Miss Conner was certainly outnumbered by the group that went in, wasn't she? And you fellows were a lot bigger than she was, weren't you?"

"Yes, but we're teddy bears," Jerry answered.

Our next witness, Lynn Mills, testified to converting Debra Henry, a clinic worker from her hometown in Livonia, Michigan, to the pro-life cause. We spent much of our case showing the jury that we weren't in the business of harassing abortion providers. We wanted to help them get out of the industry.

Our worst day of the trial was the day I took the stand. Prior to the trial, Tom had been desperate to find other attorneys to help with the case, and a few days in, Richard Caro, a seasoned litigator from New York, approached Tom and offered his services.

Conscious of the judge's animosity, Tom thought it best to have Caro handle the direct examination. I took the witness stand at 2:45 on April 6. Caro led me through a short history of activism. He asked if I was familiar with PLAN, and I talked about how and why it formed. As everyone involved in PLAN testified, I explained that it was never an entity with a budget, authority, or an organizational structure. Caro went through a series of things that organizations do, both legal and illegal, and asked whether PLAN had done any of them. He asked if PLAN or I ever gave anyone any orders. I spent several minutes delivering a number of variations of "no."

Caro asked about my first sit-in. I said that during my college days I worked for a construction company and that the workers went on a sit-down strike. Clayton immediately objected. Then I described my time in Montgomery, Alabama, with Dr. Martin Luther King Jr. Again, Clayton objected.

Caro inquired if I'd been in Wichita during the Summer of Mercy, whether I went near Tiller's clinic, and whether I'd met Tiller. I told about the time we shared a cab in New Orleans and the invitation to his clinic.

My business card was displayed again, and Caro asked if I recognized it as the one I left at a clinic.

"I've left a lot of cards around," I answered. "When I go to visit somebody and they are not there, I write a little note on the back and leave it. I don't remember that specific card."

"Was this intended to be a threat?"

"Not at all."

"Objection," said Clayton. "The witness doesn't recall it."

"Well," Judge Coar said, "if he knows, he can answer."

"I've been in this courtroom," I said, "and I know I am supposed to have left it in Pensacola. It certainly would not have been a threat. Why would I threaten someone to choose life?"

"We've had testimony concerning statements you made about not condemning bombings of clinics. Do you approve the bombing of clinics?"

"Absolutely not," I answered. "It is one of the most ridiculous things anybody can do."

"You have been quoted as saying that you don't mourn the loss of bricks and stones," Caro said. "Can you explain that?"

"I place human life above material goods. When a 747 goes down, I know that's a very expensive plane, but I'm concerned about the number of lives that were lost. And that's how I feel about abortion."

Caro went on to my comments about admiring some of the extremists' zeal and asked me to explain myself.

"I admire zeal," I said. "I have told Bill Baird, who ran four abortion clinics and used to picket us at our rallies and meetings, I admired his zeal. I admire anybody who believes strongly enough in something to do something about it. I admire the zeal of people who follow up their beliefs and their commitments. It doesn't mean I necessarily agree with the way they express that zeal."

I took the stand again the following day. On cross-examination, Clayton eagerly returned to my comments on zeal. She brought out a letter I'd penned to imprisoned arsonist Curtis Beseda.

"You tell him here that you admire his zeal, right?" she asked.

"Fay," I said, "I admire *your* zeal."

"I am not asking about mine," she said. "I am asking about the convicted arsonist's."

"Yes," I said. "I admire zeal—even misdirected."

A series of questions followed about the Wilmington and Pensacola stories that I'd described on direct examination and had been told by various witnesses from both sides at least half a dozen times already. Clayton showed a clip from *Holy Terror* featuring the Appleton convention, and we rehashed the firecracker name tag episode.

My appearance on the stand had been tolerable up to that point, but when Caro began his redirect, it quickly became unbearable. He had joined our team after the trial had already started. Ann had prepared detailed accounts for him of what we expected NOW to pursue, but he brought along a large pile of papers and documents. He kept sifting through these, sometimes unable to find the one he wanted.

I sat through an eternity of silence, waiting for the redirect to begin while he ruffled through his papers. He didn't give me anything to talk about while he was searching, so I sat in agony. Silence was far worse than Clayton's barbs. It was by far my worst moment.

When the redirect was over, Clayton came back with a brutal recross, asking for details of specific events over the years. After twenty-five years of activism, with hundreds of trips, pickets, rescues, and talks, I had only vague recollections. There was no way to recall details from every meeting and action. Too often my responses were "I can't say for sure" or "That could be." She was relentless, and Judge Coar said as long as I wouldn't answer directly, she could be argumentative. And so it went, on and on.

After the recross ordeal, our lawyers called a young woman named Lilliana to the stand. Sidewalk counselors at Chicago's Albany Clinic helped her decide to keep her child, and she stayed in contact with Tim Murphy after her baby boy was born. Debbie Fischer asked her if Tim was in the courtroom. She pointed to Tim. He stood up, holding Lilliana's little boy. Clayton and Sachnoff were outraged, claiming it was staged.

I wish we'd been that clever. Jerry Horn had been holding the boy, but the child was squirming for his mom, and Jerry handed him to Tim because he knew the boy. Judge Coar wasn't happy. He said the scene was "too cute" and should not be repeated.

To his credit, Judge Coar was good with the children in his courtroom. Tim brought his nephews one day, and the judge let them sit in his chair. He did the same with my grandson Nate Scheidler and for other young people who came to see the proceedings.

Our first witness the next day, April 7, was Sandra Cano, the "Doe" in *Doe v. Bolton*. Cano never had an abortion and never wanted one—her case had been used by abortion supporters to change the law, and she spent the rest of her life trying to undo that damage. Judge Coar ruled she couldn't identify herself as the *Doe* plaintiff, so there was a tight limit on what she could do to help us. Norma McCorvey returned to take the stand on the Wednesday before Easter that year. That day is called Spy Wednesday in recollection of the deal Judas Iscariot made to betray Jesus. While "Roe" testified on our behalf and betrayed NOW's cause, I wondered if the significance was lost on them.

No mention of McCorvey's role in *Roe* was permitted, but before becoming pro-life, "Miss Norma" worked as the marketing director for a Dallas clinic in the early 1990s. She testified about the police brutality she witnessed against demonstrators.

Tom asked her what other jobs she had over the years.

"I've worked in a carnival," she answered. "I was a painting contractor for a long time. I even sold used cars."

Clayton loved that. On cross, she asked, "Miss Norma, were you any good at selling those used cars?"

"Yes, actually," McCorvey replied. "I sold a truck one night that didn't even have a motor in it. Well, we pushed it off the lot. The guy was happy."

That got a laugh from the gallery. The jury wasn't allowed to know who Miss Norma or Sandra Cano really were, but the media knew, and they surrounded the two women in the lobby, clamoring for interviews.

That evening, I left the depressing atmosphere of the courtroom to attend Tenebrae, the Divine Office that anticipates the Triduum—Holy Thursday, Good Friday, and Holy Saturday—at St. John Cantius Church.

Back in the courtroom on Holy Thursday, Judge Coar ruled that Clayton had succeeded in damaging my reputation enough that he agreed to let Tom produce a character witness: Illinois Congressman Henry Hyde.

Once again, we weren't allowed to tell the jury *who* was testifying, so the congressman went by "Mr. Hyde." But when Tom asked him his occupation, he answered that he was a member of Congress and chairman of the House Judiciary Committee. Tom's direct examination was brief and to the point, verifying my reputation for honesty.

Sachnoff tried to trip up Hyde on cross.

"You have supported Mr. Scheidler wholeheartedly, haven't you?"

"He has the guts I wish more of us had," Hyde replied.

Sachnoff tried to object, but Hyde stopped him short. "You opened the door."

Sachnoff still thought he could pull off a coup. He asked Hyde, "If you knew Mr. Scheidler was advocating breaking the law, you wouldn't want to have anything to do with him, would you, Mr. Hyde?"

"I can't conceive of a circumstance in which I wouldn't want to have anything to do with Joe Scheidler."

Sachnoff still persisted. He brought up Hyde's oath to defend the Constitution and the laws of the land. "And the opinions of the Supreme Court of the United States," Sachnoff asked, "are part of the law of the land, sir?"

"I never agreed with Dred Scott," Hyde replied drily.

An exchange over the Dred Scott ruling continued until the judge intervened and got the case moving again.

"Mr. Hyde," Sachnoff asked, "would you vouch for the character or the integrity of anyone who openly proclaimed that he would not obey the laws of the land?"

"Absolutely," Hyde answered. "Absolutely. If the law of the land is immoral and condemns unborn children, I think that's heroic."

On redirect, Tom returned to the question of my integrity. "He is a man of strong core beliefs, a man of deep principle," the congressman told the jury. "He believes fervently, as I do, that these abortuaries are killing defenseless unborn children."

Sachnoff was apoplectic, but it was about to get worse. Tom asked how Hyde could square his belief in my integrity with the fact that I advocated civil disobedience.

"There are some people with more courage than others," the congressman answered. "Had people feeling as does Mr. Scheidler surrounded and even obstructed the entrance to Dachau or Auschwitz, there may have been fewer people incinerated there." The courtroom erupted in applause.

"Ladies and gentlemen," said Judge Coar, "if there is a repeat of that, I will clear the courtroom. This is a court of law. It is not a street demonstration. Now there will be no repetition of that conduct."

Sachnoff moved to have the answer stricken from the record, but amazingly, Judge Coar refused. It was our best day in court.

We broke for the Easter weekend. It was a relief to be able to focus on the Passion, death, and resurrection of Jesus Christ instead of the petty foolishness of my RICO trial. Ann and I hosted the whole family that Sunday for an Easter egg hunt in the backyard.

The next day, however, is the day I call "Black Monday." My daughter Cathy's family had been living with us for nearly a year as Cathy's husband completed his prerequisites for chiropractic training. It was a joy to return home to my two-year-old grandson Aaron each evening after a long day in court. Having such a vibrant child in the house continually reminded me of why we kept fighting.

Cathy's husband, Waide, finished his preliminary course that month and had been accepted to continue his studies in St. Louis. That Monday was the day their family moved out of our house. Before I left for court, I took Aaron out to the backyard and we sat in the swing together. He was playing with a little football. Cathy picked him up and he waved bye-bye as they rounded the corner. He'd left his little ball on the grass. I cried for the first time in years to see him leave. I left the little football in that spot on the grass for days. I couldn't move it.

For the seventh week in a row, Monday meant another day in court. Sachnoff, furious that Henry Hyde's comparison of abortion clinics to concentration camps had made headlines in newspapers all over the country, asked that Judge Coar tell the jury to ignore Hyde's remarks. He insisted they were prejudicial to his clients. Judge Coar refused.

We still had a few more witnesses. The judge allowed NOW to introduce a photograph that John Leonard from Maryland Right to Life had taken of a pro-life group, including me, in front of a bombed-out clinic in Maryland in 1984. Kathleen Sweet had attended that meeting, and she testified that the conference was held in *opposition* to the bombing.

Tim's detective work on the testimony of Ms. Wichita and the third anonymous witness was still far in the future. The best we could do to counter their testimony was call Jeff White, a pro-lifer who had attended both incidents. He had organized the Pico Boulevard rescue and was present for the Summer of Mercy demonstrations.

Because we added him to the witness list at the last minute, the plaintiffs tried to get him barred, but Judge Coar let him testify. Jeff testified that I had obeyed the Wichita injunction and hadn't gone near any cars making their way into the clinic.

He told the jury that he had seen the third anonymous witness on the day of the 1989 rescue she described. She was standing by her car, he explained, talking with people holding the round, blue-and-white "Keep Abortion Legal" signs. The clinic was closed that day. With no patients going in, Jeff testified, there were no escorts present. He moved his protesters to another clinic.

On cross, Clayton tried to get Jeff to admit that there were escorts at the Pico Boulevard clinic that day, to prove the clinic had been open and to verify her witness's testimony. She produced the orange vest again.

"You've seen vests that look something like this, haven't you, at a lot of the rescues?" she asked.

"We wear them," Jeff replied. "They wear them. Everybody wears orange vests."

"You've never seen an anti-abortion—an abortion opponent—wearing one that says 'escort,' have you?"

"Actually, I saw Joe Scheidler in one, once."

Clayton wasn't expecting that. At a demonstration at Chicago's Albany Clinic some years earlier, someone handed me an escort vest. The police were separating the abortion supporters from the pro-lifers, so I put the vest on and went to stand with the escorts to hear what they were saying. They complained, and the police moved me to the other side and confiscated the vest.

"Miss Clayton," Judge Coar interjected, "let's move the examination along, please."

The remaining testimony was more of the same. Witnesses claimed what the other side had said wasn't true, and six weeks of testimony was rehashed again and again.

Tom wanted to ensure that key details that did not come up through other testimony could be presented to the jury. Since Ann had been my partner in pro-life work from the beginning, Tom included her on the witness list at the start of the case. Near the end of the trial, he told the judge she would be on the stand for thirty to forty-five minutes. But the plaintiffs objected to her being a witness, and Judge Coar was inclined to agree.

"What could you possibly have to ask Mrs. Scheidler that is going to take a half-hour to forty-five minutes? What we have done so far has been so much fluff, I can't imagine it could be meaningful to this case."

In the end, Ann was allowed twenty minutes. She testified to editing *CLOSED*. Tom asked her about the phrase "Choose Life" and the League's activities: debates, leafleting, meetings, sidewalk counseling, and our outreach to abortion providers. Sachnoff objected to nearly every question, and Judge Coar sustained nearly all of his objections.

NOW put two last witnesses on the stand. Diane Strauss, who ran the Cherry Hill, New Jersey, clinic, claimed to have been grabbed and thrown to the ground during a rescue. NOW vice president and air force colonel Karen Johnson was their last witness. When Congressman Hyde took the stand, the judge had ordered that he be called "Mr. Hyde," but the witness for the plaintiffs was addressed as "Colonel Johnson." She testified to seeing me at a NOW march in Cincinnati and that she recognized my white suit and hat. That concluded the trial's testimony. Closing statements would be heard the next day, and the jury would begin deliberations.

That evening, I took Jerry Horn and Jeff White to dinner at Monastero's. I got home late and endured a sleepless night. I expected the worst. I knew we'd lost. The next morning, April 15, was the anniversary of the sinking of the RMS *Titanic*. That morning, I clipped a small picture of the ship from the newspaper. Underneath, I wrote, "They had a bad night, too."

## CHAPTER 37

# Judgment

On April 15, 1998, Judge David Coar gave instructions to the jury in *NOW v. Scheidler*. He explained the five elements that had to be satisfied in order to find a violation under the RICO statute: whether PLAN was an enterprise; whether it affected interstate commerce; whether we, the defendants, had knowledge of PLAN's "illegal activities" as defined by the RICO statute; whether we formally or informally directed PLAN; and whether PLAN or its associates had committed two or more of those illegal acts.

Judge Coar defined "enterprise" so loosely that it could apply to just about any group of people who agreed on anything. The "illegal activities" could certainly include bombing and murder, but NOW's real charge was that blocking clinic doors, an activity already a federal crime under FACE, violated federal extortion law: the Hobbs Act. The judge explained that extortion involves using threats of violence to obtain property and instructed the jury that property includes the right to perform or obtain abortions. But he added: "It does not matter whether or not the extortion provided an economic benefit to PLAN. Any fear involved must be reasonable under the circumstances. Fear includes not only fear of physical violence but fear of wrongful economic injury. Exploitation of the victim's reasonable fear constitutes extortion regardless of whether or not the defendant was responsible for creating that fear and despite the absence of any direct threats." Susan Hill feared her clinic would lose business if her patients' names, found with the bodies taken from the Vital Med loading dock, were published. This, in a nutshell, was extortion. Kansas City's clinics voluntarily closed rather than face a possible sit-in: extortion again. "Even a few hours of deprivation of legal rights will satisfy the RICO act of extortion," Lowell Sachnoff reminded the jury in his closing statement.

When Fay Clayton delivered her closing statements, she argued that our annual activist conventions proved that PLAN was an organized, decision-making body, that PLAN invented Operation Rescue, and that the rescues took place proved PLAN was an illegal enterprise. Both Clayton and Sachnoff stressed that the case wasn't about abortion—in fact, they said, they applauded the public debate on abortion.

We took a break after Clayton's closing statement. I went to lunch with Richard Caro, who advised me to declare bankruptcy immediately. He said that once the verdict came down, it would be too late.

I felt panic—how do you declare bankruptcy? Where do you begin? Did Tom know this? Fortunately, Debbie Fischer had just researched that aspect of the law and assured me we'd have three weeks after the verdict to decide whether to declare bankruptcy. What a relief.

When we got back to the courtroom, Judge Coar called the attorneys into his chambers. One juror had been looking sickly for the past couple of days and had been sitting at the edge of the jurors' box in case she needed to make a quick exit. The juror's illness turned out to be serious, and Judge Coar determined that she'd be unable to concentrate during deliberations. He excused her. Our third alternate had been seated two weeks earlier when a travel agent on the jury was excused for financial hardship. We'd lost four of our original six jurors and now had to seat the final alternate.

Finally, back in court, it was Tom Brejcha's turn for a closing statement. The issue at hand, he reminded the jury, *was* a matter of life and death. Tolerance is a virtue, he told the jury, but tolerating evil turns that virtue into vice. Protesters tried to save human lives, and at times, they turned to civil disobedience to accomplish that task. He asked the jury to consider the First Amendment.

"Keep in mind," he said, "that unity, joining associations, trying to persuade people, uniting together, is the very cement of political groups. It's the way minorities become majorities. It's the way people in this country get a voice and get power. If it's frustrated through the application of racketeering laws in a way that is contrary to those laws, which [is why] we say this prosecution of this civil lawsuit is, it's antithetical to that fundamental purpose of our democratic politics."

Tom pointed out that despite the delays, the two patients NOW put on the stand ultimately had their abortions. "Where was the deprivation of choice here?" Tom asked the jury. "It's really tantamount, we would urge, to a few hours' reprieve in a capital punishment situation—"

Sachnoff objected, and Judge Coar sustained.

Tom moved to civil disobedience:

> We urge, as part of your common sense, that you consider and recall the legacy we have in this country of other people and other groups who, regarding other issues, but of equally deep moment, gravity, and concern, have had occasion to speak up, speak out, and on occasion to engage in violations of law.
>
> The question in this case is not whether law violations occurred. Again, the question here is whether these law violations were violations of the specific laws invoked by the

plaintiffs: the racketeering law, the extortion law, and the other laws they've cited under the umbrella of racketeering laws.

Those groups include all kinds from the civil rights activists, the Underground Railroad, the anarchists, socialists, communists, pacifists, anti-nuclear activists, Greenpeace—you could go on—and the feminists. The National Organization of Women itself has said it engages in civil disobedience, or its members do.

Clayton objected.

"Sustained."

Tom continued by noting that words like "radical" and "extremist" had been used throughout the trial, and he quoted from Dr. Martin Luther King Jr.'s "Letter from a Birmingham Jail":

> Though I was initially disappointed at being categorized as an extremist, as I've continued to think about the matter I gradually gained a measure of satisfaction from the label.
>
> Was not Jesus an extremist for love: "Love your enemies, bless them that curse you, do good to them that hate you, and pray for them which despitefully use you, and persecute you.". . . . And Abraham Lincoln: "This nation cannot survive half slave and half free.". . . . And Thomas Jefferson: "We hold these truths to be self-evident, that all men are created equal. . . ."
>
> Will we be extremists for the preservation of injustice or the extension of justice? In that dramatic scene on Calvary's hill, three men were crucified. We must never forget all three were crucified for the same crime, the crime of extremism.[1]

---

1    Martin Luther King Jr., "Letter from a Birmingham Jail," *Stanford University Martin Luther King Jr. Research and Education Institute,* https://kinginstitute.stanford.edu/king-papers/documents/letter-birmingham-jail.

"These are grave and serious matters. We would urge you that a verdict for the plaintiffs in this case would turn our legacy of liberty on its head. It would cast a cloud over grassroots protest from now and henceforward. It would spread from this issue, troubling as it is, to protest on all varieties of issues."

Yet if the jury did feel that their instructions to them required them to rule for the plaintiffs, Tom said, to paraphrase Eugene Debs: "That would bring new honor to the terms 'extortionist' and 'racketeer.'"

It would have been fitting to end on Tom's eloquent summary, but the plaintiffs were entitled to the last word. "Let's look at what the two sides of the debate are doing," Clayton said. "Our side is holding signs, chanting, trying to protect people, even with our small bodies sometimes, trying to help them get in to exercise their constitutional rights. We are being lawful. We are exercising the right the law gives us. What are they doing on the other side of the debate? They are being bullies and brutes. They are beating on our patients, they're blowing up our clinics or telling us that our clinics may be blown up the next day if we don't close." Tom objected to that, and Judge Coar sustained the objection.

Clayton invited the jury to read my book on activism. Sachnoff's closing words reminded the jury of its title: *CLOSED: 99 Ways to Stop Abortion*. "The hundredth way to stop abortion," he said, "isn't in his book, but what they do day in and day out to the clinics and women in this country. The hundredth way Mr. Scheidler didn't put in his book, but wrote privately to his friends and his radical leaders, are the forcible blockades."

I wish he'd read *CLOSED*. That was chapter 32.

The trial was over. The jury retired and deliberated for two days. On April 20, Monday morning, we got a call that they had a verdict. We rushed downtown, but by the time I got to the courtroom, I was already a convicted racketeer. We left the Dirksen Building, but the media outside kept us occupied for a while.

I soon discovered that life as a racketeer wasn't much different from normal life. I left for Philadelphia a couple of days after the verdict to give a talk, then flew to Minneapolis. Thankfully we'd planned a trip to St. Louis on the weekend to visit Cathy's family and spend time with little Aaron. What a blessing that reunion was. Aaron hadn't forgotten me—he came running up to hug his old pal. Now I could go home and move that little football off the lawn. God is good.

Two and a half months later, on June 30, all parties returned to Judge Coar's courtroom for an injunction hearing. Judge Coar (no jury—they were done) would hear arguments on whether he should issue a nationwide injunction against me and the other defendants.

NOW put Susan Hill back on the stand to testify as to why they needed a national injunction and how the FACE Act prohibitions didn't go far enough. Tom put Tim Murphy on the stand to make it clear that FACE put the brakes on the rescue movement and that there was no need for a RICO injunction.

After two days of hearings, Judge Coar proposed an idea. "I told my law clerk there was a solution to a lot of what goes on in this trial," he said. "We need to bring back dueling. I will supply the pistols. We'll get it all done. What do you say, Miss Clayton?"

"I think it's a great idea," she replied.

On the last day of the hearing, Ramsey Clark joined our defense team. Clark had been attorney general under President Lyndon Johnson, and he'd been in charge of enforcing federal law during Martin Luther King Jr.'s march from Selma to Montgomery. Clark sparked interest from the local media, and soon *NOW v. Scheidler* was back in the news.

We also brought a writer and peace activist from the Catholic Worker Movement, James Douglass, to the stand. He testified to the chilling effect a nationwide injunction under RICO would have on free speech. Douglass was from Birmingham, Alabama, and it turned out he was from the same parish as Judge Coar and knew the judge's mother, who had been an active parishioner at the church where the judge himself had been an altar boy. The two had a lengthy discussion off the record of the people and places they knew in Birmingham.

In her own conference with the judge, Fay Clayton announced that she intended to present a fundraising letter I'd just sent out that emphasized we were out of funds. It was true—we were. She wanted to use the letter to show we were trying to profit from the case, whereas NOW wasn't seeking any money damages from pro-lifers. We were certain she'd call me to the stand that afternoon. It seemed prudent for me to avoid the courtroom for the remainder of the proceedings, so I spent the afternoon in the Harold Washington Library, taking in an exhibit of clothing styles from the Roaring Twenties.

Though Clayton repeatedly stated that her client, NOW, was not seeking damages, Sachnoff's clients—Susan Hill's clinics—certainly were. Despite the various dates set for summer and fall in 1998, Judge Coar didn't issue his final opinion, with the injunction and the monetary damages, until more than a year later, on July 16, 1999.

Everything went against us. The damages assessed amounted to more than a quarter of a million dollars. The appeal process began.

The judge accepted our offer to put up our house as the appeal bond, provided that we also came up with seventy-thousand dollars in cash. That was a challenge, but we were able to find some friends who helped out. We had the house appraised to ensure it could cover the full value of the bond. Clayton didn't like the appraisal our man came up with, so she sent her own appraiser. He loved our house. I don't know what figure he came up with, but I suspect it was higher than our original appraisal.

On August 6, we filed an appeal with the Seventh Circuit Court of Appeals and waited to see if they'd grant us a hearing. It was more than a year until we had oral arguments in September 2000. For years, the district court had insisted that our case wasn't about abortion, but when we stepped off the elevator on the twenty-seventh floor of the Dirksen Building for our appeal hearing, the marshal asked, "You here for the abortion case?"

Two weeks later, the Seventh Circuit affirmed the district court's ruling. I remained a federal racketeer. We appealed to the full Seventh Circuit panel of judges. It took them only a few weeks to turn us down.

So it was on to the US Supreme Court. Tom Brejcha saw that we needed appellate experience in order to succeed at that level, so he recruited Alan Untereiner of a prestigious Washington, DC, firm, who was excited about the prospect and was well acquainted with the legal issues involved.

We filed our petition for certiorari, the writ asking for judicial review, in January 2002. It was granted in April. In December, we returned to the Supreme Court for oral arguments.

On February 26, 2003, the court announced its ruling. We won, 8–1. Only Justice John Paul Stevens from Illinois voted against us. In June, we held a huge celebration in Federal Plaza across the street from the courtroom where the seven-week federal trial had taken place. The rally was followed by a gala banquet at the Congress Hotel. Pro-life leaders from across the country came to celebrate with us. Nearly a thousand attended—we had three tiers of head tables. The upper galleries were packed. There were speeches and music and a well-earned celebration.

Naturally, NOW refused to accept the verdict. They insisted that the court overlooked four acts or threats of violence, but they couldn't say what those acts or threats were because the jury hadn't been required to specify what alleged crimes they thought had been committed—what, when, where, and by whom—in order to find us guilty of extortion.

So it was back to the Supreme Court. Miraculously we were once again granted certiorari. It was the first time a case had ever gone to the Supreme Court three times. In this third instance, even Justice Stevens voted in our favor. On February 26, 2006, the court announced its unanimous ruling in our favor.

That should have ended it. But it was another eight and a half years until NOW finally lost their final appeal from our modest award of court costs, in June, 2014. The court of appeals ended our many years of legal battles on the right note, rejecting NOW's vain objection to our award of costs as "preposterous."

My youngest son, Matthias, was four years old when I was sued by NOW and the abortion clinics. He was thirty-two when the case was finally over.

## CHAPTER 38

# Passing the Torch

In the fall of 2014, Ann and I spent a morning walking the Magnificent Mile in downtown Chicago passing time before a luncheon. As we passed the high-rise that houses the Lakefront campus of Loyola University, we noticed an advertisement for an exhibit at the Loyola art museum covering the history of Jesuit activity in the Chicago area. Admission was free that afternoon, so we decided to check it out.

Sections of the exhibit were devoted to the founding of St. Ignatius College Prep and Loyola University, and there was a whole room devoted to Mundelein College, Ann's alma mater, which had been absorbed by Loyola in 1991. One of the photos in that room showed a group of students and chaperones in front of a chartered bus in Montgomery, Alabama, in 1965. It was the bus that Ann had arranged for the Mundelein group to join Dr. King's march from Selma. I was in the picture. We talked to the museum curator, and she agreed to send us a copy.

Some weeks later, Jeff White invited Eric and me to speak at the International Pro-Life Youth Conference in Corona, California. Eric and I were originally scheduled to deliver a short talk each, but

Eric decided it would be more interesting to interview each other. It was—our talk got a standing ovation.

Eric is good with modern technology. He assembled a cluster of pictures so we could have graphics during our talk, projected behind us on two screens as we interviewed each other. The first photo on the screen behind me was of the Mundelein bus, and Eric asked me about my early activism in the civil rights movement. I said that even before we were married, Ann and I fought against injustice, and now we were spending our lives working against the greatest civil rights project of our time: the defense of the unborn child.

While I interviewed Eric, a picture flashed up of our backyard in Chicago. I was working at the PR firm at the time, and my colleague Mike Sitrick snapped the photo of Ann and me and our three boys, Eric, Joe, and Peter, just weeks before Ann and I took the boys to attend our very first pro-life rally. The next picture that came up was the famous garbage bag shot from the Toronto hospital—the picture I saw at that rally that launched me into pro-life work.

I asked Eric about his introduction to pro-life work, and he told the audience that he'd attended his first pro-life rally in 1972, before *Roe* was ever decided. I'd forgotten that Ann and I had brought him along that day. It struck me, listening to him talk, how much our activist work involved our children. My son Joey was the first custodian and mailroom clerk at the first Pro-Life Action League office. Cathy and Annie wrote for *Action News*. Annie also founded Generations for Life, which specializes in youth outreach. She worked out of our Pro-Life Action League office for years, while my daughter Sarah worked for both the Pro-Life Action League and the Thomas More Society. Matthias works on the Face the Truth Tours. Peter does as well—and he helped me compose this memoir.

In the summer of 1985, when the *Chicago Tribune* featured me in their Sunday Magazine section, they used a picture of me in my familiar white suit and bullhorn on the cover. Part of the focus of the article was the pro-life family.

"Two of the boys leave for their weekend jobs," it reads. "Two of the little girls grab their Cabbage Patch dolls and snuggle up on a couch in the family room. Mom is in the kitchen. All seems right with the world. Son Eric, home from the University of Illinois where he is studying literature and rhetoric, sits with his father reviewing tapes of Scheidler's performance the previous night on a local television talk show."

That particular show featured four guests: myself, the Chicago director of Planned Parenthood, a NOW representative, and a counselor from a local clinic.

"Eric breaks in," the *Tribune* story continues. "'Why do they have *three* abortionists against you? I'm surprised they don't have ten. The media is so biased.' Father and son then join the Joe Scheidler on the TV screen to argue against the three pro-choice advocates."

Eric went back to the University of Illinois and then on to the University of Georgia to teach rhetoric and earn his MA in English. He returned to Chicago, married his college girlfriend April, started a family, and taught English and composition at local colleges. He left teaching in 1999 to work with the Gift Foundation, an organization dedicated to building strong, holy marriages by spreading the principles of John Paul II's *Theology of the Body*. One of his projects there was to present the link between artificial contraception and abortion, an area where many pro-life groups fear to tread.

I was extremely proud of Eric's work with the Gift Foundation, and I recruited him to help with some of the League's projects. In 2004, he left the foundation to join us full time as the Pro-Life Action League's new communications director. He created our website, wrote for and edited *Action News*, and ran our Face the Truth Tours. In 2009, he took over as executive director. I became the national director and founder. The League moves forward in its fight to save lives and souls under the direction of my son, with whom I was happy to defend the unborn in the '80s and whom I'm thrilled to see taking leadership in the pro-life movement today.

In 2005, Eric moved to Aurora, Illinois, a town about forty miles west of Chicago. Planned Parenthood, coincidentally, intended to build the largest abortion facility in the country in Aurora at that time. They had created a shell company called Gemini Office Development to purchase the land and contract with firms. Gemini, the astrological sign of the twin, claimed not to know that the new building's tenant would be their corporate twin, America's number-one abortion provider: "Abortion Incorporated," as Eric called them.

A contractor looking over the plans for recovery rooms, surveillance cameras, and bulletproof glass rightly concluded the building's gristly purpose. He discussed the matter with his pastor, who tipped off the Pro-Life Action League about the facility. When their scheme was made public, Steve Trombly, the regional Planned Parenthood director, admitted in a July 27, 2007 *Chicago Tribune* article to being surprised that they were able to keep their plans a secret for so long.

Eric led the fight to keep the Planned Parenthood facility from opening its doors. He organized a round-the-clock prayer vigil at the site for fifty-two days before its scheduled opening. He traveled around the Fox Valley area hosting numerous community forums and attending city council and zoning board meetings. Planned Parenthood responded by hiring a call center to tell residents they represented "your church" and to get lawn signs to set up around town supporting Planned Parenthood. They also purchased ads in the *Aurora Beacon News* that made accusations about the Pro-Life Action League and claimed that their opposition had a well-documented history of advocating violence.

This was precisely the kind of allegation NOW had tried to introduce at my trial and that Judge Coar had rejected as nonsense. They had tried to claim violence again before the Supreme Court, which was once more quashed by the justices. Now Planned Parenthood tried to use these claims to defraud a community that didn't want an enormous abortion fortress opening in their area.

The litany of deceit eventually went far enough. Eric and eighteen other community members filed a defamation lawsuit. Planned Parenthood's lawyers once again set out to get the legal system to work on their behalf, but just weeks before Eric and his allies filed their suit, the Illinois General Assembly passed the Citizens Protection Act. The act was designed to protect grassroots groups from large corporations who could threaten lawsuits to silence opposition to their projects.

When the Fox Valley Families Against Planned Parenthood, led by Eric, filed their suit, Planned Parenthood's lawyers countersued under this brand new state law, positioning their organization as the poor aggrieved community group and the pro-lifers as the aggressive corporate entity.

History was repeating itself. I had spent twenty-eight years defending myself in court against pro-abortion forces, and now the abortion conglomerates were going after Eric. The entire industry's very existence relies on turning the legal system to their benefit, and their strategies have served them well. But with the legal expertise of the Thomas More Society, Eric was able to defeat Planned Parenthood's misuse of the Citizens Protection Act. Meanwhile, his own suit against Planned Parenthood is still making its way through the courts.

But perhaps someday Eric will tell that story in his own memoir. I've often remarked that I'd only pass on the torch when it was pried from my cold, dead hand. I'm not there yet, and I'll continue to battle abortion as long as the Lord gives me life and strength. But as Eric has competently moved into a leadership position in the pro-life movement, I've begun to loosen my grip, confident that the work is in good hands.

# TIMELINE

| | |
|---|---|
| September 7, 1927 | Joe Scheidler born |
| March 1, 1932 | Lindbergh kidnapping |
| December 7, 1941 | Pearl Harbor attacked |
| May 1945 | Joe graduates from Hartford City High School |
| May 1945 | Joe joins the US Navy |
| August 1946 | Joe discharged from the navy |
| September 1946 | Joe enrolls at Notre Dame University |
| May 1950 | Joe graduates from Notre Dame University |
| June 1950 | Joe and three classmates take biking trip through Europe |
| September 1950 | Joe takes a job at the *South Bend Tribune* |
| September 1951 | Joe enters Our Lady of the Lake Seminary, Wauwausee, IN |
| September 1952 | Joe attends St. Meinrad Seminary in Southern Indiana |
| August 1954 | Joe joins the Benedictine monastery at St. Meinrad |
| September 1958 | Joe works at the St. Thomas Aquinas Center at Purdue University in Lafayette, IN |
| September 1959 | Joe takes a teaching job at Notre Dame University in the Department of Communication Arts |

| | |
|---|---|
| September 1962 | Joe attends a one-year master's degree program at Marquette University in Milwaukee, WI |
| September 1963 | Joe begins teaching journalism and theology at Mundelein College in Chicago, IL |
| March 25, 1965 | Dr. Martin Luther King Jr. marches from Selma to Montgomery |
| September 4, 1965 | Joe Scheidler marries Ann Crowley |
| June 1966 | Joe takes a job with the city of Chicago Department of Youth Welfare |
| June 1972 | Joe takes a public relations job with Selz, Seabolt and Company |
| January 22, 1973 | *Roe v. Wade* decision handed down |
| March 1973 | Joe starts the Chicago Office for Pro-life Publicity |
| January 1974 | Joe hired by the Illinois Right to Life Committee |
| Summer 1978 | Joe and Father Charles Fiore found Friends for Life |
| May 1980 | Joe and Ann found Pro-Life Action League |
| March 1986 | Protest at the Ladies Center in Pensacola |
| April 1986 | Joe and three pastors visit WHO abortion clinic in Wilmington, DE |
| June 7, 1986 | Joe is served with notice of *NOW v. Scheidler* under Sherman-Clayton Antitrust laws |
| June 12, 1986 | Joe is arrested in Denver on charges from Pensacola |
| October 17, 1986 | *NOW v. Scheidler* refiled in Chicago |
| February 2, 1989 | NOW files amended complaint adding RICO violations |

| | |
|---|---|
| May 28, 1991 | Federal District Court Judge James Holderman dismisses *NOW v. Scheidler* |
| 1992 | Seventh Circuit Court of Appeals affirms dismissal |
| November 1992 | NOW appeals to US Supreme Court |
| December 8, 1993 | Oral hearings before US Supreme Court |
| January 24, 1994 | US Supreme Court rules 9–0 that RICO can be applied to protesters in *NOW v. Scheidler* |
| April 1997 | Abramson & Fox withdraws from defense team<br>Pro-Life Law Center, Thomas More Society founded |
| March 2, 1998 | Trial begins in *NOW v. Scheidler* |
| April 20, 1998 | Jury finds Scheidler guilty in *NOW v. Scheidler* |
| July 16, 1999 | Judge David Coar issues injunction and opinion |
| October 2, 2000 | Seventh Circuit Court of Appeals affirms the District Court finding that Scheidler is guilty under RICO |
| December 4, 2002 | Oral hearing in *NOW v. Scheidler* before US Supreme Court |
| February 26, 2003 | US Supreme Court finds 8–1 in favor of Scheidler |
| November 30, 2005 | Third oral hearing at US Supreme Court |
| February 28, 2006 | US Supreme Court issues unanimous decision in favor of Scheidler |
| June 26, 2014 | NOW finally issues a check for the costs in the *NOW v. Scheidler* litigation |

# ACKNOWLEDGMENTS

My wife, Ann, introduced me to pro-life activism when she asked me to attend an Illinois Right to Life rally in Chicago in 1972. A photo of aborted babies in a black plastic bag jolted me into awareness of the reality of abortion and prepared me for the full-time battle. Ann also suggested that I write this book. My seven children encouraged me to put my life experiences in writing. I hope they enjoy reading this memoir and see their years growing up in a new light.

My son Peter was an invaluable partner as coauthor of *Racketeer*. His enthusiasm for research and diligence in reading most of my pro-life library brought the book a level of accuracy I could never have matched on my own. My son Eric, an accomplished writer and editor, contributed important insights and recommendations.

My dear friend Monica Miller, a veteran pro-life activist and "partner in crime," did a yeoman's job of checking facts in my early draft and making valuable suggestions. Dinesh D'Souza called Monica's book *Abandoned* "the best book ever written on abortion." It is.

Tim and Bea Murphy read *Racketeer* and helped me get names and places right. Tim's infallible memory was a godsend. Tom Brejcha and John Jakubczyk, my attorneys, helped get the legal facts right. I checked details many times with Jack Ames, John Ryan, Randy Terry, Dr. Eugene Diamond, Jerry Horn, Andy Scholberg, John Mackey, Pat Trueman, Sam Lee, John Cavanaugh O'Keefe, Dan Gura, Cathy Mieding, Mary Anne Hackett, and Lynn Mills.

Corrina Gura Conczal and Beverly Geck spent hours speed-typing my stories as I related them. Ralph Rivera was my legislative advisor.

John Brick, who had worked with Monica on *Abandoned*, helped us reduce the book to a readable size and added a professional touch. He was a delight to work with. The editorial and production team at TAN books, especially Rick Rotondi and John Moorehouse, brought *Racketeer* to fruition.

There are others who contributed to this book who have requested that their names not appear, and I honor that request.

# INDEX

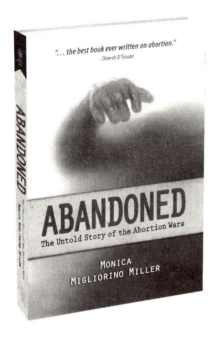

"... the best book ever written on abortion."
—Dinesh D'Souza

# The definitive memoir of the Pro-Life Movement

### Monica Migliorino Miller

Heartfelt, honest, and unflinching, *Abandoned* is Miller's first-hand account of the Pro-Life movement. At turns profound, breathtaking, and daring, this is not simply the story of one woman, it is an oral history of the Pro-Life movement, a true-life tale of life and death, and a plea for the protection of the innocent children threatened by abortion.
978-1-61890-394-5 • *Hardcover*

# Rock solid arguments why abortion should be ended now

### Janet Morana

In *Recall Abortion*, author Janet Morana exposes the myriad ways abortion exploits women, and calls for a national recall of this deadly procedure. She documents the way abortion risks and degrades women's health. And she exposes the false promises and lies by which it is pushed and sold. Morana also investigates abortion's debilitating after-effects, and gives a voice to those women who have chosen abortion and have regretted it.
978-1-93530-127-9 • *Hardcover*

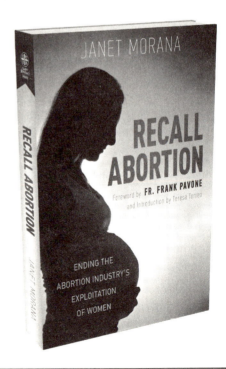

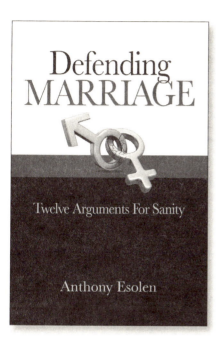
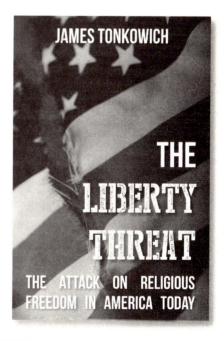

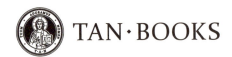 **TAN·BOOKS**

TAN Books is the Publisher You Can Trust With Your Faith.

TAN Books was founded in 1967 to preserve the spiritual, intellectual, and liturgical traditions of the Catholic Church. At a critical moment in history TAN kept alive the great classics of the Faith and drew many to the Church. In 2008 TAN was acquired by Saint Benedict Press. Today TAN continues to teach and defend the Faith to a new generation of readers.

TAN publishes more than 600 booklets, Bibles, and books. Popular subject areas include theology and doctrine, prayer and the supernatural, history, biography, and the lives of the saints. TAN's line of educational and homeschooling resources is featured at TANHomeschool.com.

TAN publishes under several imprints, including TAN, Neumann Press, ACS Books, and the Confraternity of the Precious Blood. Sister imprints include Saint Benedict Press, Catholic Courses, and Catholic Scripture Study.

For more information about TAN,
or to request a free catalog, visit
TANBooks.com

Or call us toll-free at
(800) 437-5876